TECHNIQUES AND PROCI

CRITICAL CAﾚﾚ

Robert W. Taylor, M.D.

Associate Professor of Medicine, Baylor College of Medicine;
Director, Medical Intensive Care Unit
The Methodist Hospital, Houston, Texas

Joseph M. Civetta, M.D.

Professor of Surgery, Anesthesiology, Medicine, and Pathology
University of Miami School of Medicine;
Director, Surgical Intensive Care Unit
University of Miami/Jackson Memorial Medical Center, Miami, Florida

Robert R. Kirby, M.D.

Professor of Anesthesiology
University of Florida College of Medicine, Gainesville, Florida

With 24 additional contributors

TECHNIQUES AND PROCEDURES IN CRITICAL CARE

 J. B. Lippincott Company   *Philadelphia*

Grand Rapids   New York   St. Louis   San Francisco   London   Sydney   Tokyo

Acquisitions Editor: Nancy Mullins
Indexer: Ann Cassar
Production Manager: Janet Greenwood

Production: Ruttle, Shaw & Wetherill, Inc.
Compositor: Ruttle, Shaw & Wetherill, Inc.
Printer/Binder: R. R. Donnelley & Sons

1 3 5 6 4 2

Library of Congress Cataloging-in-Publication Data

Techniques and procedures in critical care / [edited by] Robert W.
   Taylor, Joseph M. Civetta, Robert R. Kirby; with 24 additional
   contributors.
       p.   cm.
     Includes bibliographies and index.
     ISBN 0-397-51029-2
     1. Critical care medicine.   I. Taylor, Robert W. (Robert Wesley),
   1949–   . II. Civetta, Joseph M.   III. Kirby, Robert R.
     [DNLM: 1. Critical care—methods.   2. Intensive Care Units.   WX
   218 T255]
   RC86.7.T43   1990
   616'.028—dc20
   DNLM/DLC
   for Library of Congress   89-12638

The authors and publisher have exerted every effort to ensure that drug selection and dosage set forth in this text are in accord with current recommendations and practice at the time of publication. However, in view of ongoing research, changes in government regulations, and the constant flow of information relating to drug therapy and drug reactions, the reader is urged to check the package insert for each drug for any change in indications and dosage and for added warnings and precautions. This is particularly important when the recommended agent is a new or infrequently employed drug.

CONTRIBUTORS

Michael J. Banner, RRT, Ph.D.
Associate in Anesthesiology
Department of Anesthesiology
University of Florida College of Medicine
Gainesville, Florida

Tina Banner, R.N., M.N., CCRN
Assistant in Anesthesiology
Department of Anesthesiology
University of Florida College of Medicine
Gainesville, Florida

Mark B. Berger, M.D.
Clinical Professor of Medicine
Baylor College of Medicine
Houston, Texas

Philip G. Boysen, M.D.
Professor of Anesthesiology and Medicine
University of Florida College of Medicine
Chief, Respiratory Therapy, VAMC
Gainesville, Florida

David L. Brown, M.D.
Chief, Department of Anesthesiology
Virginia Mason Medical Center
Clinical Associate Professor
Department of Anesthesiology
University of Washington School of Medicine
Seattle, Washington

Joseph M. Civetta, M.D.
Professor of Surgery, Anesthesiology, Medicine
and Pathology
University of Miami School of Medicine
Director, Surgical Intensive Care Unit
University of Miami/Jackson Memorial Medical
Center
Miami, Florida

Cheryl A. Clark, M.D.
Assistant Professor of Medicine
University of South Florida
Tampa, Florida

Howard G. Dubin, M.D.
Clinical Assistant Professor of Medicine
Brown University Program in Medicine
Providence, Rhode Island
Director, Intensive Care Unit, Memorial Hospital
of Rhode Island
Pawtucket, Rhode Island

Gregory R. Flick, M.D.
Assistant Professor of Pulmonary Medicine
University of Texas Medical Branch
Galveston, Texas

James F. Flynn, M.D.
Assistant Professor of Anesthesia
Memorial University of Newfoundland
Staff Anesthesiologist/Director, Pain Clinic
Health Sciences Centre
St. John's, Newfoundland, Canada

Gary W. Gammage, M.D.
Anesthesiology
North Florida Regional Medical Center
Gainesville, Florida

Reed M. Gardner, Ph.D.
Professor of Medical Informatics
University of Utah
Co-Director of Medical Informatics
LDS Hospital
Salt Lake City, Utah

Eloise M. Harman, M.D.
Professor of Medicine, Pulmonary Division
University of Florida, College of Medicine
Chief, Medical Intensive Care Unit
Shands Hospital at the University of Florida
Gainesville, Florida

James R. Higgins, M.D.
Associate Clinical Professor of Medicine
University of Oklahoma School of Medicine and
Tulsa Medical College
Director of Electrophysiology
St. Francis Hospital
Tulsa, Oklahoma

Judith A. Hudson-Civetta, RN, MSN, CCRN
Research Associate
Division of Surgical Intensive Care
Department of Surgery
University of Miami School of Medicine
Miami, Florida

William Kaye, M.D., F.A.C.P.
Associate Professor of Surgery and Medicine
Brown University
Director of Critical Care Medicine and Intensive
Care Unit
The Miriam Hospital
Providence, Rhode Island

Philip D. Lumb, M.D.
Professor of Surgery
Albany Medical College
Chairman, Department of Anesthesiology
Albany Medical Center
Albany, New York

John J. Marini, M.D.
Professor and Director of Critical Care
Department of Medicine
University of Minnesota
Director of Pulmonary and Critical Care Medicine
St. Paul-Ramsey Medical Center
St. Paul, Minnesota

Loren D. Nelson, M.D., FACS
Associate Professor of Surgery and Anesthesio-
logy
Director, SICU
Vanderbilt University Medical Center
Director, SICU
Nashville VA Medical Center
Nashville, Tennessee

Scott H. Norwood, M.D., FACS
Assistant Professor of Surgery
University of Illinois College of Medicine
Director, Critical Care and Trauma Services
Carle Foundation Hospital
Urbana, Illinois

Robert A. Smith, RRT, FCCM
Assistant Professor of Anesthesiology
College of Medicine
University of South Florida
Tampa, Florida

Andrew F. Stasic, M.D.
Assistant Professor
Department of Anesthesiology
University of South Carolina School of Medicine
Attending Anesthesiologist
Richland Memorial Hospital
Columbia, South Carolina

Robert W. Taylor, M.D.
Associate Professor of Medicine
Baylor College of Medicine
Director, MICU
The Methodist Hospital
Houston, Texas

Arthur P. Wheeler, M.D.
Assistant Professor
Division of Pulmonary Medicine and Critical Care
Vanderbilt University
Vanderbilt University Medical Center
Nashville, Tennessee

Neil S. Yeston, M.D.
Associate Professor of Surgery
Dept. of Surgery, University of Connecticut
School of Medicine
Director, Division of Critical Care Medicine
Hartford Hospital
Hartford, Connecticut

PREFACE

For the new practitioner, the first image of intensive care usually involves invasive monitoring and "high tech" equipment. The opportunity to place catheters and tubes fits with the drama that pervades (often superficially) the modern ICU. Actually, proper placement, though admittedly important, is but one step of a complicated process that transforms physiology into bedside measurements. In addition, this process must be maintained over time, verified, and validated if the "numbers" are to have meaning. Finally, much technical information is necessary to ensure that the relevant data are interpretable and accurate.

Although technical, practical, and concrete, these aspects of critical care are as vital to successful practice as knowledge of pathophysiology and therapy. Although, perhaps, a lesser intellectual stimulus, these techniques and procedures form the foundation upon which cognitive functions are based.

The role of the practitioner is not even limited to technical skills and cognitive knowledge. We realize that the caregivers are involved in iatrogenesis, beyond just errors of technique. Technology is inherently dependent upon correct methodology and interpretation. Erroneous "numbers" may directly harm patients, as they often give rise to inappropriate therapeutic interventions. Finally, the caregivers are, themselves, susceptible to risks and subject patients to additional risks. Thus, aseptic technique has implications for patients and caregivers alike.

Accordingly, we have tried to group together relevant topics, not just insertion techniques though, of course, these are featured. Accordingly, we have incorporated chapters on measurement, maintenance, and function to provide a single source of information helpful in ensuring that the link between physiology and technology is sound.

Robert W. Taylor, M.D.
Joseph M. Civetta, M.D.
Robert R. Kirby, M.D.

CONTENTS

PART ONE

TECHNIQUES

CHAPTER ONE

CLINICAL ASSESSMENT IN THE ICU

Philip D. Lumb

Armstrong and Aldrin did it right the first time. (No second chances!) But despite all their careful mathematics it turned out there was one hell of a big rock in their way. Sheer virtuosity and a hatful of fuel bought them a landing they could walk away from. (If they had not had the hatful of fuel left, would space travel have been delayed half a century or so? We don't honor our pioneers enough).

—Robert A. Heinlein, The Cat Who Walks Through Walls

Although the above account appears in a work of fiction, it is factual. The guidance equipment on the Apollo 11 spacecraft and the lunar lander were undoubtedly the finest available in 1969, but success was measured in human ability. This ability was all the more remarkable because automated guidance systems were overridden and the lunar lander placed, with no reserve fuel, onto an alien surface. Experience, skill, and "feel" were all required for success. Although the landing would not have been possible without enormous technological backing, the ultimate decisions were made by skilled professionals who were able to integrate data in a fashion that the machine could not duplicate. This chapter stresses the importance of two aspects of critical care medicine: one that relies on the clinical approach to patient care, and the other that requires the integration of the former with technologically derived data (usually invasively obtained) to provide a treatment plan for the critically ill patient. Indeed, it is inappropriate to consider critical care medical practice without using all available data. Therefore, equally it is inappropriate to exclude the value of a well-performed clinical evaluation and concentrate solely on the flow sheet, usually found at the foot of the bed or in the hallway outside the patient's room.

Additionally, controversies surrounding the accuracy of currently available techniques make it imperative that careful clinical assessment be used to correlate with invasive measurements whenever possible. For example, the differences noted between invasive and noninvasive blood pressure measurements are well documented and have led to the perception that "at times, the reading, which is considered the more 'normal' of the two or more in keeping with the patient's clinical condition, is chosen to represent arterial pressure."[1,2] Also, inaccuracies associated with the measurement of pulmonary artery pressures are reported[3] that make clinical correlation and integration of data vitally important. The care and the setup of electronic equipment require time and precision if accurate and reproducible results are to be recorded (See Chapter 4, "System Concepts for Invasive Pressure Monitoring"). Of concern in modern intensive care units (ICUs) is the apparent lack of similar precision in the performance of a clinical examination. Proper lighting, patient position, equipment, and, perhaps most important, time are required to make appropriate judgments. The early morning rounds scarcely allow enough time to read the enormously detailed flow sheet and fail to provide for appropriate patient evaluation.

In direct contrast to these comments are the findings by Del Guercio and Cohn that clinical assessment in the preoperative, elderly patient cannot approach the accuracy of invasive monitoring and that more refined monitoring of selected patients would be expected to decrease mortality of some surgical procedures and could alter the proposed treatment in others.[4] The inaccuracy of clinical impression is also addressed by Connors and co-workers, who demonstrated that experienced observers were no more likely to predict correctly the results of right-heart catheterization than were medical students and first-year residents.[5] It is perhaps easy to understand how invasive monitoring has begun to supplant clinical assessment in critical care medicine: it is recognized as being accurate and reproducible—therefore, it must be good. Unfortunately, this is too great a leap forward and the conclusion may not be justified. Undoubtedly a balanced approach benefits patients the most. One without the other represents an uncritical reliance on either system and is not best for patient care and assessment.

PERCEPTIONS OF CLINICAL EVALUATION

The clinical evaluation of critically ill patients has been relegated to a secondary position over the last few years. In part, this is due to the commonly perceived superiority of invasive measurements. However, and perhaps as importantly, the increased rapidity of ward rounds, with less care and time spent on each patient, has added to the increasing reliance on digital reflections of the patient's state. A complete clinical examination of the cardiovascular or respiratory system begins with an appropriate, insightful history followed by a careful, history-guided physical examination. A former teacher and cardiologist stated that 90% of all diagnoses were made before the physical examination, and he proved this one day by diagnosing correctly the condition of every patient on a morning ward round—despite the fact that his senior registrar had stuffed his stethoscope with cotton wool. In a grand and good-natured tutorial over tea following this experience, he chided his listeners that it is not what passes into the ears that matters so much as the substance lying between them and the interpretations that subsequently are made on all available data. The time taken in performing these clinical activities can best be evaluated in the following description: "The right ventricular filling pressure (RVFP) has traditionally been estimated by observation of the jugular venous pulse. Elevation of the jugular venous pressure (JVP) is best appreciated with the patient lying in repose at a 45° angle with tangential light across the neck so that fluctuation of blood in the internal jugular vein can be observed. The height of the column of blood in the jugular vein is measured vertically above the sternal angle, which by convention is taken as being 5 cm above the middle of the right atrium. Another zero reference point is taken as the midway position in the anteroposterior diameter of the chest in the fourth or fifth intercostal space."[6] In either case, the clinical evaluation is not expected to be accurate in the absolute sense but rather to provide an approximation of the patient's condition. On the other hand, the measurement, when associated with manometer or transducer, develops a veracity out of keeping with its value, especially when measurement protocols require specific positioning of the patient so that the "zero reference point" will remain constant. Additionally, it has been shown that the ability of nurses to locate reproducibly a reference point is poor and that relatively large changes in recorded central venous pressure (CVP) are sometimes due to changes in transducer or manometer position.[7] These discrepancies relate only to the most basic consideration and in no way incorporate the additional considerations of length and type of connective tubing and system frequency response characteristics.

Another common feature of critical illness is the dependence on mechanical life-support devices. Routinely, patients are placed on ventilators, receive continuous infusions of vasoactive medications, neuroleptic agents, and muscle relaxants, and often have organ-supporting devices such as artificial kidneys or intra-aortic balloon pumps. In different ways, each of these interventions affects the practitioner's perception of the patient and requires appropriate integration of data and clinical condition to arrive at an appropriate conclusion. For example, the rise in CVP measured during mechanical ventilation inspiration is, in fact, accompanied by a decrease in right atrial volume as blood is forced out of the chest. Obviously, this is a paradoxical relationship and, as such, could be misinterpreted and ultimately cause a mistaken treatment plan to be undertaken. Although this is a well-known problem, others involving pulmonary artery pressure measurements and arterial measurements are also described.

Therefore, if the patient is paralyzed, intubated, and narcotized, of what value is the clinical examination? Is it indeed appropriate to assume that an approach to clinical management can be based successfully on the provision or the reflections of physiology as represented by routine hemodynamic and ventilatory data? Obviously, the answer is no. Indeed, as described by Goldenheim and Kazemi, "Critically ill patients require frequent monitoring of their vital signs, which, in addition to providing important data about cardiopulmonary function, brings a member of the health care team into close contact with the patient. This permits frequent observation of the patient's sensorium, skin temperature and color, and respiratory effort."[8] Obviously, the intent is to integrate the objective with the subjective—the so-called "feel" of the experienced ICU nurse or clinician. This subjective information must be added to the data base, which provides the foundation for therapeutic decisions.

MONITORING

As a definition, it is notable that "monitor" is perceived as both noun and verb. A monitor (noun) is a "person or thing which warns or instructs or a device for observing a biological condition or function." The verb may "keep track of, regulate or control the operation, or watch, observe or check, especially for a special purpose."[9] Similarly, the types and sophistication of available monitoring systems must be understood before data derived from them are interpreted and applied. The data can be divided into one of four overlapping groups, each of which has a different implication with respect to interpretation. Quantitative data are of the highest order of accuracy, both in terms of reproducibility and signal acquisition. Examples of this level are results obtained in the cardiac catheterization laboratory in which special tranducers and tubing systems are used and a small number of staff deal with the setup and quality assurance of all procedures performed. This is contrasted with qualitative data, which are more generally available in the ICU setting. Reproducibility and absolute accuracy are both reduced because of an increased variability in nursing and support staff, a decreased precision of equipment and subsequent lack of specificity in obtaining any measurement, a much increased frequency of data acquisition, and a greater likelihood of random oscillation around any value obtained. Simple errors including variability in establishing an appropriate zero reference point, nonuniform balancing and checking transducers, and neglected clearing pressure tubing of air bubbles all decrease the accuracy of any particular measurement. For the most part, however, many of these errors cancel, and this degree of accuracy is sufficient to follow trend values over time. That is, is the patient staying about the same, or do we see an overall change that leads to the suspicion that a major deviation is occurring or has occurred? Other subtle changes in the electronics of the monitoring devices also change a quantitative data point into a qualitative one. For example, the diagnostic or unfiltered mode on an EKG signal may be unacceptable for clinical use because of random interference in the monitoring location. On the other hand, in "monitor mode" the additional frequency filtering may render a clean trace but one that can no longer produce true diagnostic information, especially in situations in which two simultaneously recorded leads are being electronically compared. Similarly, rollover frequency modulators are seen in pressure transducers. Therefore, before equipping an ICU, it is important to know the specific characteristics of all devices. Most equipment can and does work well as long as its limitations are understood from the outset and the data are not overinterpreted.

Two other classes of information are primary and derived. Primary information is, as implied, unaltered and uninterpreted. Other than the reservations expressed previously, primary data fall into degrees of accuracy that we interpret as either diagnostic or monitoring, almost synonymous with quantitative and qualitative. Perhaps the most misleading and yet some of the most widely used data are derived. Certainly since the 1970s, mathematic manipulation of physiologic data has been accepted into critical care medicine, and it is important to realize the lack of precision that occurs when doubtful data are multipled by other inaccuracies or constants in order to derive a third number on which treatment is to be based. Again, a great deal of value can be obtained from following the trends of these data as long as the absolute number is not believed to be of diagnostic quality. To summarize, then, it must be remembered that data collection and interpretation are subject to multiple fixed and variable inaccuracies. Appropriate management decisions can be based on interpretation of these numbers, but only as long as the deficiencies of the methods are understood. Unfortunately, in many ICUs the need for critical appraisal voiced herein is not recognized, and absolute management plans are based on noncritical interpretation of erroneous data. This tendency, in the absence of a clinical impression of the patient's progress, can lead to inappropriate diagnosis and care.

To this point, the major focus of the discussion has centered on hemodynamic monitoring and interpretation because of the prevalence of these devices in all ICUs. In fact, and probably inappropriately, intensive care areas have become equated with intensive monitoring areas. Indeed, it has been said that for most areas, with the exception of the coronary care unit, a primary change in the EKG is the least likely event to predict or precede a major change or deterioration in a patient's condition. An important feature of intensive care is the documentation of progress that occurs in the nurses' and physicians' notes written on a shift or day basis. It is in the activities implicated by this documentation that a definition of intensive care can be found. For example, the number of times a patient receives endotracheal suctioning, is turned, receives a dressing change, has splints applied, is fed, or is changed—the list is long—implies an important feature of the illness and its severity. These aspects of care are often overlooked by the busy rounding team in their review of the apparently more important, and certainly technologically more advanced, data from the monitors, prominently displayed on the flow sheet and now even more impressively displayed in various ways on the monitor screen at the touch of one or two keys on a soft pad. The transition of the ICU into the era of "microwave oven controls" has seemingly done little for patient survival, and the mortality of many diseases remains unchanged. In fact, in an NIH consensus conference on critical care medicine in 1983, it was surprising that final conclusions in defense of the enormous efforts in time, energy, and resources were made by consensus opinion of already committed practitioners rather than by a statistical analysis of success. Perhaps this is a reminder that the emphasis in the profession is on care rather than monitoring.

OVERALL ASSESSMENT

Another important observation is that in most ICUs with experienced nursing staff, patient outcome is usually as well predicted by the head nurse and his or her senior associates as it is by any of the more sophisticated scoring systems, which tend to be based either on interventions (usually invasive) or physiologic data points that are accurately charted. The most striking deviant from this tendency comes in the neurologic assessment. The experience of the observer is key in interpreting the small changes in condition that may signal a totally different plan for the patient. Again, the personal appraisal and the physical examination of the patient are the most important indications. There is a well-known perception that if a patient has cold feet, then he may be prone to having cold feet. On the other hand, if his knees and feet are both cold, then the likelihood is that he is in a low output state associated with poor distal perfusion. This observation was formalized by Henning and associates, who showed the validity of assessing the temperature of the great toe and measuring the gradient between this temperature and ambient temperature. It was shown that this gradient is a useful and reproducible measurement for assessing tissue perfusion.[10] In a simplistic way, this demonstrates the important relation between a recognized clinical observation and a subsequent "flow sheet" correlate; it does seem unfortunate, however, that the hand of the experienced observer is now replaced with a temperature probe. Similarly, although the pulse oximeter is a highly accurate and useful device, it must not replace clinical observation of skin color. This was highlighted some years ago during the treatment of a young trauma victim, who, after a long illness, became increasingly hypoxemic despite escalating ventilatory support. As the Pa_{O_2} and saturation continued to fall, the bedside nurse believed that something was wrong because the patient "didn't look as bad as the numbers." A subsequent arterial blood gas determination from a different site confirmed the nurse's suspicion, and a small amount of contrast medium revealed evidence of an arteriovenous fistula. This example demonstrates that knowledgeable observation can prevent the nurse from embarking on an erroneous therapeutic course based entirely on the "gold standard" of blood gas analysis.

The basic questions about any patient can be stated simply: Is the patient all right? Is he better or worse than several minutes, hours, days ago? What can we predict about future course of the acute illness and ultimate prognosis? These questions are common to the practice of medicine and do not reflect only in the events within the ICU. The questions also demonstrate the important implications of trained, integrated observation and data review to produce an accurate diagnosis, a short-term detailed inventory of signs and symptoms that allow the available trend data to be analyzed and placed appropriately into the progress assessment of the patient, and the ability to predict the future. The last ability does not imply unnatural talent, but it does require several components that are not always available in the ICU. Most critical care physicians and nurses are justifiably proud about their charting and other recording abilities, and these abilities are usually excellent for an individual patient. However, acquisition of data on all patients that are then integrated into an appropriate database is more difficult to obtain. Without adequate archival information, appropriate prognoses cannot be made because the future is merely an accurate reflection of the past in the short term. True, the advent of major breakthroughs in therapy such as the discovery of penicillin will acutely change prognoses, but, for the most part, even with the changes in mechanical ventilatory techniques, mortality from respiratory failure remains high if associated with adult respiratory distress syndrome (ARDS). On the other hand, appropriate application of technology and subsequent integrated management seem capable of reducing the incidence of perioperative myocardial infarction. It is important to realize that monitoring alone is not beneficial or protective, but rather the integration of the data with the knowledge of the observer who subsequently must alter management if outcome is to be affected. This concept is noted by Rao and colleagues, who demonstrated that active management of operative patients with previous myocardial infarction decreased the incidence of repeat perioperative infarction when compared to previously reported data.[11] Of interest is the need to control multiple variables rather than focusing on one or two isolated areas that logically may appear related to the problem but which may not be the primary cause. Again, the importance of experienced observer interaction with, and manipulation of, the data is highlighted. The nurse and clinician must have a high degree of suspicion and be able to recognize errors when it comes to the appropriate use of the commonly available hemodynamic and respiratory variables.

An insidious aspect of critical care medicine that has received much attention is the patient depersonalization that occurs during a long, critical illness. As important and less publicized is the change in physicians who work in ICUs, especially those who rotate through in learning rotations. Most become content to watch the patients' progress by remote control, and few are willing to question the validity of the data. In part, this can be explained by the overwhelming volume of information that becomes available on a daily, if not hourly, basis. It becomes much easier to concentrate on numbers, and during this process clinical skills appear to be devalued by members of rounding teams. Hopefully, critical care physicians more familiar with the environment develop different reflexes and priorities that permit integration of all aspects of care. A major component of critical care management is in providing respiratory support and mechanical ventilatory assistance. Unfortunately, the uninitiated regard the simplicity of the ventilator's controls as representing a lack of sophistication in the machine and, by inference, a device that is physiologically benign. Obviously, this is untrue, and the clinical evaluation of all patients who require ventilatory assistance is a mandatory exercise for all ICU participants. Minimal standards of care in the operating room for anesthetized (narcotized and hypnotized) and paralyzed patients require the continuous presence of either an anesthesiologist or a certified registered nurse anesthetist.[12] This should be contrasted to the sometimes cavalier assumption made in some ICUs that the ventilator alarms are sufficient to warn of impending tragedy and that, like a telemetered EKG, the patient's safety can rest in the "hands" of mechanical monitoring. The reverse is true.

RESPIRATORY ASSESSMENT

Clinical assessment of the respiratory system begins with a good history. Many patients are placed in the ICU following some catastrophic event that may have been followed by aspiration of stomach contents. Additionally, postoperative and post-traumatic conditions are common in surgical units, whereas pneumonias and generalized infections are seen frequently in medical areas. In all cases, although the primary diagnosis is of concern, the ICU staff are usually as concerned with the appropriate support of the failing lung as with treatment of the underlying condition. Additionally, clinicians should always attempt to wean patients from mechanical support whenever possible, and the following discussion addresses the clinical correlates of appropriate pulmonary function and support.

The patient who is *seen* to be breathing is in respiratory failure until proven otherwise. As an axiom, this statement is useful because it draws attention to the obvious: the use of accessory muscles of respiration and (in adult patients) rates greater than 30 per minute indicate respiratory insufficiency. The blood gases may appear adequate, and, in some cases, patients may tolerate the condition well. In the long term, however, the likelihood is that the patient will require some intervention.

Another observation that is misinterpreted often concerns the patient who is "fighting the ventilator," that is, the patient's breathing pattern is asynchronous with ventilator efforts, and the patient and care team are uncomfortable. Normally, this observation should be interpreted that the patient is not receiving adequate ventilatory support rather than that the patient's efforts are inappropriate. A normal ventilatory pattern is one that is unobtrusive to the observer, that is, each inhalation is followed by passive exhalation, with a pause before a subsequent breath. Tachypnea in adults (rates above 28–30 breaths per minute) is usually an indication of respiratory distress. In fact, newer ventilatory support modes (mandatory minute ventilation, pressure support) are often adjusted in an attempt to control respiratory rate rather than an attempt to provide either a specific tidal volume or inspiratory pressure. Another important feature of patients receiving mechanical ventilation is the appropriate auscultatory clinical examination. Too often, respiratory rate is counted by placing a hand on the abdomen and counting the number of times per minute that the abdominal effort is sensed. Unfortunately, although respiratory effort is initiated during this maneuver, gas passage into the lungs is often asynchronous and does not necessarily equal the abdominal effort. The appropriate way to count respirations in any ICU or recovery room setting is by placing a stethoscope over the lung fields and auscultating each breath. In this fashion, a disparity between heard breaths and counted breaths is often apparent, which should not be surprising to the practitioner who is used to counting the difference between the apex beat and the peripheral sensation of transmitted pulse waves at the radial artery. Similarly, respiratory paradox can be uncovered and needs treatment. In many instances, the paradox is due to a supraglottic obstruction or an inappropriate ventilator setting. In all instances, corrective actions should be taken immediately. Under no circumstances should the number appearing on the ventilator or the flow chart be regarded as truth until clinical assessment has confirmed the digital output of the ventilator sensors, which may underestimate the number of breaths in the patient with low tidal volume and high rate. This is especially important if energy requirements are being estimated because in this setting the caloric cost of breathing can approximate 20% of the total caloric requirement.

Another feature of respiratory/ventilator interaction with which the intensive care physician needs to be familiar involves the residual effects of muscle relaxants used either in the operating room or primarily in the ICU. On many occasions, a patient will appear to be agitated and apparently out of synchrony with the ventilator. In some instances, this may be due to residual muscle paralysis and, in fact, the patient's condition mimics that of a myasthenic. In this setting, simple clinical assessment helps to determine causes of agitation, and the patient's ability to lift his head off the pillow and to exhibit adequate grip strength helps determine a correct diagnosis. Additionally, small jerking motions and a worried facies help confirm the diagnosis. In cases of extreme doubt, the use of a peripheral nerve stimulator and assessment of the "train of four" response confirm the diagnosis. Commonly, those individuals whose weakness is caused by the presence of one of the nondepolarizing muscle relaxants exhibit post-tetanic facilitation and fade following a supramaximal stimulation of the ulnar nerve at the wrist and elbow.

An additional influence of clinical evaluation is seen in the often difficult decision of whether to intubate a patient. Certainly, arterial blood gases are a poor indicator, and all students are warned of the possibility that a normal P_{CO_2} may be a reflection of inadequacy rather than appropriate gas exchange. This is true in patients who initially hyperventilate but then tire and develop normocapnia which, if not treated, rapidly leads to decompensation. The clinician can often decide on intubation by observing the patient, noting the degree of respiratory effort, and counting breaths. In adults, rates greater than 30 are poorly tolerated and should signal caution. Also, the patient's ability to converse provides an indication of air hunger. The individual should be asked to breathe in and then count aloud on exhalation. Patients who cannot count beyond five or ten are at extreme risk and should be monitored closely in an environment in which intubation facilities are available instantly. Below five, prophylactic intubation is indicated, and in the gray zone of five to ten many would advocate mechanical support. Although not particularly scientific, these guidelines often help in a doubtful patient who demonstrates acceptable "numbers."

HEMODYNAMIC ASSESSMENT

Some of the problems of invasive hemodynamic monitoring have been mentioned already, and it is in this area that careful clinical examinations are often omitted. Assessment of the circulatory system should not be left to cardiac output and blood gas evaluations. Again, simple clinical assessment often helps to determine the volume status of a patient, and, although clinical prediction of invasively obtained filling pressures may be low, it is unwise to hesitate in providing appropriate therapy while waiting for invasive monitoring to be established. Certainly, patients can indicate their volume status in answer to the simple question of "are you thirsty," which often helps to clarify an otherwise confusing situation. Patients who are truly thirsty, can differentiate the sensation of thirst from that of a dry mouth. Often a low intravascular volume and associated high serum osmolarity are reflected clinically as thirst. On the other hand, patients who are satisfied with a sponging of the mouth to alleviate dryness usually do not demonstrate signs or symptoms of a low intravascular volume. Unfortunately, urine output and concentrating ability do not always reflect accurately intravascular volume because of coincident hormonal abnormalities associated with anesthesia or stress. Many patients in the postoperative ICU and recovery room are found to have glycosuria with elevated or even normal serum glucose. This reflects a change in the tubular threshold for glucose and is indicative of stresses associated with the perioperative period. In fact, many patients coming to the operating room are relatively hyperglycemic, and the operative period exacerbates this condition. In the recovery room, it is not unusual to see a nondiabetic patient with a blood glucose in the 200 to 300 mg/dl range. Treatment, if any, should be gentle because these patients tolerate exogenous insulin poorly and generally correct spontaneously without intervention. Additionally, glycosuria promotes an osmotic diuresis, and inappropriate intravascular depletion may occur unless the clinician is aware of the phenomenon and checks the urine for the presence of glucose and ketones.

In addition, other indicators of hemodynamic stability are the rate of temperature restitution after surgery and the changes in blood pressure associated with rewarming. Certainly, patients who return to the recovery room or ICU at 34°C may exhibit hypertension and tachycardia. As they are rewarmed, it is not unusual to see marked decreases in blood pressure associated with continued tachycardia. This should not be surprising because of the increased intravascular space made available by peripheral vasodilation, and appropriate volume resuscitation should be anticipated during this period. On the other hand, these changes may be minimized by using vasodilating drugs such as nitroprusside during the operative stage, which may prevent vasoconstriction and enable adequate maintenance of intravascular volume. Clinically, the speed at which a patient rewarms and the degree of hemodynamic instability encountered are often indicative of the relative state of intravascular volume and hemodynamic compromise. Patients with low filling pressures and cardiac outputs tend to require a longer time for rewarming associated with a metabolic acidosis and large swings in pressure as the temperature rises. In addition, the requirement for passive heaters is greater than that seen in patients with adequate preload and stable cardiac output.

IATROGENIC CONCERNS

Perhaps the most important aspect of clinical evaluation in critical care medicine—the prevention of iatrogenesis—is often overlooked or undervalued. A morning rounding challenge for all critical-care-based physicians should be to determine the number of mistakes and potential mistakes that are evident in the setup of the patient's monitoring equipment, ventilator, or associated addenda such as chest tubes and urinary catheters. In addition, charting errors and numbers of medications should be noted. In all instances, recorded data should be scrutinized and the patient's environment checked for hazards. For example, inappropriate ventilator settings may provoke respiratory paradox and a worsened patient condition. Problems may be as simple as an inappropriately set peak flow rate or inspiratory sensitivity, either of which can provoke an apparent paradox between patient and machine. In addition, calibration constants on cardiac output computers, location of flow-through temperature probes, attention to details of injectate volume, and zero reference points for transducers can all affect the perceived appropriateness of care. All clinicians should become familiar with the noises of the ICU, and the sounds of a ventilator that works under stress should be distinguished from those of one that is working comfortably. In the former situation, give careful attention to the patient and make appropriate adjustments to the mechanical device. Usually the patient and his condition determine the ventilatory requirement, rather than *vice versa*. In addition, the amount of data recorded on most patients is extensive, and clinicians must not get overwhelmed by a regurgitation of normal data that obscure the critical points; rather, detailed appraisal of appropriate abnormalities should be routine for all rounding teams. In this way, the subtle areas of ICU practice may be exposed. For example, the suddenly abnormal blood gas may be due to inappropriate sampling, with excess heparin remaining in the sample syringe, rather than to sudden deterioration of the patient's condition. Appropriate critical and clinical appraisal of the patient may keep the clinician aware that although subtle changes may be reflected only by sophisticated monitoring techniques, major changes are unusual without some form of clinical manifestation. In many instances, the clinician works outside the conventions of normal numbers and purely within the boundaries of clinical intuition and careful physical examination. For these techniques to be valuable, repeated assessment is as important for clinical decision-making as it is for trend monitoring and interventional management techniques.

CLINICAL CARE AND THE ROLE OF THE INTENSIVE CARE UNIT

In March 1983, the NIH sponsored a Consensus Panel discussion to address the benefits and successes of critical care medicine. The basic feeling of the participants at the end of the conference was that the information, staffing, and care in ICUs were beneficial, but the only area in which this feeling was documented to improve outcome was in the area of coronary care. Certainly, in this environment, dysrhythmia monitoring and prophylaxis or treatment is associated with improved survival. In the surgical and medical units, efficacy is more difficult to demonstrate and success more a matter of faith. The interesting feature of this conference was that no one felt particularly uncomfortable with this conclusion, nor with joining the sentiment and agreeing with the conclusion that care was better and had improved considerably over the past several years because of the expert care rendered. Considering that intensive care medicine is increasingly criticized as being overly expensive and for its technology "running wild," the future challenge appears to be the correlation of a clinical intuition with objective, prospective outcome data to prove the conference's hypothesis. This is extremely important because, in this manner, a method may be developed that will help relate the clinical experience and bias with the scientific outcome data that are needed so badly. In fact, any discussion about clinical care in a critical care environment is already hampered by the lack of objective data to demonstrate effectiveness. The medical and nursing professions have become so used to discounting clinical input and relying on monitor-derived patient assessment that quantitative clinical assessment is underemphasized.

On the other hand, even the most sophisticated units often ignore data that are readily available. For example, mixed venous oxygen saturation monitoring has been described and used clinically for the past decade. Over the past several years, technology has permitted the continuous measurement of this variable, and overall oxygen balance can be easily assessed for any patient. In this fashion, an assessment of the adequacy of cardiac output is possible as a more appropriate patient evaluation. It is likely that as monitoring techniques become more intelligently applied, their interpretation will begin to approach the accuracy of clinical intuition. It is probably a waste of a pulmonary artery catheter to use it for pressure and cardiac output monitoring only. The purpose of cardiac output is oxygen delivery, and the efficiency and appropriateness of delivery should be assessed in all cases. Only in this way is it possible to determine the adequacy of cardiac output. In addition, if it is remembered that the determinants of mixed venous saturation are arterial oxygen saturation, hemoglobin concentration, cardiac output, and metabolic rate, interesting therapeutic options become available that may have been overlooked.

Certainly, the burden of proof for the efficacy of critical care medicine is on the ICUs, and it will be interesting to see whether the creation of step-down units will have any impact on the common perception that ICUs have been created at the expense of routine care units. There is a feeling that routine ward care has suffered since the advent of critical care units because of the placement of the nurses with knowledge and experience in great numbers in the ICU. There have, however, been suggestions that a large bulk of the work done in the ICU is related to documentation and that actual contact with the patient is not as great as initially thought. On the other hand, often the routine wards are nowhere near as well staffed, especially during the night, so that medications and other ordered interventions may not be given at the prescribed time or may even be omitted. Perhaps the advent of the ICU has merely provided a certain group of patients with accurate and timely nursing care while it has diminished care in other areas. If this is true, then perhaps the clinical judgment that is applied to patient care should be directed at selecting the appropriate patients to receive critical care.

Although these comments may appear outside the context of a chapter on clinical evaluation in the ICU setting, they are not far off the subject. Admission criteria to critical care units differ from institution to institution, and outcome with respect to diagnosis may well be related to the severity of illness of the admitted patients. This subject was recently addressed by Pollack and colleagues in an article that studied outcome of illness between various ICUs. It was noted that outcome was related to severity of illness at the time of admission to the unit, and not the diagnosis *per se*.[13] Certainly, the present diagnosis-related grouping (DRG) reimbursement system needs to be modified if appropriate distribution of health care allocations are to be made between competing institutions. This argument is paraphrased in an accompanying editorial by Schroeder[14] in which he points out the importance placed on outcome monitoring by review bodies such as the Joint Commission on Accreditation of Hospitals (JCAH). In this setting, it becomes apparent that simple mortality statistics cannot be used to compare overall effectiveness of hospitals because of the difference in the patient population between the institutions. Indeed, the mortality statistics corrected for severity of illness are usually similar, and it is only in the study by Knaus and co-workers[15] that actual differences in the apparent quality of rendered care are noted. The implication of all these comments is that ICU admission policies may well determine patient mortality, that reimbursement may be allocated unfairly to hospitals with a lower acuity value for a given diagnosis, and that JCAH accreditation policies may discriminate unfairly against more sophisticated units in which more complicated cases are managed. It should be obvious that the clinical input into the management and classification of these cases will become increasingly important and that a more appropriate database than is currently available will be necessary. Current data collection and analysis lack discrimination, and true outcome data are unknown despite their being used as a grading tool and perhaps ultimately being used as a quality assurance tool. As Schroeder questions, are we ready?[14]

SUMMARY

A primary problem in critical care medicine is that clinical examination and diagnostic conjectures have been undervalued over the past several years and clinical intuition has been largely discounted. The objective of the preceding discussion is to reintroduce clinical skepticism and judgment into any therapeutic decision involving the critically ill patient. Certainly the stated bias is to decrease dependence on information obtained uncritically from invasive monitors and to increase clinical interpretation and application of all information, including the reports of ancillary and nursing personnel and their subjective impressions of the patient's progress and ultimate prognosis. This should not be construed as advocating a democratic approach to management, but rather a situation in which the clinician avails himself of all available information. This attitude is also important in choosing between available therapeutic regimens or deciding that the initial choice is suboptimal, which is often difficult and inappropriately implies mistaken judgment rather than a failed clinical trial. In fact, an important component of critical care medicine is the environment in which it is practiced. In no other hospital setting are trained observers ready to interpret the results of any drug combination and deal with the possible consequences of therapy.

The implications of a diagnosis are enormous, and the ways in which patients are managed vary. More difficult, perhaps, is the application of pharmacologic principles to the management of problem cases. Infrequently, a practitioner admits to a lack of sophistication with newer agents. More commonly, minimal understanding associated with apparent success in carefully selected cases creates a sense of false optimism that leads to overprescription of a specific therapy. In this fashion, protocols and traditions are born.

Into this difficult arena the clinician brings the pharmacologic knowledge of the therapeutic preparations and the expected and desired physiologic responses. It is his job to provide the clinical background for, and outcome assessment of, individual therapies in an attempt to titrate care appropriately. This individual is the true arbiter of the critical care process: by making the diagnosis, he assigns the denominator against which therapy will be judged; by prescribing care, he accepts the responsibility of pharmacologic manipulation; and by determining outcome, he forces the system to accept statistical probability for cure that is artifact and varies between institutions, as demonstrated by the difficulty encountered in comparing results between ICUs.

This problem has been addressed by those who use the various scoring systems to assess patient condition and progress of disease. Unfortunately the language of clinical assessment does not always translate between observers, and there is a lack of precision even in the most "accurate" invasive measurements. As previously stated, the first response after admission of any patient into the ICU or emergency department is for a rapid initial assessment followed by resuscitation based on a priority system aimed at preserving vital organ function. In the case of cardiac life support, the sequence of airway, breathing, and circulation is well established. Also, the trauma life support teaching courses stress this orientation with the addition of the primary and secondary assessments supplementing the initial evaluation. Familiarity with these techniques increases their usefulness, and in the case of neurosurgical nursing the following comments are illustrative.

But as the critical care nurse begins to use these basic techniques with each new neurosurgical patient, a "feel" for the neurological assessment begins to develop and will become part of the nurse's physical assessment routine. Also, to really understand what is happening to the neuro-surgical patient, a good knowledge of the anatomy and physiology of the nervous system is necessary . . . These same difficulties are the critical care challenges which become easier with experience, but for those interested in neurosurgical critical care, not less stimulating.[16]

Much of the activity of the rounding critical care physician can be described as integrated control coupled with a capacity to assimilate all of the available information. Evaluation of a conversation with a colleague provides a comprehensive neurologic assessment of the individual only if the listener becomes a critical observer as well as the recipient of information. The same is true for the physician who evaluates a critically ill patient with attention focused not only on the flow sheet, but also on the nursing report, patient appearance, respiratory effort, ventilator synchrony, presence of dysrhythmias, family evaluation of progress, and so on. As previously stated, not only is a critical patient assessment required, but also a review of the technology should be performed in conjunction with patient care. Too frequently, over-reliance on mechanical support devices leads to tragedy, and the unattended patient becomes one at unacceptably high risk if survival depends on the exemplary technologic function.

This philosophy can be stated differently: "The collection and recording of basic physiologic variables (such as temperature, pulse, and blood pressure) by the nursing personnel, although important, serve the additional and perhaps more important function of bringing the nurse or physician to the patient's bedside at regular intervals,"[17] an attitude reminiscent of Goldenheim and Kazemi.[8] Indeed, a worrisome trend in the middle to late 1970s was the creation of units designed in such fashion that the nurse was removed from direct patient contact and relegated to the position of a monitoring technician.[18] Recent developments in unit design and the interest in patient data management systems seem to have reversed this trend, and now the concern is in making individual bedsides functionally independent so that all data processing can be accessed by the care nurse without having to go to a central work station. This development, in part due to increased sophistication and miniaturization of computer equipment, should provide critical care practitioners with the next step in management. It should also make data acquisition and processing easier for the clinician and decrease the tendency to make mistakes when multiple therapies are used and occasional drug interactions are overlooked. In addition, this is a development that parallels the clinicial development of a nurse or physician, that is, the ability to integrate the complexities of the patient's clinical situation and associated physiologic information into an appropriate management plan. Hopefully, data processing in the ICU will replace the current data overload that has done little to alter outcome in most of the studies quoted in the recent literature.

CONCLUSION

The skill and experience of the medical and nursing staff are the factors that have the greatest impact on the quality of monitoring and treatment of the critically ill surgical patient. Basic determinations at the bedside together with periodic evaluation of the whole patient by the medical staff may, in selected cases, be supplemented usefully by more invasive monitoring techniques. The specific complications and technical pitfalls of these techniques should be known, and caution should always be exercised that the values provided are not misinterpreted.[17]

The focus of this discussion has been on the relationship between the clinical assessment of patients in the critical care environment and the commonly used adjuncts of diagnosis and care. Too frequently, reliance on the invasively obtained hemodynamic parameters or other laboratory data have reduced the importance of the clinical information derived by patient examination and observation. Also, the importance of communication between the nursing staff, the physicians, ancillary personnel, and the patient's family has been stressed as has the importance of repeat examinations accomplished with a high level of suspicion and integrated with all ancillary data. Sibbald and associates address this issue by stating "The ability to distinguish noncardiac pulmonary edema from cardiac pulmonary edema is vitally important since management, beyond initial stabilization, is radically dissimilar."[19] They then proceed to describe this process by dividing the discussion into pathophysiology, etiology, clinical distinction between cardiac pulmonary edema (CPE) and noncardiac pulmonary edema (NCPE), and conclusions. Of relevance to this discussion, however, are his clinical subdivisions, which include physical examination ("In contrast to CPE, NCPE is usually a hyperdynamic illness, clinicially apparent as a warm, vasodilated periphery"[19]), laboratory examination, chest radiography, indices of the metabolic rate of the illness, pulmonary edema fluid and complement analysis, radiotracer techniques, and measurement of extravascular lung water.

This approach stresses the integrational responsibility of the rounding physician. In addition, it broadens the traditional definition of clinical assessment to include laboratory and other diagnostic, supportive, and therapeutic techniques that are perhaps more traditionally regarded as monitoring devices. The clinical assessment does not end with the documentation of the physical examination; rather, the complete clinical work-up must integrate the pathophysiology of the underlying process with the appearance of the patient and results of bedside examination and the special investigations deemed appropriate. Subsequently, an appropriate conclusion and plan of treatment based on a priority listing are formulated. In this fashion, the clinician re-establishes his role in the ICU and provides integrated patient care of the highest order. Future development of therapy depends on this support but is impossible if the physician does not play an active role in the clinical management of critically ill patients.

REFERENCES

1. Chuyn DA: A comparison of intra-arterial and auscultatory blood pressure readings. *Heart Lung* 1985; 14:223
2. Venus B, Mathru M, Smith RA, et al: Direct versus indirect blood pressure measurements in critically ill patients. *Heart Lung* 1985; 14:228
3. Nadeau S, Noble WH: Misinterpretation of pressure measurements from the pulmonary artery catheter. *Can Anaesth Soc J* 1986; 33:352
4. Del Guercio LRM, Cohn JD: Monitoring operating risk in the elderly. *JAMA* 1980; 243:1350
5. Connors AF, McCaffree DR, Gray BA: Evaluation of right heart catheterization in the critically ill patient without acute myocardial infarction. *N Engl J Med* 1983; 308:263
6. Holder DA: Does hemodynamic monitoring complement conventional methods of assessment in the critically ill cardiac patient? *Can Med Assoc J* 1979; 121:895
7. Drake JJ: Locating the external reference point for central venous pressure determination. *Nurs Res* 1974; 23:475
8. Goldenheim PD, Kazemi H: Cardiopulmonary monitoring of critically ill patients: I. *N Engl J Med* 1984; 311:717
9. *Webster's New Collegiate Dictionary*, Springfield, Massachusetts, G & C Merrian, 1977
10. Henning RJ, Wiener F, Valdes S, et al: Measurement of toe temperature for assessing the severity of acute circulatory failure. *Surg Gynecol Obstet* 1979; 149:1

11. Rao TLK, Jacobs KH, El-Etr AA: Reinfarction following anesthesia in patients with myocardial infarction. *Anesthesiology* 1983; 59:499
12. Eichorn JH, Cooper JB, Cullen DJ, et al: Standards for patient monitoring during anesthesia at Harvard Medical School. *JAMA* 1986; 256:1017
13. Pollack MM, Urs ER, Getson PR, et al: Accurate prediction of the outcome of pediatric intensive care. *N Engl J Med* 1987; 316:134
14. Schroeder SA: Outcome assessment 70 years later. Are we ready? *N Engl J Med* 1987; 316:160
15. Knaus WA, Draper EA, Wagner DP, et al: An evaluation of outcome from intensive care in major medical centers. *Ann Intern Med* 1986; 104:410
16. Miller L: Neurological assessment: A practical guide for the critical care nurse. *J Neurosurg Nurs* 1979; 11:2
17. Allardyce DB: Monitoring of the critically ill patient. *Can J Surg* 1978; 21:75
18. Maloney JV: The trouble with patient monitoring. *Ann Surg* 1968; 168:605
19. Sibbald WJ, Cunningham DR, Chin DN: Noncardiac or cardiac pulmonary edema? A practical approach to clinical differentiation in critically ill patients. *Chest* 1983; 84:452

CHAPTER TWO

CLEAN AND ASEPTIC TECHNIQUE AT THE BEDSIDE

Judith A. Hudson–Civetta
Joseph M. Civetta

Sepsis is recognized as a significant cause of death or a major complicating factor in most intensive care units (ICUs) today. Because of the risk of nosocomial infection, a great deal of attention must be focused on sterile technique and on maintaining a sterile interface at insertion sites of vascular catheters, particularly in the long-term ICU patient. The three relevant factors in the development of a clinical infection are the host, the organism, and the environment. Although powerless to influence the process at present, we are well aware that the patient with multiple system dysfunction who remains in the ICU for protracted periods becomes increasingly susceptible to nosocomial infection due to compromise in immune function, both cellular and humoral elements. Malnutrition and liver dysfunction potentiate the process because of diminished production of acute phase reactive proteins. Evidence for depressed immune function may also be inferred from the types of organisms creating late nosocomial infections. *Staphylococcus epidermidis*, a ubiquitous skin organism, may be isolated from a high percentage of catheter-related infections.[1] Opportunistic or superinfections commonly occur; however, the bacteria isolated are not "super" organisms but organisms that usually cannot colonize a patient with normal symbiotic flora and normal immune function. With respect to the environment, we shall describe methods for skin preparation and creation of a sterile field during insertion as well as the types of dressings used to maintain sterility during the period of catheterization. Although there are some individual variations, the basic principles used in creating the field and constructing the dressings are remarkably similar in many articles and textbooks today. We shall describe the variations in terms of the usually advanced rationales and the procedures themselves in sufficient detail to guide a novice or to serve as a starting point suitable for "customizing" in your own unit.

Notwithstanding the focus and attention placed on the techniques, everyone agrees that the *care-giver* plays the major role in transmitting nosocomial infection. In terms of generating innovative countermeasures, however, the effect of this knowledge appears to be quite limited. Everyone acknowledges the role of care-givers with the usual admonishment— "wash hands between each patient contact." But this appears to be the extent of control, and as soon as administrative interest flags, there is progressive apathy in the care-givers themselves. In a way, this situation seems analogous to the sporadic public outcry against the ongoing carnage due to trauma or the immense impact on public health caused by smoking. In truth, we must maintain "eternal vigilance" at the bedside. Each must be responsible for his or her actions *and* watch the other members of the team as well. We should remember the words of James Cabell, Professor of Anatomy, Physiology, and Surgery at the University of Virginia who, in speaking about peripheral infection at the 1882 meeting of the American Surgical Association said, "The source was to be found in the hands of the medical men in attendance."[2] These remarks, issued during the "Listerian" debates of the early 1880s, were not the only point of view and many distinguished leaders of American surgery disagreed. J. W. S. Gouley, Professor of the Diseases of the Genitourinary Tract of the College of Physicians and Surgeons in New York City, said in 1882, "Listerism (anti-sepsis) is dead." Claudius Mastin, a later president of the American Surgical Association, proclaimed, "Not a single surgeon in the state of Alabama uses the Lister method."

Physicians still tend to retain a certain disbelief that, after all their years of medical training, bacteria could or would actually be transmitted through their ministrations. Let us examine the role of the physician care-givers, to determine why the admonition "wash hands between each patient contact" is so easy to express, so universally acknowledged, yet so difficult to practice. We must first examine the cast of usual ICU characters. First, attendings know the dangers of person-to-person contamination and the risks of such infections to the compromised patient. They understand the value of limiting contact to the extent that they rarely touch patients. Nurses know the dangers and are constantly aware, given a two-patient assignment, that they must frequently move between patients; hand-washing becomes second nature. On the other hand, because nurses limit their contact to their assigned patients, the risk of cross-contamination is also limited. Physicians outside the unit staff see only their own patients, but again have a limited opportunity to spread organisms throughout the ICU. On the other hand, surgeons may need to examine open wounds or do other bedside procedures. Although the use of sterile technique is second nature, remembering to stop at the sink after visiting each bed would require a special conscious effort, because this is not universal practice during rounds outside the ICU.

Technicians and therapists are usually aware or reminded by the patient's nurse of the risks of nosocomial infection. Although they may be exposed to a greater number of patients, their physical contacts with the patients are, perhaps, more limited and away from the actual sites of catheterization.

In fact, the group at highest risk is the ICU team of physicians. They have the most direct contact with the most ICU patients. Furthermore, given rotations of relatively junior personnel, they may be less knowledgeable with respect to risks of nosocomial infection, aseptic technique, and the technical procedures themselves. It is also truly a herculean task to remember handwashing between each patient contact because of the sheer number of patient contacts during their tour of duty. Also, it is extremely difficult to place handwashing at the top of the list when suddenly called to assist in an emergency. Thus, there are many realistic reasons why the ICU physicians are the care-givers most likely to transmit infection.

There are, in addition to these realistic factors, other beliefs (read "delusions"). Although no one has actually ever expressed these, we have observed behavior that seems to indicate their presence: [1] bacteria honor emergency situations. This is somehow conceived to be similar to workers honoring a picket line. In any case, personnel who ordinarily carefully wash between each patient contact may rush from one patient to another because of a crisis and omit this step; [2] physicians, similar to the international diplomats, have been given a certain type of immunity. For physicians, this immunity renders them free from bacterial contamination. We assume that this belief must have motivated the physician whom we observed performing barehanded endotracheal suctioning; [3] the admonition "Wash between each patient contact" really is akin to the admonition that you must attend each class during college and medical school. Because no one really takes attendance, you can skip a few without "hurting anyone." Thus, washing, most of the time, is sufficient; and [4] paraphrasing "Cleanliness is next to godliness," to be "*goodliness* is just like cleanliness." In other words, bacteria respect good intentions. If you work hard and are generally nice, it is not as necessary to concentrate on such mundane details as handwashing.

Perhaps these beliefs do not exist even in an unexpressed form; however, in a busy ICU, it is extremely difficult to adhere absolutely to the simple precept to wash each time between each patient contact as well as between different procedures on the same patient. The difficulty does not diminish the importance of doing so. Perhaps this can be best emphasized by understanding the magnitude and importance of the problem of nosocomial catheter sepsis.

IMPORTANCE OF NOSOCOMIAL INFECTION

Catheter-related septicemia is among the more serious complications of intravenous therapy and affects an estimated 50,000 patients in the United States each year.[3] This complication of catheter-related septicemia represents 8% of the total complications of intravenous infusion therapy.[4] In contrast to the infection rates related to intravenous infusion therapy in general, investigations in the literature report rates of pulmonary artery (PA) catheter-related infection that vary widely from 8%[5] to 29%.[6] Reports of the rate of PA catheter-related septicemia vary from 3%[6] to 11%.[7]

Regardless of the variable percentages of catheter-related infection and catheter-related septicemia, the infectious complications represent a serious risk to the safety of the ICU patient. The source(s) of the bacteria that contaminate or infect catheters and that may also predispose to catheter-related septicemia are many. The following factors have been implicated by investigations in the literature:

1 length of catheterization;[4-9]

2 direct entry of bacteria into the bloodstream from contaminated or infected intravascular catheters;[4,8,9]

3 bacteria on the patient's skin near the site of catheter insertion;[4,6,8]

4 contaminated transducer-pressure-monitoring systems attached to the catheter;[8,10]

5 another source of infection in the patient coexisting with the catheter;[4,7-9,11]

6 excessive time intervals between replacement of the catheter's dressing, stopcocks, transducer, or infusion fluid.[8,12]

This list has a common denominator: the care-giver who maintains and uses the catheterization-monitoring systems.

SOURCES OF BACTERIA

There are three sources of the bacteria: the patient's own skin; the care-giver; and other sites in the patient. With respect to the patient's own skin, antisepsis will be discussed in the section on preparation. Remember, however, that skin cannot be permanently sterilized because bacteria colonize hair follicles and sweat glands. Even if the surface is rendered sterile temporarily, regrowth occurs over time from the depths of the skin appendages, the indication for repeating sterilization techniques at specified intervals. The importance of maintaining surface sterility can be recognized from Sitzman's study in which there was an 8% incidence of positive catheter segment cultures in patients who had negative cultures of the skin site compared to a 50% rate of positive catheter segment cultures in patients who had positive cultures from the skin.[13] Thus, the skin surrounding the insertion site is an obvious source of bacteria. If bacteria growth flourishes, organisms can gain entrance through the skin puncture site and grow in the subcutaneous tract; this growth is usually termed colonization. Subsequently, this may lead to either signs of local infection or bacteremia if bacteria enter the bloodstream through the perforation in the vessel wall caused by catheterization.

The care-giver might also be the source of the bacteria ultimately responsible for nosocomial infection. Common sites of transmission include the skin (especially the hands), hair, nose, and mouth. It is for these reasons, obviously, that gloves, caps, and masks are used.

Other sites in the patient, the final source of nosocomial infection, include open wounds and drains, the lungs, urinary tract, and perineum. There are two potential pathways for transmission, difficult to study and difficult to separate. The first is an exogenous pathway. Bacteria from the primary patient source arrive at the catheter insertion site through some intermediate step or steps. For instance, bacteria in tracheostomy secretions may penetrate the dressing overlying a subclavian catheter, or a person wearing sterile gloves during a dressing change may reach up to reconnect the ventilator tubing that "popped off" the endotracheal tube. In doing so, the operator's gloves are accidentally contaminated and, if they are not changed, will contaminate the catheter insertion site. During subsequent manipulations of the catheter to perform a cardiac output, bacteria can be transferred to the stopcock used for injection of the indicator for determining cardiac output.

The second mode of organism spread from one site in a patient to another can be termed endogenous. After the development of bacteremia from a distant source (abscesses or pneumonia), organisms may lodge in a fibrin sheath surrounding the intravascular portion of the catheter. This fibrin sheath is more common with the usual central venous and PA catheters; the use of less reactive materials such as silicone elastomers and the incorporation of heparin into the catheter surface are attempts to decrease this sheath formation. Bacteria in the arterial circulation may lodge in the wound (hematogenous spread) produced by the insertion of the vascular catheter. A cause-and-effect relationship to demonstrate endogenous transmission is difficult for many reasons. Peripheral bacteremia may not be detected, removal of the catheter may strip the fibrin sheath, and culture of the catheter tip (often performed, but on an incorrect specimen) that has only briefly traversed the catheter wound may not reveal the organism. For both physiologic and methodologic reasons, this mode of transmission may be difficult to document or to infer the correct sequence of events.

Because many similar terms are used, and definitions often vary, we shall try to establish some restricted meanings for commonly used terms for purposes of discussion here.

Sterile. No growth of microorganisms or a technique that is presumed to be free of microorganisms.

Contamination. Bacteria are introduced into a sterile area or onto the surface of components that were previously sterile. This term probably should not be used in a quantitative sense to distinguish a small from a large amount of bacterial growth on the surface of a monitoring catheter. Some studies refer to "infected" catheters, signifying large growth and "contaminated" catheters if only a few organisms are present.

Colonization. Bacteria growing in a host without evidence of infection. The obvious normal example is the gastrointestinal tract; it may be applied to a catheter's subcutaneous *tract* if there is no evidence of local infection.

Infection. Probably should not be applied to an inanimate object. Infection represents reaction of the host to bacterial growth. Some would, therefore, prefer the term catheter-related infection to catheter infection.

Positive component or catheter segment culture. Because there is no agreement, terms such as contaminated, colonized, and infected have different meanings when used by different people. Perhaps the term "positive component culture" could be used to describe inanimate objects, and we should limit the use of infection to gross signs or the numerical definition,[4] greater than 15 colonies on semiquantitative culture of the catheter segment, which is commonly quoted.

Catheter-related bacteremia. Bacteria of the same species are recovered from the blood and culture of the catheter. The implication is that bacterial growth from the catheter site was the source of the bacteremia. However, fibrin may collect around an intravascular catheter. Bacteremia may originate from pneumonia or abscess. Bacteria may lodge and multiply in this fibrin sheath. This may be termed secondary seeding of the catheter. The subcutaneous tract might be seeded hematogenously from a distant source as well. Because it may be impossible to differentiate, use of the term "synchronous bacteremia" may be preferable, which assigns a temporal but not causal relationship to the isolation of bacteria of the same species simultaneously from peripheral blood and a catheter segment culture.

INSERTION PROTOCOLS

Usual written descriptions and even a quick glance at an ongoing insertion procedure in the ICU provide a view that seems reasonably similar to sterile technique in the operating room (OR). Many limiting factors make this appearance quite deceiving. First, the patient is usually not asleep so that the field itself does not remain stationary. All of us have experienced unexpected "help" as the patient frees his arm and a hand suddenly enters the sterile field. The actual physical isolation of the sterile area from nonsterile areas is much more difficult than in the OR because they must overlap during continued treatment of the patient. To achieve this separation and isolation in the OR, separate sterile and nonsterile teams are necessary. It is a far cry from the OR team of a surgeon, assistant, scrub nurse, technician, and one or two circulating nurses to the team in the ICU, which is usually limited to the fellow or resident and nurse. Training in sterile technique is limited in many of the individuals involved in sterile procedures in the ICU *and* there are fewer "watchdogs," those in the OR assigned to keep an eye on the inexperienced (usually) medical students and junior residents during their first exposures to sterile technique. The time factor must also be considered—in the OR the need for sterility ends with the end of the procedure; in the ICU, the efforts to maintain sterility must be maintained for all of the days of monitoring. Finally, there are some hard data on handwashing. Universally considered one of the most basic and vital infection control measures,[3] handwashing is done infrequently after contact with high-risk patients, estimated at less than one third of the time in the U.S. centers.[14] In the operating room, everyone scrubs for 5 to 10 minutes, even three or four times a day. In studies of comparative handwashing, the duration studied and found to be effective has been 30 to 60 seconds, considered *impractically long* and unlikely to be accepted by busy hospital personnel. Yet, handwashing with antiseptic-containing agents effectively reduced counts of microorganisms, more so than do nongermicidal soaps.[15,16] Disturbingly, after a *typical 7- to 10-second* handwashing, the number of organisms that can be transmitted from the person's hands often increases significantly.[15–17] Apparently, then, we have a difficult environment, busy personnel, inadequate education and training, less supervision, and hurried techniques. These factors, more than any specific technical detail of the insertion procedure, are probably responsible for the high incidence of catheter-related infection.

A PRACTICAL BEDSIDE APPROACH

Before describing the physical steps of preparation and dressing, we should consider some general concepts. There is universal agreement that masks and gloves should be used because hands and the upper airways are common sources of pathogens in hospital personnel. Shoe covers would appear to be of no benefit unless there are strict rules and strict enforcement applied *across the board.* Even in operating areas, it is common to see the orderly leave the operating suite to pick up a new patient and, because time is important, fail to change the shoe covers each and every time the operating suite is entered again. It is almost impossible to conceive that better discipline would be maintained in an ICU. Caps should be used for the restraint of hair when appropriate. The use of gowns appears to be a matter of personal taste. Because of the space limitations, on the one hand, it is impossible to keep the gown as sterile as in the operating room. On the other hand, it does limit the possibility of inadvertent contamination of the longer catheters. Try to establish separate sterile and nonsterile work areas. A small table can be used for kits and the additions necessary. For the sterile field, try to create as large a covered area as possible. Remember to talk to the patient ahead of time to provide reassurance and explanations. Remember not to underestimate the duration of the procedure or to minimize the discomfort that the patient might experience. When things do not proceed as quickly as hoped, anxiety may be *created*; do not gloss over or minimize the time and pain to "spare" the patient. Sedation may be necessary and restraints should be used. Work through as small an opening in the sterile drapes as possible to avoid inadvertent contamination with other pieces of equipment surrounding the patient. Use prepackaged kits whenever possible. They are easier and faster to assemble and more likely to contain the "right" components; however, the major advantage is that each preassembled connection eliminates another potential source of contamination by the care-giver during assembly. We prefer using the closed cardiac output injectate systems and continuous measurement of mixed venous oximetry instead of the intermittent syringe injection system or aspiration of mixed venous blood gases. Again, each intermittent technique is an additional opportunity for transmission of organisms.

In invasive catheterization, the focus usually is on the actual insertion procedure. In fact, the physician asks to be called when everything is ready and leaves when the catheter is in place. There is a much broader focus, which we believe is necessary to understand the complete process, many days in duration. From this perspective, the nurse in the ICU is charged with the responsibility of maintaining and caring for the catheter before, during, and after insertion as well as assessing the patient for signs and symptoms of infection.[18] His or her responsibilities include the following activities in caring for the critically ill patient:

1 assembling the transducer-pressure-monitoring system with sterile technique;

2 ensuring proper cleaning of the transducer between use;

3 assembling the equipment needed for insertion of the catheter using sterile technique;

4 testing the patency and function of the catheter;

5 maintaining sterile technique during insertion;

6 monitoring the patient's physiologic status during insertion;

7 applying the sterile, occlusive dressing and changing the dressing every 48 hours or when soiled, saturated, or disturbed;

8 assessing the catheter–skin interface for signs of inflammation;

9 obtaining pressure measurements from the catheter as the patient's physiologic needs indicate;

10 calibrating the transducer on a periodic basis;

11 obtaining blood samples as indicated;

12 infusing intravenous fluids and medications; and

13 obtaining cultures of blood, urine, tracheal aspirate, and wound as indicated for patients with a known or suspected source of infection.

All of these responsibilities are included in either prevention, detection, or amelioration of focal or contextual stimuli that affect the patient's healing process.[19] The list of nursing responsibilities emphasizes the importance and the magnitude of the nursing interaction required for a patient with an invasive catheter.

PREPARATION OF SITE AND DRESSING

Preparing the insertion site with antiseptic solutions appears to be an area of little controversy, not even discussed for future research.[3] We will present what is commonly accepted, with variations and comment.

Shaving before elective surgical operations used to be done the night before. However, nicks and scratches became reddened, and it was noted that if shaving was performed too early, an increased incidence of wound infection resulted.[20] Because sterilization of the site is necessary for days, shaving for the purpose of adding sterilization would not be advisable. However, in hirsute patients, shaving may be necessary to enable a dressing to be fastened securely. If necessary, shaving should be done lightly and repeated when necessary. Various solutions have been proposed in various combinations. Acetone is often used first, to remove old tape and otherwise debride. Another common indication is to "defat" the skin, although we cannot find any published advantage of lean skin. Alcohol is an excellent antiseptic if the time of contact is 2 minutes or longer. Iodine is used in two forms, the traditional tincture of iodine or, more commonly today, povidone–iodine. Tincture of iodine is effective but can be irritating, and if it is used, it is usually removed at the end of the procedure. Part of its effect may be due to the alcohol, which is used as the vehicle. Organic iodine solutions need to stay in contact with the skin for at least 2 minutes, and usually the recommendation is to let the skin dry before the insertion technique is begun. It is often difficult to wait; do not estimate the time—look at a clock. These organic solutions are often removed at the end of the procedure to prevent skin irritation from prolonged contact under the airtight dressing. Description of the actual skin preparation and the final catheter dressing range from nonexistent to brief at best, because we tend to concentrate our attention on the details of the technical procedure of catheter insertion. Because these features are discussed in detail for each procedure in other chapters, we will reverse the process and concentrate on the preparation and dressing.

TECHNIQUE OF SKIN PREPARATION

Each catheter should be inserted by use of a prepackaged kit containing all essential sterile components assembled by a central supply department or by a manufacturer (Figure 2-1). The individual catheter and the solutions used for preparation of the skin are added after the sterile field is formed.

Figure 2-1 A prepackaged insertion kit is opened, creating a sterile work area on a bedside table. Not only are these kits faster and easier to use, but also they contain all of the proper elements needed.

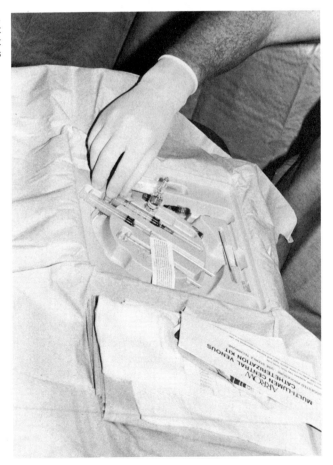

The kit should be placed on a clean, dry surface. After the outer wrapper is opened, masks and gloves are distributed to the involved personnel at the bedside before the inner kit is carefully opened. Masks should decrease the transmission of oral and nasal flora onto the sterile field and should be worn by everyone at the bedside (including an extubated patient). In intubated patients, the exhalation port of the ventilator should be directed away from the field.

The physician dons sterile gloves and prepares the kit contents for the procedure. An assistant pours the two solutions used for preparation of the skin: acetone (or alcohol) and povidone–iodine. Preparation of the skin should be done according to a defined protocol to prevent bacterial contamination from both the patient's skin flora and the equipment. The physician begins preparing the skin, first applying acetone with a soaked sterile gauze sponge (4 × 4 in), folded twice and clamped in forceps. Prepackaged swabs may also be used. The skin is briskly scrubbed in an expanding circular manner, beginning at the proposed insertion point and reaching a diameter of approximately 6 inches. The forceps and gauze (or swab) are changed, and the cleansing process is repeated in the same manner a second and third time with the povidone–iodine solution. The final application is allowed to remain in contact with the skin for at least 2 minutes to allow its antimicrobial action to occur and to provide residual activity.

The surrounding skin is covered by sterile drapes, and a sterile sheet is placed over the remainder of the patient's body. (*Note:* A sterile sheet is used only for insertion of the PA catheter.) The sterile drapes provide a large sterile working area to prevent contamination of the equipment used in insertion (Fig. 2-2). The combination of drapes and sheet is used for the insertion of the PA catheter because a large sterile area is needed for handling the unwieldy equipment. After the preparation has been completed, the catheter is introduced according to defined technique. When the catheter is in correct functional position, it is attached to the appropriate connection, and the povidone–iodine solution is removed by cleaning with sterile normal saline to prevent possible burning of the patient's skin (Fig. 2-3). Antimicrobial ointment is then applied to the site of insertion on the skin (Fig. 2-4). Povidone–iodine ointment has been recommended for use by Maki and Band.[21] The method used to secure the placement of the catheter varies according to the type of catheter. A sterile sleeve used with PA catheters is attached to the hub of the introducer and is fixed 20 to 30 cm along the catheter body. This leaves a segment enclosed in the sheath so that it can be manipulated later if the tip of the catheter must be readjusted to maintain proper position. The introducer is usually sutured to the skin. Arterial and central venous catheters commonly have flanges for anchoring skin sutures as well. The surrounding skin is dried and then sprayed with tincture of benzoin. The dressing is completed with occlusive tape (Fig. 2-5) and then sealed with clear, waterproof tape (Fig. 2-6). The occlusive tape prevents entry of bacteria that are airborne, and the waterproof tape prevents oral or tracheostomy secretions and any other moisture from saturating and contaminating the dressing. The date and time are written on the surface of the dressing. A chest radiograph is obtained to verify the position of the catheter and to rule out complications such as pneumothorax.

Catheters for parenteral nutrition (PN) should never be connected to pressure monitoring equipment for verification of position in order to reduce possible contamination; we consider verification by radiography the only means of establishing the correct position of the catheter tip. Until the correct position is known, 5% dextrose in water should be infused slowly at a "keep-open" rate. This precaution prevents the concentrated dextrose solution

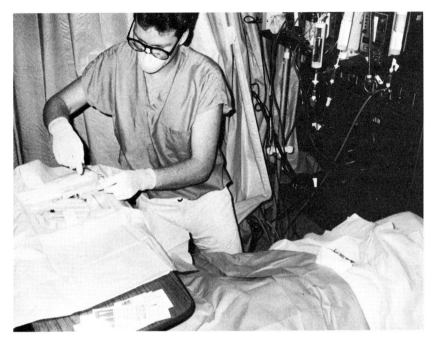

Figure 2-2 After preparation of the skin, the proposed insertion site is covered with a fenestrated drape. A sterile sheet is spread over the patient's body, providing a continuous sterile work area from the insertion site to the insertion kit.

from being infused into a noncentral vein and should lessen the incidence of thrombotic complications that may result.

Our final connection to the catheter for central venous and arterial catheters is a T-connector. We prefer the T-connector to the stopcock, both for the patient's safety and to minimize the risk of microbial contamination. Catheters for PN are connected to a "final" filter (0.22μ) before infusing the nutritional solutions. After the PN catheter is connected to the appropriate filter, tubing, and solution, the system must never be interrupted except to change the dressing, the intravenous tubing, and the final filter. The catheter is never used to infuse medication or withdraw blood samples for routine laboratory studies or cultures. Substances are not added to the solution after its preparation in the pharmacy. These precautions have been recommended to prevent bacterial contamination.

MAINTENANCE OF INTRAVASCULAR CATHETERS

DRESSING CHANGES

All dressings on invasive intravascular catheters should be handled in a similar manner. We currently change them every 48 hours or more often if soiled, saturated, or disturbed to minimize the growth of microorganisms.[11,22] The dressing should be changed by competent personnel who have been certified in the prescribed technique.

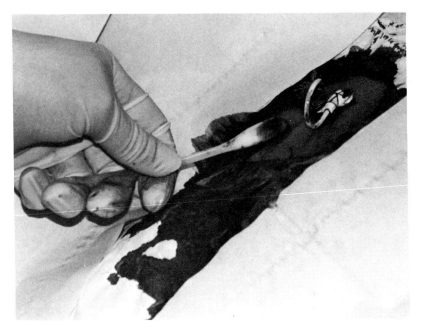

Figure 2-3 After insertion, the area is again cleansed with povidone-iodine, which is removed with an alcohol swab. This process should remove any inadvertent surface contamination during the insertion process.

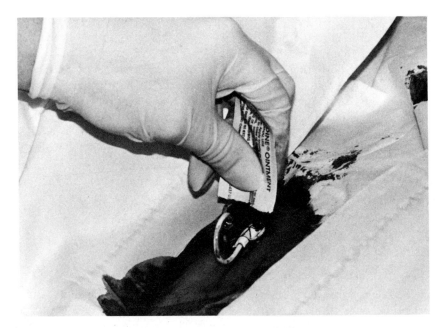

Figure 2-4 Povidone-iodine ointment is applied after the catheter has been sutured in place. The skin surface should be dry, and there should be no bleeding from the insertion site or sutures. Sterile gauze is then applied.

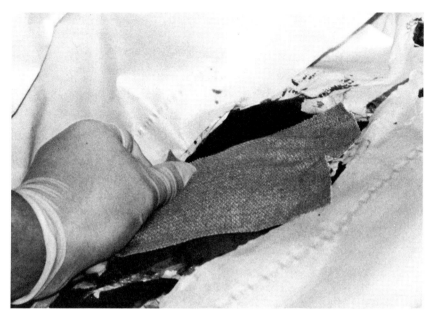

Figure 2-5 Elastoplast tape is applied after tincture of benzoin spray.

We use dressing kits prepackaged by the hospital or commerically available because they facilitate the process and prevent use of scattered available components that may be undesirable. The ready availability of all sterile components decreases the possibility of "breaks" in technique.

The dressing change kit is placed on a clean, dry surface; the outer package is opened; the packages of gloves, masks, and sterile occlusive tape are removed; and the mask is donned by the practitioner. The inner package is opened, and the practitioner dons sterile gloves and arranges the contents of the kit to position the receptacles for the skin cleansing solutions. The currently recommended solutions are acetone or alcohol and povidone–iodine.[11,22] The gloves are discarded, the solutions are poured, povidone–iodine ointment to be used in the new dressing is squeezed onto a sterile gauze square, and the old dressing is removed. After donning a new pair of sterile gloves, the cleansing process is begun. The process is identical to that previously described for inserting a catheter. Care must be taken not to dislodge any catheter that is not sutured.

After the acetone has been applied and the povidone–iodine ointment removed, the site should be visually inspected and palpated for indications of infection. Specifically look for exudate around the site of insertion, redness, or edema, and then palpate for tenderness or warmth. If any abnormal sign is noted, the catheter should be removed and cultures taken.

After the cleansing process has been completed, the ointment is applied and a new occlusive dressing secured. Quality assurance and surveillance must be maintained routinely by the charge nurse or the infection control nurse to check the dressings (noting date and time of change and appearance) and, on a more formal basis, through the quarterly use of a process audit tool designed by the ICU personnel. The audit can be designed to measure the

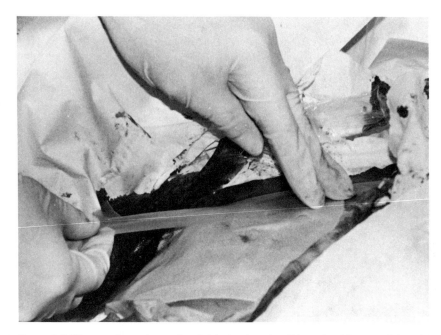

Figure 2-6 Waterproof tape is used to finish the dressing. We prefer this type of dressing to transparent dressings for reasons outlined in the text.

presence or absence of specific procedures related to the care of intravascular catheters: frequency of dressing change, frequency of change for pressure monitoring and intravenous tubing and solution change, rate and type of positive cultures, and so on.

Intravenous tubing, fluid, filters, and other paraphernalia used without pressure monitoring equipment should be changed every 48 hours.[11,12,23] The fluid, connecting tubing, and filters should be replaced every 24 hours for PN catheters (glass bottles of PN solutions are changed every 12 hr). On the basis of a recent study, we use the external system for pressure monitoring for 72 hours.[24] Any equipment must be replaced if known or suspected contamination has occurred.

We have not adopted the use of transparent polyurethane dressings. The potential advantages are described as visibility of the insertion site, a watertight seal, and an extended time (5–7 days) between dressing changes, resulting in sufficient savings in materials and nursing care to offset the higher initial cost. However, permanent sterilization of the skin cannot be achieved. In one study, transparent dressings had a higher rate of site colonization than sterile gauze.[25] No antibiotic or antimicrobial ointment was used in either group. Additionally, there was a higher rate of bacteremic arterial catheter-related infection when transparent dressings were used. In a later study, either a polyantibiotic or povidone–iodine ointment significantly reduced colonization, although the rate was higher in the polyurethane dressing control group.[26] We had difficulty maintaining the seal if ointments were used; thus, dressing changes were necessary more frequently than 5 to 7 days. In most of our patients, monitoring is finished or catheters are changed on the third and fourth day. Positive catheter segments often occur without visible signs of infection; thus, we found that none of the proposed advantages actually did apply to our population.

TWO SEMIQUANTITATIVE CULTURE SPECIMENS
USING GUIDEWIRE EXCHANGE

The technique was devised to avoid problems in interpreting cultures of a catheter withdrawn through a subcutaneous tract and submitting the tip alone for culture. This technique can be used only when a catheter (usually PA) has been placed through an introducer. If only a catheter (PN, double or triple lumen) is present, the only proper and necessary culture specimen is the intracutaneous segment. The tip should not be cultured because it does not add meaningful information and may underestimate the number of colonies present.[4,24] Further, if the catheter with any fibrin or organisms on its surface is withdrawn through the introducer, it should provide a specimen that is protected from contact with the subcutaneous tract. Any organisms then cultured should represent those on the intravascular portion of the catheter. The intracutaneous portion of the introducer should be cultured separately to derive information on bacterial growth in the subcutaneous tract. These general considerations led to the development of the following technique.

The dressing is removed, including any remaining antibacterial ointment. The insertion site is scrubbed with povidone–iodine solution for 2 minutes and then prepared with alcohol. This method attempts to sterilize the skin before the intracutaneous segment is removed and to remove existing skin bacteria as a source of contamination of the introducer segment to be cultured. However, for investigative purposes, recognizing the importance of maintained skin sterility with respect to positive catheter segments, a culture of the skin can be taken before the preparation as well.[13] Preparation should include the introducer from the insertion site to the end of the hub, including the tubing of the sidearm. After the skin and introducer have been prepared, the hub is detached from the introducer, and the hub and catheter are removed together. The catheter is *not* withdrawn through the diaphragm of the introducer hub since this would defeat the purpose of a separate culture of the tip by stripping the fibrin from the surface of the catheter. A syringe is placed temporarily into the introducer to prevent backbleeding. The 3-cm segment of the distal catheter tip is grasped in sterile forceps and cut free using a sterile scissor. Alternatively, the operator can don a new sterile glove (Fig. 2-7) and grasp the end of the catheter. The catheter tip is placed on a blood agar plate (Fig. 2-8) and rolled once back and forth across it. The use of a new sterile glove is recommended to decrease the likelihood of contamination of these all-important cultures. Although the entire procedure is held to be sterile, the semiquantitative culture method is sensitive, and the gloved hand usually has handled connections, gauze, and may be blood-spotted from the manipulation of the catheter. The catheter tip is pushed lightly into the agar without breaking it. The plate must be rapidly transported to the microbiology laboratory. Even a 1-hour delay in incubation can invalidate the results by underestimating the number of bacteria present. The syringe is removed from the end of the introducer and a guidewire inserted (Fig. 2-9). The introducer is removed; note or mark the skin insertion site. A gauze sponge may be placed over the site and gentle pressure applied if there is any backbleeding. Another sterile glove or sterile forceps is used to grasp the intracutaneous segment. The introducer is cut just below the level of the skin insertion site (Fig. 2-10) and again 3 cm more distally with sterile scissors to obtain a segment of the introducer that lay in the intracutaneous tract. This segment is cultured on a blood agar plate similar to the method described for the catheter tip. The gauze is removed and a new catheter placed over the guidewire. Alternatively, the introducer may be placed in a sterile area of the prep tray (Fig. 2-11). The new catheter may be inserted (Fig. 2-12). A new glove is then donned or the introducer held in a sterile forceps, and the segment of the introducer can be removed for

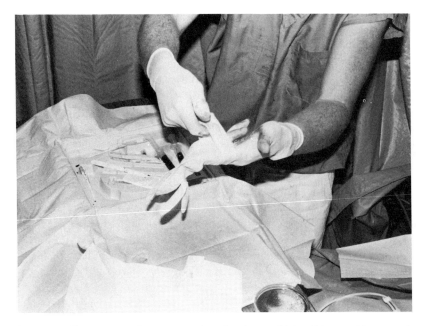

Figure 2-7 The operator dons a second sterile glove, which will be used to grasp the tip of the catheter and to roll it across the culture plate. The initial glove is usually visibly stained with solutions, blood, and the like and may have been contaminated.

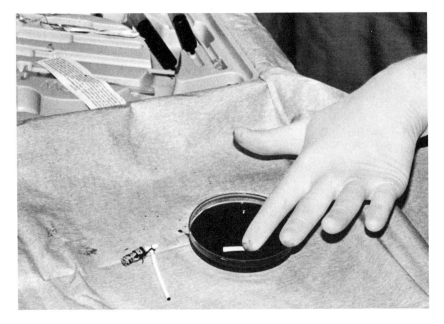

Figure 2-8 The tip of the catheter is rolled across-and-back the surface of a blood agar culture plate. It is then pressed into the agar gently without breaking the surface. The plate must be incubated as soon as possible.

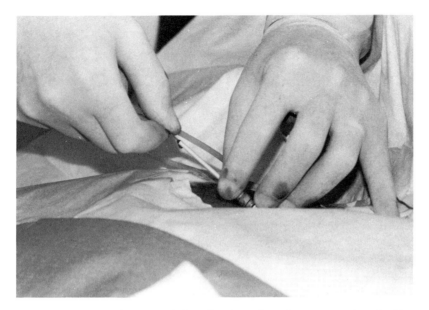

Figure 2-9 After the introducer hub and catheter have been removed, a flexible J-tip guidewire is advanced through the introducer. It should enter the lumen freely, but only 15 to 20 cm should be inserted to avoid perforation or dysrhythmias. The guidewire serves to maintain continuity between skin and interior of the vessel, and a great length is not necessary.

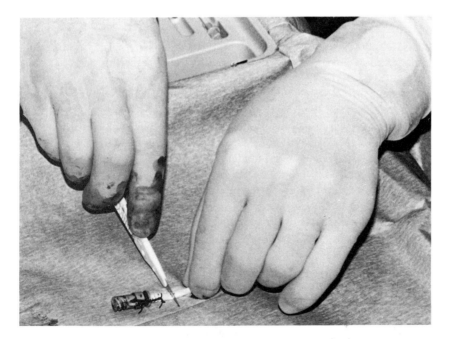

Figure 2-10 The introduer, touched only by the newly gloved hand, is positioned on a sterile portion of the insertion kit cover. A 3-cm length of the segment previously beneath the skin surface is isolated by severing the hub-end just below the point of skin insertion and then cutting off the excess on the other end.

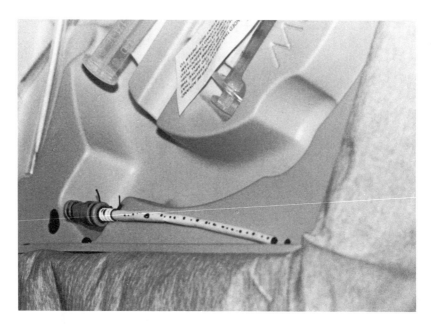

Figure 2-11 The introducer has been removed, leaving the guidewire in place. The operator wishes to insert the new catheter and then perform the culture of the intracutaneous segment. The introducer can be placed in an undisturbed section of the insertion tray temporarily. The new catheter can be placed. The operator can then put on a second sterile glove or grasp the intracutaneous segment with a sterile forceps, sever the outer and inner portions with sterile scissors, and plate the segment for culture.

culture. The guidewire is removed and the catheter attached to the appropriate tubing. The catheter should be sutured in place, and a dressing is fashioned as described above (Fig. 2-13).

It is essential to develop a system in conjunction with the microbiology laboratory by which specimens are logged in, cultured, and results recorded in easily accessible fashion. These catheter segment cultures must be checked on a daily basis. Normally, growth occurs at 24 hours or not at all. In perhaps only 1 of 50 segments, growth will be reported as negative at 24 hours yet positive some time later. However, depending on the time of day that the catheter segment is initially cultured, a negative result the next day may reflect only an insufficient time for growth. We check the cultures for 2 days to be sure. These seemingly trivial details are necessary to preserve the utility of guidewire exchanges for reasons of decreasing the risks of second insertions and the costs associated with them, yet avoiding catheter-related infection.

GUIDELINES FOR THE USE OF GUIDEWIRES

Because the risk of infection of the catheter wound increases with duration of catheterization and there is a significant risk of bacteremia without necessarily any external signs of infection, the "proper" duration of catheterization would be difficult to assess based on clinical observation alone. A second insertion procedure contains both risks and added

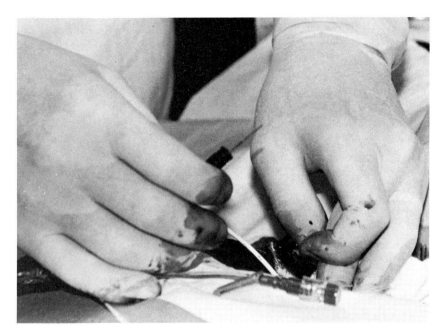

Figure 2-12 The new catheter—in this case, a triple lumen central catheter—is advanced over the guidewire until the flange is in proper position and the tip of the guidewire emerges from the end of the new catheter. The guidewire can then be removed.

expenses. Exchanging a catheter over a guidewire is a method of separating the catheters with significant bacterial growth from those without, yet maintaining continuity of the tract to avoid the risk of a new insertion procedure. Guidelines for the use of guidewire techniques and careful technique for culturing the removed catheter segments are both mandatory for this approach to be practical. Currently, we use the following schema. There are three exclusions: signs of local inflammation, a previous positive catheter segment culture from the same site, and a previous guidewire change. We found that second guidewire changes were used infrequently and had no bacteriologic culture success so we no longer permit a second exchange.[27] Technical problems often develop, particularly with multifunction, multilumen catheters. These catheters may be exchanged within the first day through the same introducer.

If patients develop a temperature approximately 2°F above their normal highest daily temperature, the catheter should be changed over a guidewire. The purpose, once again, is to obtain specimens for culture. The introducer would then be removed and its intracutaneous segment cultured separately. This would determine whether organisms are present within the catheter tract. If culture results are positive (the next day), the replaced catheter should be removed, and a new catheter must be inserted in a new site. If culture results are negative and the fever resolves, the replaced catheter may be left in place. If the culture results are negative and fever persists, however, we would consider catheter-related sepsis to be less likely and would continue an investigation to determine the source of the fever. The patient would have been spared the risk of a second insertion in this case.

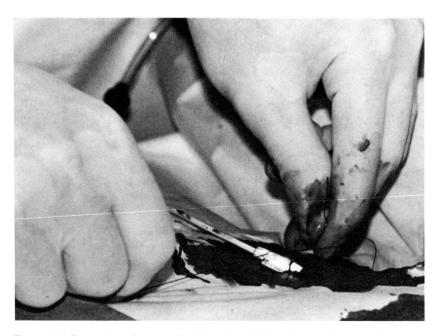

Figure 2-13 The catheter is sutured in place through the perforated flanges adjusted to lie near the point of insertion.

We do not believe that the duration of PA catheterization should be continued indefinitely in either "clean" patients or those with a known source of infection. In "clean" patients, we found an increase in positive segment cultures when duration was extended to 6 days compared to 4 days. Accordingly, if monitoring must be continued or if we wished to continue to use the access, the existing catheter may be changed over a guidewire at 4 days. Certain specific factors such as coagulopathy or anatomic distortions due to massive edema or subcutaneous emphysema may be so severe that we wish to delay change or removal of a catheter. In these situations, the risk of insertion to the patient is considered of greater magnitude than the risk of catheter-related infection and bacteremia. The prevalence of positive catheter segments is much higher than either clinical infection or catheter-related bacteremia. There are positive segment cultures in about 33% of patients at 6 days, but the prevalence of *sterile* catheter segments is still 67%. Of course, even in the face of these reasons for extension, should bacteremia be suspected or local infection appear, the catheter must be removed. A new catheter may remain in place only if the removed segments are negative on culture. The guidewire may be used only once. After 8 days, a new site must be used.

In patients with a known source of infection, we limit the duration of initial PA catheterization to 3 days. Catheters may be changed over a guidewire at that time, giving a 6-day continuum using the original insertion site. Again, the exchanged catheter may remain in place only if the removed segments remain negative on culture.

With the tremendous variety of catheters now available, as the need for monitoring

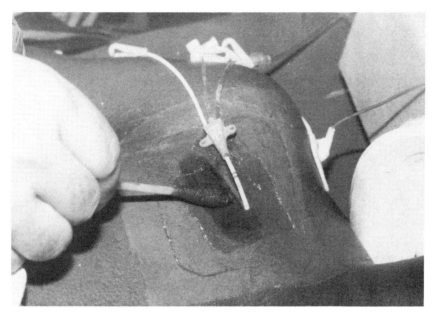

Figure 2-14 After the dressing has been removed, wipe away any ointment that remains at the skin insertion site. Acetone may be used first to aid in the removal of the ointment. Povidone-iodine swabs are then used to sterilize completely both the skin surface and the external portion of the catheter.

and routes of fluid infusion change, so too will the type of catheter desired. Staying within the same guidelines for total duration of catheterization, PA catheters may be changed to triple lumen catheters, or *vice versa*.

The technique should be performed as follows:

1 Prepare the skin and surface of the catheter to be removed (Fig. 2-14).

2 Drape the area, leaving only a small access area (Fig. 2-15). Because venous access has been previously attained, a larger area for manipulation and palpation of landmarks is not necessary.

3 Disconnect IV tubing. Introduce guidewire (Fig. 2-16). Remember that only the tip need extend into the vein. Avoid the tendency to introduce a larger length, which may lead to puncture of the vein or even the heart.

4 Remove the existing catheter while holding the guidewire (Fig. 2-17). As soon as the distal end of the catheter exits the skin, grasp the guidewire at the skin end and remove the catheter from the guidewire completely.

5 Take appropriate sections for culture if indicated.

6 Thread new catheter over guidewire.

7 Remove guidewire.

8 Aspirate new catheter to be sure its tip is in an intravascular position (Fig. 2-18).

9 Suture the new catheter in place (Fig. 2-19).

10 Cover insertion site with povidone-iodine ointment and cover with dressing.

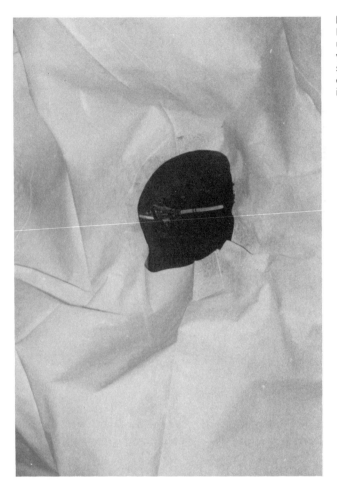

Figure 2-15 The area is draped in sterile fashion. During primary insertions, individual towels may be used to produce a larger sterile field. Because the vein has already been cannulated, such a large sterile field is not necessary during a guidewire exchange. A drape with a small central cut-out area is satisfactory.

When monitoring is finished and patients are ready for transfer to the ward, again, central access is often considered desirable. In "clean" patients, PA catheters or introducers may be changed to a single, double, or triple lumen catheter over a guidewire. However, we believe it is important that the ICU team remain responsible for determining whether the culture of the removed segment is negative. If significant growth is detected, we must ensure that the replaced catheter is removed. It must be remembered that this is a practice of convenience and can be used only if the ICU team uses both surveillance and authority to supervise the subsequent care of catheters placed in the ICU.

Recently, a compressed collagen silver treated cuff* was developed to be placed around the catheter or introducer and positioned just below the insertion site. The objective is to provide a physical and physiological barrier to the ingrowth of bacteria from the skin. In preliminary studies we have not seen the usual increase of positive catheter segments with increased duration of catheterization. Because the original and guidewired catheter wih the

*Vitacuff, Vitaphore Corp.

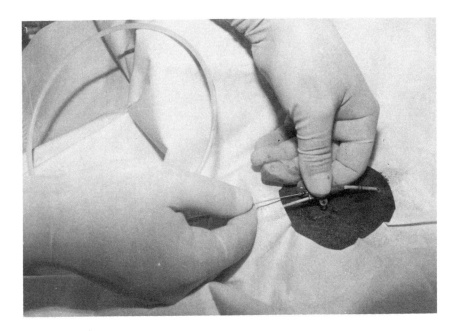

Figure 2-16 Grasp the exiting catheter and insert the guidewire approximately 15 cm. When 2 to 3 cm of catheter are visible, approximately 15 cm of guidewire will traverse the subcutaneous area and extend into the venous lumen far enough to ensure continued venous access when the catheter is removed. It is not necessary to insert the guidewire beyond the tip of the existing catheter and, in fact, this would only increase the risk of complications.

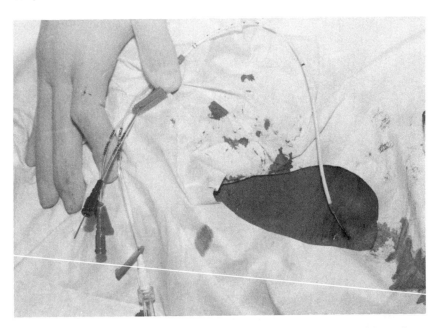

Figure 2-17 Holding the guidewire in a stationary position, withdraw the exiting catheter. As the catheter hub approaches the portion of guidewire in the fingers, move the fingers backward while advancing the catheter, thus keeping the position of the guidewire constant in relation to the patient. As this maneuver is continued, the end of the catheter will become visible at the skin insertion site. Grasp the guidewire at this site and remove the catheter.

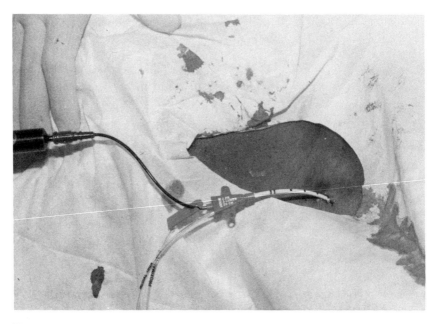

Figure 2-18 After the new catheter has been advanced into position and the guidewire removed, attach a syringe to the end of the new catheter and aspirate. Blood should be obtained easily.

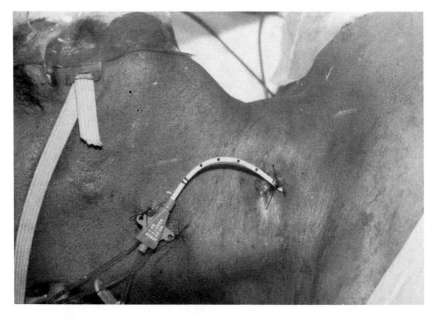

Figure 2-19 The catheter should be advanced approximately 15 cm from the right internal jugular and right subclavian positions and approximately 5 cm further when the procedure is performed from the left side.

cuff can be left in place longer, the infection rate should be lower than the cumulative rate of most first and second duration limited catheterizations. This would then enable us to leave the original catheters in place longer with greater prevention of infection and catheter insertion complications as well as cost savings.

CONCLUSION

Clean and aseptic technique, when applied to invasive catheterizations, is a complex subject in the ICU. The battle against bacteria is not glamorous but must be never-ending. Many factors in the environment, in the host, and in the organisms themselves tend to favor infection rather than sterility. We have focused on details beyond the technical aspects of insertion because most physicians seem concerned with the vascular cannulation and seem to consider placing the catheter as both the beginning and the end of their role. For long-term catheterization of patients who remain critically ill, this approach is too limited. We can expect further progress in the study of catheter-related infections especially with respect to techniques to maintain sterility in the ICU. There is another avenue that may also be fruitful.[28] Given the difficulties in creating an OR-type sterile environment in the ICU, an innovative approach is to eliminate the exposure of the catheter to contamination during insertion through the use of a cassette which may be attached directly to the hub of an introducer. The catheter itself is never touched by the operator nor exposed to potential contamination during insertion. This would remove another source of contamination similar to the substitution of closed cardiac output systems and continuous measurement of mixed venous saturation. It will not, of course, address the problem of skin organisms gaining access to the subcutaneous tract traversed by the introducer, likely to be the most important route for catheter-related infection.

Ultimately, the success of invasive catheterization depends on a maintained process of clean and aseptic technique. Scrupulous and persistent attention to detail are the only forces sufficiently powerful to keep the enemy at bay.

REFERENCES

1. Haslett TM, Isenberg HD, Hilton E: Microbiology of indwelling central intravascular catheters. *Interscience Conf. Antimicrobial Agents and Chemotherapy* 1987; 27:383
2. Ravitch M: *A Century of Surgery 1880–1980.* Philadelphia, JB Lippincott, 1981
3. Maki DG: Skin as a source of nosocomial infection: Directions for future research. *Infect Control* 1986; 7:113
4. Maki DG, Weise CE, Sarafin HW: A semiquantitative method for identifying intravenous catheter-related infection. *N Engl J Med* 1977; 296:1305
5. Sise MM, Hollingsworth P, Brimon JE, et al: Complications of the flow-directed pulmonary artery catheter: A prospective analysis in 219 patients. *Crit Care Med* 1981; 9:315
6. Pinnella JC, Ross DF, Martin T, et al: Study of the incidence of intravascular catheter infection and associated septicemia in critically ill patients. *Crit Care Med* 1983; 11.21
7. Caruthers TE, Reno DJ, Civetta JM: Implications of positive blood cultures associated with Swan–Ganz catheters. *Crit Care Med* 1979; 7:135
8. Maki DG, Hassemer CA: Endemic rate of fluid contamination and related septicemia in arterial pressure monitoring. *Am J Med* 1981; 70:733
9. Applefeld J, Caruthers T, Reno D, et al: Assessment of sterility of long-term cardiac catheterization using the thermodilution Swan–Ganz catheter. *Chest* 1978; 74:377
10. Donowitz LG, Marski FJ, Hoyt JW, et al: *Serratia marcescens* bacteremia from contaminated pressure transducers. *JAMA* 1979; 242:1749
11. Maki DG, Weise CE, Rhame FS: Infection control in intravenous therapy. *Ann Int Med* 1973; 79:867

12. Centers for Disease Control: *National Nosocomial Infections Study Report, Annual Summary 1979*, March 1982
13. Sitzmann JV, Townsend TR, Siler MC, et al: Septic and technical complications of central venous catheterization: A prospective study of 200 consecutive patients. *Ann Surg* 1985; 202:766
14. Larson E: Handwashing and skin physiologic and bacteriologic aspects. *Infect Control* 1985; 6:14
15. Dineen P, Hildick–Smith G: Antiseptic care of hands. In Maiback HI, Hildick–Smith G (eds): *Skin Bacteria and Their Role in Infection*. New York, McGraw Hill, 1965
16. Maki DG, Zilz MA, Alvarado CJ: Evaluation of the antibacterial efficacy of four agents for handwashing. *Interscience Conf. Antimicrobial Agents and Chemotherapy* 1980; 20:1089
17. Lowbury EJL, Lilly HA: Use of 4% chlorhexidine detergent solution (Hibiscrub) and other methods of skin disinfection. *Br Med J* 1973; 1:510
18. Kenner CV: Multisystem failure. In Kenner CV, Guzzetta CE, Dossey BM (eds): *Critical Care Nursing: Body-Mind-Spirit*. Boston, Little Brown & Company, 1981
19. Roy C Sr: The Roy adaptation model. In Reihl JP, Roy C (eds): *Conceptual Models for Nursing Practice*, 2nd ed. New York, Appleton–Century–Crofts, 1980
20. Seropian R, Reynolds BM: Wound infection after preoperative depilatory versus razor preparation. *Am J Surg* 1971; 121:251
21. Maki DG, Band JD: A comparative study of polyantibiotic and iodophor ointments in prevention of vascular catheter-related infection. *Am J Med* 1981; 70:739
22. Hudson–Civetta J, Caruthers Banner TE: Intravascular catheters: Current guidelines for care and maintenance. *Heart & Lung* 1983; 12:466
23. Ryan JA, Abel RM, Abbott W: Catheter complications in total parenteral nutrition. *N Engl J Med* 1974; 290:757
24. Hudson–Civetta JA, Civetta JM, Martinez OV, et al: Risk and detection of pulmonary artery catheter-related infection in septic surgical patients. *Crit Care Med* 1987; 15:29
25. Maki DG, Will L: Colonization and infection associated with transparent dressings for central venous, arterial, and Hickman catheters—A comparative trial. *Interscience Conf. Antimicrobial Agents and Chemotherapy* 1984; 24:993
26. Maki DG, Will L: Study of polyantibiotic and povidone–iodine ointments on central venous and arterial catheter sites dressed with gauze or polyurethane dressing. *Interscience Conf. Antimicrobial Agents and Chemotherapy* 1986; 26:287
27. Civetta JM, Hudson–Civetta JA, Nelson D, et al: Utility and efficacy of guidewire changes. *Crit Care Med* 1987; 15:380
28. Lynn LA, Braun SR: Personal communication, 1987

CHAPTER THREE

PRECAUTIONS FOR CAREGIVERS

Robert W. Taylor

A 34-year-old man was admitted to our critical care unit with hypothermia, altered mental status, and presumed sepsis. No family member or friend accompanied him and no prior hospital records could be located. He was emaciated, had evidence of prior radical neck surgery, and had a tracheostomy tube in place (metal, 6 Fr, non-cuffed).

During the first minute of evaluation the patient sustained a respiratory arrest. His metal tracheostomy tube was not adaptable to the standard 15-mm couple of the resuscitation bag. The metal tube was removed, but the ostomy site would not accept a 7 Fr cuffed tracheostomy tube or a 7 Fr endotracheal tube. A smaller tube was not immediately available. The critical care fellow in attendance initiated mouth-to-stoma rescue breathing with good results as measured by symmetrical chest expansion and improvement in cyanosis. The patient became more arousable and coughed, expelling several milliliters of mucus into the fellow's mouth. After approximately 1 minute a 6 Fr endotracheal tube was located and successfully inserted into the ostomy site. Ventilation was continued with 100% oxygen and a resuscitation bag.

Blood was being drawn by a nurse during the respiratory arrest. As the phlebotomy needle was withdrawn she was accidentally jostled, causing the exposed needletip to puncture her bare left palm.

A finger-stick glucose determination (later confirmed by the laboratory—glucose 24 mg/dl) suggested the patient was markedly hypoglycemic. The patient was given intravenous thiamine and glucose, after which he became alert. The laboratory reported significant bacteriuria and pyuria, and intravenous antibiotics directed toward gram-negative rods were instituted. His urine and blood cultures grew *Escherichia coli* on the second hospital day. The patient recovered nicely and was discharged from the critical care unit on day 3. He related that his radical neck operation had been performed because of laryngeal carcinoma at another institution 2 years earlier. The patient returned home after a 10-day course of intravenous antibiotics.

The critical care fellow and nurse were relieved to learn that the patient's RPR and hepatitis B serologies were negative and that no acid-fast organisms (*Mycobacterium tuberculosis*) were seen on sputum stain. Cold chills ran up and down both spines, however, when they learned that the patient was a homosexual intravenous drug abuser. Many sleepless nights followed the report of the patient's positive human immunodeficiency virus (HIV) test.

Can this happen to you? What are the risks? Are you concerned? Do you know how to protect yourself?

INTRODUCTION

Universal precautions for prevention of transmission of HIV, hepatitis B virus (HBV), and other blood-borne pathogens in health care settings have recently been updated by the Centers for Disese Control (CDC) in Atlanta.[1,2] In 1983, it was suggested by the CDC that blood and body fluid precautions be undertaken for patients with known or suspected blood-borne pathogens. The frightening escalation of HIV dissemination since that time has called for the application of blood and body fluid precautions to *all* patients irrespective of suspicion of prior infection.[2]

This chapter defines which organisms are of most concern to the caregiver, identifies which body fluids are dangerous, and outlines precautions to be taken to prevent transmission of disease.

ORGANISMS OF CONCERN

While health care workers may be at a slightly increased risk for transmission of pneumonia, meningitis, tuberculosis, syphilis, herpetic whitlow, and other diseases, the blood-borne pathogens HIV and HBV are by far of greatest concern. The epidemiology of HIV infection is similar to that of HBV.[3,4] Both diseases are spread by exposure to blood and by intimate personal contact. Although HIV infection has recently received far more public attention than HBV, the latter is in fact more highly infectious.[5–8]

Data suggest that transmission rates of both diseases are low, but that acquisition of disease by work-related accidents does occur.[3,6] Approximately 95% of health care workers with acquired immunodeficiency syndrome (AIDS) admit to engaging in high-risk activities such as anal receptive intercourse and illicit intravenous drug use.[9] In the absence of direct parenteral inoculation of blood, over 1600 hospital workers were exposed to patients with AIDS and potentially infected body fluids without documented seroconversion.[9]

Although the risk to caregivers is slight, it is real. Curran and co-workers reported the occurrence of HIV infection in three of 351 health care workers following needlestick exposure to the blood of an HIV-positive individual.[3] The risk of HIV infection among laboratory workers may be even higher.[10] Transmission of HIV infection to health care workers following the exposure to infected blood of open skin lesions or mucous membranes is thought to be rare,[11,12] but has occurred.[3]

BODY FLUIDS

Both HIV and HBV occur in a variety of body fluids (Table 3-1).[13–20] Blood exposure is most dangerous for health care workers. Universal precautions apply to semen and vaginal secretions, although caregiver exposure to these fluids is unusual and no cases of disease transmission via these fluids have been reported in health care workers. HIV and/or HBV have

TABLE 3-1 RISK OF PRESENCE OF HIV AND HBV IN BODY FLUIDS

I. Fluids Associated With HIV and HBV Infections
   Blood
   Breast milk
   Semen
   Vaginal secretions

II. Fluids Possibly Associated With HIV and HBV Infections*
   Cerebrospinal fluid
   Synovial Fluid
   Peritoneal fluid
   Pleural fluid
   Amniotic fluid

III. Fluids Not Implicated in HIV and HBV Infections†
   Saliva
   Feces
   Nasal secretions
   Sputum
   Sweat
   Tears
   Urine
   Vomitus

*HIV and HBV have been isolated from these fluids, but the risk of disease transmission is not known.
†Although HIV has been isolated from some of these fluids, the risk of disease transmission is believed to be low or nonexistent.

been isolated from cerebrospinal fluid, synovial fluid, peritoneal fluid, pleural fluid, and amniotic fluid. The risk of disease transmission by these fluids to the caregiver is unknown. Because these fluids are often encountered by the caregiver in the presence of sharp instruments and needles, however, universal precautions apply.

HIV has been isolated from tears and saliva;[9] however, the risk of transmission of infection is felt to be low or nonexistent. Feces, sputum, sweat, urine, and vomitus are probably noninfectious unless mixed with blood.[20] No specific recommendations are made regarding waste management. Institutional policies regarding collection, decontamination and disposal of waste products should be followed. Although HBV and HIV have been found in breast milk, transmission to health care workers via exposure to this fluid is unlikely.[17,21] HBV and possibly HIV have been occupationally transmitted to dental workers.[8,22,23] Blood, rather than saliva, is the likely vehicle. In summary, universal precautions apply to the body fluids listed in Table 3-2.

PROTECTIVE METHODS

Gowns, gloves, masks, and protective eyewear should be used by health care workers during times of possible exposure of the body fluids listed in Table 3-2. Clinical judgment is important in estimating risk of exposure since no guideline can cover every possible situation. Particular care should be taken when handling sharp instruments. Needles should be disposed of immediately after use in special puncture-resistant containers available close to patient care areas. Needles should *not* be recapped, bent, broken, or removed from the

TABLE 3-2 BODY FLUIDS REQUIRING UNIVERSAL PRECAUTIONS

Blood
Semen
Vaginal secretions
Cerebrospinal fluid
Synovial fluid
Pleural fluid
Peritoneal fluid
Pericardial fluid
Amniotic fluid

syringe as these practices increase the likelihood of needlestick injury. Prompt and thorough washing of all skin surfaces contaminated with the body fluids listed in Table 3-2 is warranted. Gloves should be worn during phlebotomy and when performing finger and heel sticks, and they should be changed between patients. Gloves should be worn by health care workers who have skin lesions on their hands prior to potential contact with the body fluids listed in Table 3-2. If the lesions are extensive or weeping, the health care worker should refrain from direct patient contact. Gloves should also be worn for procedures involving contact with mucous membranes. They should be disposed of after each use. They should not be washed or disinfected for reuse. Hands should be thoroughly washed after gloves are removed.

In high patient acuity areas such as the ICU the need for emergency mouth-to-mouth resuscitation should be minimized by the rapid availability of resuscitation masks, bags, and other airway and ventilation equipment.

IMMUNIZATION

The world anxiously awaits development of an effective HIV vaccine. However, highly effective immunoprophylaxis exists for HBV. Active immunization with hepatitis B vaccine prevents this form of viral hepatitis.[24–30] The vaccine was licensed in 1982 and has been safely given to more than 750,000 susceptible individuals. The vaccine is recommended for individuals listed in Table 3-3.

Despite documented efficacy and safety, many health care workers at risk have not been vaccinated. The prevalence of hepatitis B surface antigen (HBsAg) or antibody is 8% to 20% in medical residents and 14% to 25% in surgical residents,[31] documenting these groups to be at high risk. However, less than 50% of health care workers accept the vaccine when offered. Only 57% of individuals who received the initial dose of vaccine completed all three injections.[31]

Although the vaccine is derived from the plasma of individuals at high risk for AIDS, there is absolutely no evidence that the vaccine transmits the virus.[28,33,34] The process employed in the preparation of the vaccine inactivates HIV. Despite these facts, health care workers often voice concern about the possible transmission of hepatitis B and/or AIDS virus with the vaccine.[35] Hepatitis B vaccine contains 20 μg of HBsAg per milliliter. Normal adults receive 1.0 ml IM (each dose) in the deltoid on three separate occasions. The second dose is given 1 month after the first, and the third dose is given 6 months after the first.[36]

Health care workers with percutaneous or mucous membrane exposure to an individual

TABLE 3-3   PERSONS IN WHOM ACTIVE IMMUNIZATION WITH HEPATITIS B VACCINE IS INDICATED

Health care workers with frequent exposure to blood products
Staff of institutions for the mentally retarded
Hemodialysis patients
Homosexual males
Intravenous drug abusers
Close contacts of hepatitis B carriers
Infants born to HBsAg-positive mothers
Persons from or traveling to highly endemic areas
Prisoners

known to be HBsAg positive should be passively immunized with hepatitis B immune globulin (0.06 ml/kg IM) within 24 hours.[7,36] Vaccination would begin at the time of the initial exposure. When the index individual's HBsAg status is unknown, hepatitis B vaccine should be given (1.0 ml IM). The index individual's HBsAg status should be determined. If it is positive, then 0.06 ml/kg of hepatitis B immune globulin should also be given within 7 days of initial exposure.

SUMMARY

Blood and body fluid precautions should be undertaken for *all* patients irrespective of suspicion of prior infections. The prevention of HIV and HBV infection to caregivers is of greatest concern. Gowns, masks, gloves, and protective eyewear should be worn during any procedure placing the health care worker at risk for contamination with splattered body fluids (see Table 3-2). Gloves should be worn when performing a phlebotomy and during procedures exposing the health care worker to mucous membranes. Even though HIV and HBV are not thought to be transmissible via saliva or sputum, other diseases may be (e.g., *M. tuberculosis*). The necessity for mouth-to-mouth (or mouth-to-stoma) resuscitation should be kept to a minimum. Intensive care unit (ICU) workers are at increased risk for hepatitis B and should give strong consideration to active immunization with hepatitis B vaccine.

What recommendations do you have for the physician and nurse exposed to the HIV-positive patient presented at the beginning of this chapter?

Obviously, having the correct equipment immediately available to manage the airway would have been appropriate for many reasons. Attempts to minimize the necessity for mouth-to-mouth or mouth-to-stoma resuscitation breathing are appropriate even though saliva and/or sputum are body fluids not likely to cause HIV or HBV infection. Data suggest that the nurse, following needlestick injury, has about a 0.76% chance of becoming sero-positive for HIV.[11] She should have a baseline and follow-up HIV after about 90 days. Appropriately, she had been previously immunized for hepatitis B. Although gloves would not have prevented a needlestick, she should have been wearing them at the time of the phlebotomy.

*I am grateful to Mrs. Gail C. Frazer for guidance and technical assistance in preparation of this chapter.

REFERENCES

1. Centers for Disease Control: Recommendations for prevention of HIV transmission in health-care settings. *MMWR* 1987, (Suppl 2s)36

2. Centers for Disease Control: Update: Universal precautions for prevention of human immunodeficiency virus, hepatitis B virus, and other bloodborne pathogens in health-care settings. *JAMA* 1988; 260:462

3. Curran JW, Jaffe HW, Hardy AM, et al: Epidemiology of HIV infection and AIDS in the United States. *Science* 1988; 239:610

4. Quarterly report to the domestic policy council on the prevalence and rate of spread of HIV and AIDS in the United States. *MMWR* 1988; 37:223

5. Robinson WS, Lutwick LI: The virus of hepatitis, Type B. *N Engl J Med* 1976; 295:1168

6. Alter HJ, Seeff LB, Kaplan PM, et al: Type B hepatitis: The infectivity of blood positive for e antigen and DNA polymerase after accidental needlestick exposure. *N Engl J Med* 1976; 295:909

7. Krugman S, Overby LR, Mushahwar IK, et al: Viral hepatitis, Type B: Studies on natural history and prevention re-examined. *N Engl J Med* 1979; 300:101.

8. Department of Labor, Department of Health and Human Services. *Joint Advisory Notice: Protection Against Occupational Exposure to Hepatitis B Virus (HBV) and Human Immunodeficiency Virus (HIV).* Washington, DC, US Department of Labor. US Department of Health and Human Services, 1987

9. Friedland GH, Klein RS: Transmission of the human immunodeficiency virus. *N Engl J Med* 1987; 317:1125

10. Weiss SH, Goedert JJ, Gartner S, et al: Risk of human immunodeficiency virus (HIV-1) infection among laboratory workers. *Science* 1988; 239:68

11. Henderson DK, Saah AJ, Zak BJ, et al: Risk of nosocomial infection with human T-cell lymphotropic virus type III/lymphadenopathy-associated virus in a large cohort of intensively exposed health care workers. *Ann Intern Med* 1986; 104:644

12. Gerberding JL, Bryant–LeBlanc CE, Nelson K, et al: Risk of transmitting the human immunodeficiency virus, cytomegalovirus, and hepatitis B virus to health care workers exposed to patients with AIDS and AIDS-related conditions. *J Infect Dis* 1987; 156:1

13. Lifson AR: Do alternate modes for transmission of human immunodeficiency virus exists: A review. *JAMA* 1988; 259:1353

14. Oskenhendler E, Harzic M, Le Roux J–M, et al: HIV infection with seroconversion after a superficial needlestick injury to the finger (letter). *N Engl J Med* 1986; 315:582

15. Bond WW, Petersen NJ, Gravelle CR, et al: Hepatitis B virus in peritoneal dialysis fluid: A potential hazard. Dialysis Transplant 1982; 11:592

16. Mundy DC, Schinazi RF, Gerber AR, et al: Human immunodeficiency virus isolated from amniotic fluid. *Lancet* 1987; 2:459

17. Lee AKY, Ip HMH, Wong VCW: Mechanisms of maternal–fetal transmission of hepatitis B virus. *J Infect Dis* 1978; 138:668

18. Wirthrington RH, Cornes P, Harris JRW, et al: Isolation of human immunodeficiency virus from synovial fluid of a patient with reactive arthritis. *Br Med J* 1987; 294:484

19. Hollander H, Levy JA: Neurologic abnormalities and recovery of human immunodeficiency virus from cerebro-spinal fluid. Ann Intern Med 1987; 106:692

20. Sande MA: Transmission of AIDS: The case against casual contagion. *N Engl J Med* 1986; 314:380

21. Thiry L, Sprecher–Goldberger S, Jonckheer T, et al: Isolation of AIDS virus from cell-free breast milk of three healthy virus carriers. *Lancet* 1985; 2:891

22. Centers for Disease Control. Update: Acquired immunodeficiency syndrome and human immunodeficiency virus infection among health-care workers. *MMWR* 1988; 37:229, 239

23. Klein RS, Phelan JA, Freeman K, et al: Low occupational risk of human immunodeficiency virus infection among dental professionals. *N Engl J Med* 1988; 318:86

24. Szmuness W, Stevens CE, Harley EJ, et al: Hepatitis B vaccine: Demonstration of efficacy in a controlled clinical trial in a high-risk population in the United States. *N Engl J Med* 1980; 303:833

25. Maupas P, Chiron J–P, Barin F, et al: Efficacy of hepatitis B vaccine in prevention of early HBsAg carrier state in children: Controlled trial in an endemic area (Senegal). *Lancet* 1981; 1:289

26. Francis DP, Hadler SC, Thompson SE, et al: The prevention of hepatitis B with vaccine: Report of the Centers for Disease Control multicenter efficacy trial among homosexual men. *Ann Intern Med* 1982; 97:362

27. Szmuness W, Stevens CE, Harley EJ, et al: Hepatitis B vaccine in medical staff of hemodialysis units: Efficacy and subtype cross-protection. *N Engl J Med* 1982; 307:1481

28. Dienstag JL, Werner BG, Polk BF, et al: Hepatitis B vaccine in health care personnel: Safety, immunogenicity, and indicators of efficacy. *Ann Intern Med* 1984; 101:34

29. Beasley RP, Hwang L–Y, Lee GCY, et al: Prevention of perinatally transmitted hepatitis B virus infections with hepatitis B immune globulin and hepatitis B vaccine. *Lancet* 1983; 2:1099

30. Wong VCW, Ip HMH, Reesink HW, et al: Prevention of the HBsAg carrier state in newborn infants of mothers who are chronic carriers of HBsAg and HBeAg by administration of hepatitis B vaccine and hepatitis B immuno-globulin: Double-blind randomized placebo-controlled study. *Lancet* 1984; 1:921

31. Parry MF, Brown AE, Dobbs LG, et al: The epidemiology of hepatitis B infection in housestaff. *Infection* 1978; 6:204

32. Tong MJ, Howard AM, Schatz GC, et al: A hepatitis B vaccination program in a community teaching hospital. *Infect Control* 1987; 8:102

33. Dienstag JL: Safety of the hepatitis B vaccine (letter). *N Engl J Med* 1985; 312:376

34. Stevens CE: No increased incidence of AIDS in recipients of hepatitis B vaccine (reply to letter). *N Engl J Med* 1983; 308:1163

35. Harward MP, Kaiser DL, Fredson DS: Acceptance of hepatitis B vaccine by medical and surgical residents. *J Gen Intern Med* 1988; 3:150

36. Recommendation of the Immunization Practices Advisory Committee (ACIP): Recommendations for protection against viral hepatitis. *MMWR* 1985; 34:313

CHAPTER FOUR

SYSTEM CONCEPTS FOR INVASIVE PRESSURE MONITORING

Reed M. Gardner

Invasive pressure monitoring is now routinely performed at the patient's bedside, incorporating technology more advanced than that which, formerly, only specialized cardiac catheterization laboratories used. The monitoring enables the clinician to better understand the relation between the pressure and blood flow in the patient's cardiovascular system. However, every measuring system has the capability of producing false information. Constant vigilance and understanding of the system are currently the best prescription for ensuring acquisition of high-quality pressure monitoring information.

INVASIVE BLOOD PRESSURE MEASUREMENT

Arterial blood pressure can be measured by both invasive and non-invasive means. However, central venous pressure (CVP), pulmonary artery (PA), and pulmonary artery occlusion pressure (PAOP), at present, can only be measured by invasive means.

The invasive measurement of blood pressure allows for continuous and accurate assessment of blood pressures. Continuous pressure measurement permits detection of dangerous hemodynamic events and provides the information necessary to initiate and titrate patient therapy. Nevertheless, invasive pressure monitoring provides valuable information only when it is obtained accurately with correct technique.

EQUIPMENT

The components of an invasive blood pressure monitoring system for critically ill patients are shown in Figure 4-1.[1,2] The components known as the "plumbing system" (1–7 in the figure) must always be sterile because they come in direct contact with the patient's blood. Usually these components are disposable items and are often discarded after 48 to 72 hours to minimize the risks of infection. The other components (8–11) in the system are used for processing and displaying pressure waveforms and obtaining derived hemodynamic parameters, and they will be briefly described.

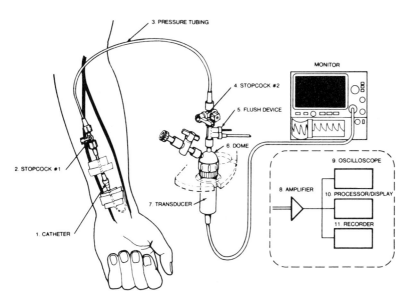

Figure 4-1 The 11 components used to monitor blood pressure directly are nearly the same independent of whether the catheter is in an artery (radial, brachial, or femoral) or in the pulmonary artery. The size of the transducer and plumbing components were enlarged for illustration purposes. (Adapted from Gardner RM, Hollingsworth KW: Optimizing ECG and pressure monitoring. *Crit Care Med* 1986; 14:651)

Catheter. Arterial and pulmonary artery catheters provide access to the patient's blood vessels to monitor intravascular pressure and to provide a site for samples for blood gas analysis and other tests.

Stopcock Number 1. This stopcock is used as a sampling site for withdrawing blood for analysis. When filling the plumbing system with fluid, precautions must be taken to be sure all central switching cavities of the stopcock are filled and that all entrapped air bubbles are removed. Because stopcocks are particularly vulnerable sources of patient contamination, they should be handled with extreme care; ports not in active use should be covered with sterile caps and the open ports should never be touched. Some prefer to eliminate the stopcock for this reason and replace it with a T connector. This permits withdrawal of specimens without opening the system but does introduce a short piece of compliant tubing.

Pressure Tubing. The catheter and stopcock are normally attached to the flush device and transducer by noncompliant pressure tubing. To optimize the dynamic response of the plumbing system, long lengths of tubing should be avoided.

Stopcock Number 2. The stopcock is usually put in place to allow disconnection of the flush device and transducer from the patient when the patient is moved or during initial filling of the system with fluid.

Continuous Flush Device. The continuous flush device is used to fill the pressure monitoring system initially and helps prevent blood clotting in the catheter by continuously flushing fluid through the system at a rate of from 1 to 3 ml/hr.

Transducer Dome. Disposable diaphragm domes have come into common use in recent years. These domes provide isolation between the transducer and the patient and permit rapid reuse of the transducer without resterilization. However, if the diaphragm domes are not properly coupled to the pressure transducer, severe waveform distortion can occur.

Pressure Transducer. Available in a variety of sizes and shapes, pressure transducers are usually resistive devices that convert the movement of their sensing diaphragm into an electrical signal. Recently standards for blood pressure transducers have been developed by the Association for the Advancement of Medical Instrumentation (AAMI) and adopted by the American National Standards Institute (ANSI).[3,4] These standards should greatly simplify transducer selection and will eventually allow the same transducer to be used interchangeably with any monitor. Several excellent quality disposable pressure transducers are now available.[5] They are smaller, have better technical qualities, and can better withstand the rigors of clinical use than the outdated reusable transducers.

Amplifier System. The output voltage required to drive an oscilloscope or strip recorder is provided by an amplifier system inserted between the transducer and display. Transducer excitation is provided either from a direct current (DC) or alternating current (AC) source at a voltage of 4 to 8 volts RMS. Most amplifier systems include low pass filters that filter out unwanted high frequency signals. Pressure amplifier frequency response should be "flat," from 0 to 50 Hz to avoid pressure waveform distortion.[1,2]

Oscilloscope. Pressure waveforms are best visualized on a calibrated oscilloscope.

Processor/Digital Display. Digital displays provide a simple method for presenting quantitative data from the pressure waveform. They are found on most modern pressure monitoring equipment. Systolic, diastolic, and mean pressure are derived from the pressure waveforms.

Recorder. Frequently strip chart recorders are used to document dynamic response characteristics, respiratory variations in pulmonary artery pressures, and aberrant rhythms and pressure waveforms.

EQUIPMENT SET-UP

Zeroing the Transducer

The accuracy of blood pressure readings depends on establishing an accurate reference point from which all subsequent measurements are made. The patient's midaxillary line (right heart level) is the reference point most commonly used. The zeroing process is used to compensate for offset caused by hydrostatic pressure differences, or offset in the pressure transducer, amplifier, oscilloscope, recorder, and digital displays. Zeroing is accomplished by opening an appropriate stopcock to atmosphere and aligning the resulting fluid–air interface

Figure 4-2 Two methods of zeroing a pressure transducer. Note the place at which the water–air interface occurs should always be at the midaxillary line when zeroing. **Top.** The stopcock is placed near the transducer at the midaxillary line. **Bottom.** The stopcock near the catheter is placed at the midaxillary line. (Adapted from Gardner RM, Hollingsworth KW: Optimizing ECG and pressure monitoring. *Crit Care Med* 1986; 14:651))

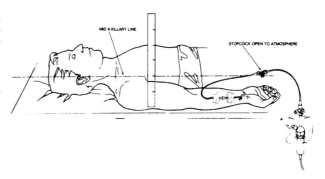

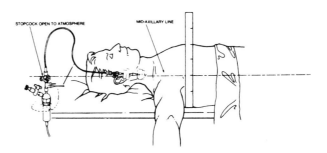

with the midaxillary reference point.[1,2,6] Figure 4-2 shows two methods which can be used to zero the transducer.[1,2]

Once the system is zeroed, the appropriate stopcock can be switched to allow the patient's waveform to be displayed. Because PA and PAOP are especially susceptible to improper zeroing, the zero should be verified, if the reading is questioned.

Verifying Sensitivity

The sensitivity of the AAMI/ANSI interchangeable blood pressure transducer is fixed at 5.0 μV/V/mm Hg and calibrated by the manufacturers to within 1%.[4] This degree of accuracy is appropriate for clinical purposes. By using transducers which meet the AAMI/ANSI interchangeability standards and monitors which also interconnect with the standard transducer, the clinician will only need to zero the system in order to obtain accurate pressure measurements. Although this simplified method is not universally applicable in 1989, it will be within a few years, and when it is, invasive blood pressure monitoring will be simpler and easier.

Checking and Optimizing Dynamic Response Characteristics

Catheter-tubing-transducer "plumbing" systems used in the intensive care unit can be characterized as underdamped second-order dynamic systems.[1,2,7,8] A second-order system can be expressed mathematically by a second-order differential equation with characteristics determined by three mechanical parameters: elasticity, mass, and friction. These same parameters apply to a catheter-tubing-transducer system in which the natural frequency (Fn in Hz) and damping coefficient zeta (Z) determine the dynamic characteristics for the plumbing system.

Dynamic response characteristics of catheter-tubing-transducer systems are expressed by two interrelated techniques: one specifies a bandwidth (frequency) and requires that the system's frequency response be "flat" up to a given frequency so that a specified number of harmonics (usually ten) of the original pulse wave can be reproduced without distortion (Fig. 4-3). The second specifies the natural frequency (Fn) and damping coefficient.[7] The resulting plot of natural frequency and damping coefficient is shown in Figure 4-4.[7] If the characteristics of the plumbing system fall in the adequate or optimal area of the graph, the pressure waveforms will be adequately reproduced. If they fall in the remaining three areas, there will be waveform distortion. Catheter-tubing-transducer plumbing systems assembled under optimal conditions are underdamped; a few fall into the unacceptable area. Methods for

Figure 4-3 Family of frequency versus amplitude ratio plots for five different damping coefficients (Zeta) and two different natural frequencies, 10 and 20 Hz. A damping coefficient of 0.1 occurs if the system is very underdamped, while a damping coefficient of 2 occurs when a system is overdamped. The dashed line shows the ideal or "flat" frequency versus amplitude response. Note that the response of the system with a 10-Hz natural frequency can be brought closer to the ideal "flat" response if the damping coefficient is between 0.5 and 0.7. However, by increasing the natural frequency to 20 Hz, the range of damping coefficients can be widened still further and give nearly the same "flat" frequency response.

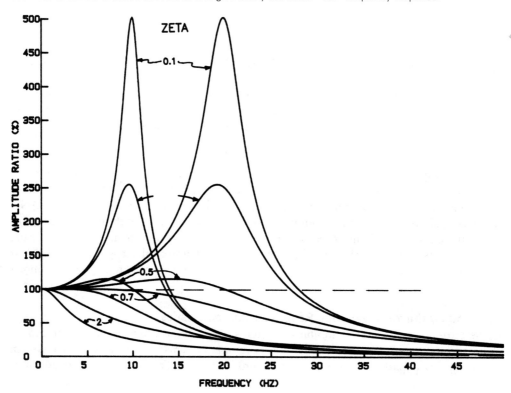

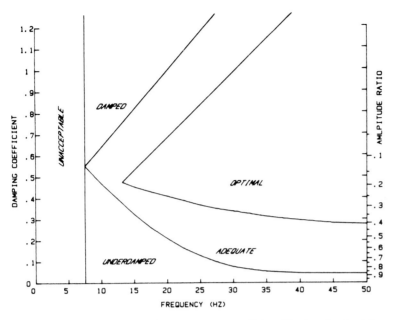

Figure 4-4 Plot shows the range of damping coefficient (Zeta) and natural frequencies outlining the regions that indicate the type distortion of the pressure wave. See Figure 28-5 for examples.

optimizing the plumbing system components have been outlined.[1,7] In the clinical setting there are dramatic differences between each patient set-up; therefore it is mandatory to test the adequacy of each pressure monitoring system. This can be done easily using the fast-flush technique. The fast-flush is produced by opening the valve of the continuous flush device (for example, by pulling and quickly releasing the pigtail on an Intraflo). The rapid closure generates a square wave, from which the natural frequency and damping coefficient of the plumbing system can be measured.

Once the fast-flush test has been executed two or three times, the dynamic response characteristics (Fn and Z) can be quickly and easily determined.[1,7] Natural frequency can be estimated by measuring the period of each full oscillation on a strip chart recorder (Fig. 4-5A) following a fast-flush, and calculating the frequency from the period. To determine the damping coefficient, any two successive peak amplitudes are measured and an amplitude ratio obtained by dividing the measured height of the lower peak by that of the amplitude of the larger peak (Fig. 4-5B). This ratio is then converted to the damping coefficient.

Once the natural frequency and the damping coefficient have been determined, these data can be plotted on the graph in Figure 4-4 to ascertain the adequacy of dynamic response. Some bedside monitors and recorders may compromise the fast-flush technique with their built-in low pass filters. These filters should be expanded to at least 50 Hz or eliminated.

Several factors lead to poor dynamic responses: air bubbles in the system, usually caused by a poor initial plumbing system set-up; pressure tubing that is too long, too compliant, or a diameter which is too small; and pressure transducers that are too compliant. The best way to enhance the system's dynamics is to maximize its natural frequency.

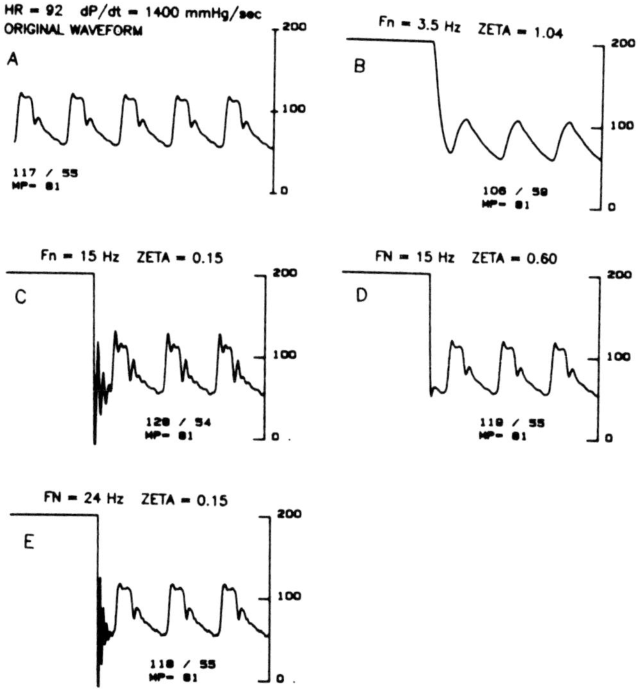

Figure 4-5 Arterial pressure waveforms recorded with different pressure monitoring systems. Patient heart rate is 92 with a maximum dp/dt of 1400 mm Hg/sec.

Panel A. The original patient waveform as it might be recorded with a catheter tipped pressure transducer. The systolic pressure is 118 mm Hg, diastolic is 55 mm Hg, and mean pressure is 81 mm Hg.

Panel B. The same patient's arterial pressure waveform recorded with an "overdamped" plumbing system. Zeta is 1.04 and Fn is 3.5 Hz. Note the "fast flush" signal *(upper left)* returns slowly to the patient waveform. Systolic pressure is underestimated at 106 mm Hg, diastolic pressure is overestimated at 59 mm Hg, but mean ressure is unchanged at 81 mm Hg.

Panel C. An "underdamped" condition with a low damping coefficient of 0.15 and a natural frequency of 15 Hz. After the "fast flush," the pressure waveform oscillates rapidly and returns to the original waveform shape quickly. Systolic pressure is overestimated at 128 mm Hg, diastolic is nearly the same as the original at 54 mm Hg, and the mean pressure is unchanged at 81 mm Hg.

Panel D. Same as in Panel C, but now a damping device has been inserted and adjusted.[1,7] The waveform is optimally damped with a damping coefficient of 0.60 and a natural frequency of 15 Hz.

Panel E. An "underdamped" condition but with high natural frequency of 24 Hz. Note the pressure waveform is only slightly distorted and the pressures are close to the true pressures.

CLINICAL VERSUS LABORATORY MEASUREMENT OF DYNAMIC RESPONSE

Several investigators have studied the dynamic response characteristics of catheter-transducer systems.[1,2,7,8–23] However, all of these studies were performed in the laboratory and not extended to the clinical setting. A recent study has determined the dynamic response fidelity of catheter-transducer systems in the laboratory *and* the clinical setting.[24]

The results of this study indicate that the simpler the mechanical plumbing set-up of a pressure monitoring system, the higher its fidelity.[24] The more complex the system, that is, the greater the number of components within the system, the greater the susceptibility of that system to giving a degraded dynamic performance. Lack of tubing and absence of the membrane dome–transducer diaphragm coupling minimized the chances of air bubble entrapment. Chances for set-up error were also minimized with simpler systems.

The dynamic response characteristics of a system that uses compliant catheters or tubing, or that contains air bubbles have large volume displacement. Systems that use long narrow catheters (such as the pulmonary artery catheter), or have long lengths of small-diameter pressure tubing, are not desirable because Fn will decrease and zeta will increase. Conversely, if the catheters and tubing are noncompliant, and short, with large diameters, and no air bubbles, then the Fn will increase and zeta decrease.

Figure 4-6 illustrates the effects of tubing length and air bubbles entrapped in the

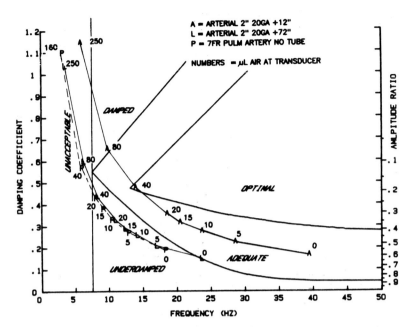

Figure 4-6 Plot of natural frequency versus damping coefficient for two arterial and one pulmonary artery pressure monitoring system shows the effect of inserting small bubbles into the transducer dome. The volumes (Vd) of air inserted in microliters are shown near the marks on the curves. The curves were generated using the modeling techniques of Taylor et al.[23] Results are presented for short radial catheters (Deseret 2") with 12" *(Index A)* and 72" *(Index L)* of pressure tubing. The results from a pulmonary artery catheter system without extension tubing are shown as *Index P.* Note that for all situations the operating point moves upward and to the left with the addition of air into the system. The best condition is always when *NO* air is in the system.

system. As the volume displacement (Vd) increases, there is a decrease in Fn and an increase in damping coefficient. The magnitude of the change is multiplied for systems with long catheters or tubing (pulmonary artery catheter and radial catheter with 72-inch tubing). For the short radial arterial catheter, the effect of tubing length is also apparent. Increasing the tubing from 12 to 72 inches with no air bubbles in the system reduces the Fn from 39 to 23 Hz. For a pulmonary artery catheter system without pressure tubing, the effect of increasing air bubble size (Vd) on the system is shown. Note in every case that the operating point moves upward and to the left. Despite what is taught in some centers, adding air to the transducer to "damp" the pressure waveform is *not* a good idea.

The use of extension tubing for PA lines was found to be especially detrimental to the system's response. The adverse effects of long tubing are compounded because of the long length of the PA catheter. The use of extension tubing, which affords greater freedom of mobility from the transducer to the catheter, seems to be contraindicated.

This same study found that each clinical catheter-tubing-transducer system must have its dynamic response verified at frequent intervals.[24] There can be a vast difference in fidelity between the ideal laboratory setting and the clinical setting, where the system is subject to changes over time, human assembly error, repeated blood sample withdrawal, and air entrapment. The fast-flush method of determining the dynamic response characteristics is a simple, rapid, and safe testing modality that can be easily incorporated clinically.[1,2,7] By performing the fast-flush testing on each clinical system, the adequacy of dynamic response can be verified and optimized if necessary. If a fast-flush testing produces dynamic response characteristics that are inadequate, the user can take the opportunity to trouble-shoot the system (*i.e.*, remove excessive tubing length, purge air bubbles, reattach membrane dome according to protocol) until acceptable characteristics are obtained.

SELECTING BLOOD PRESSURE TRANSDUCERS

The objective of the recently published AAMI/ANSI blood pressure transducer standards was to provide labeling and performance requirements, testing methodology, and terminology to help ensure that health care professionals are supplied with safe, accurate blood pressure transducers that could be used interchangeably with any monitor.[4] Unfortunately a connector change or a conversion cable adapter alone may not be sufficient to allow interchangeability with standardized transducers. To provide interchangeability the monitor must use the AAMI/ANSI standard connector; have an excitation voltage between 4 and 8 volts RMS in the frequency range of DC (0) to 5000 Hz; be able to accept a transducer imbalance in the range of ± 75 mm Hg; supply an excitation voltage and accept transducers with an excitation impedance of greater than 200 ohms; be based on a transducer sensitivity of 5 μV/V/mm Hg; and maintain accuracy when used with a transducer that has a signal impedance of less than 3000 ohms.

To ensure that the monitor has these capabilities, it is recommended that the monitor's specifications be carefully analyzed or that the monitor manufacturer be asked about any limitations which would prevent the use or accuracy of the AAMI/ANSI standard for interchangeable blood pressure transducers.

REQUIREMENTS OF THE AAMI/ANSI INTERCHANGEABILITY STANDARD

Environmental Performance: The transducer should be able to operate at temperatures between 15°C and 40°C.

Mechanical Requirements: Operate over a pressure range of −30 to +300 mm Hg, and not be damaged by overpressure of −400 to +4000 mm Hg. Luer-Lok or Linden fittings should meet the ANSI standard "Performance Standard for Medical Luer Taper Fittings."

Electrical Performance: Transducer excitation should be within 4 to 8 volts RMS in the frequency range of DC (0) to 5000 Hz. The transducer excitation impedance should be greater than 200 ohms over this same frequency range. The transducer signal impedance should be less than 3000 ohms over the same frequency range. The transducer sensitivity should be 5 μV/V/mm Hg ±1% under specified conditions. The linearity and hysteresis shall be within ±2% of the pressure reading or ±1 mm Hg, whichever is greater.

Safety Requirements: The transducer shall maintain electrical isolation between the fluid column and the case, to prevent unsafe electrical current leakage into the patient. The transducer must withstand five repeated discharges of a defibrillator.

Instruction Manual: In addition to these performance criteria the instruction manual for the transducers should contain the following information:

Information, cautions, and warnings about storage, use handling, and sterilization of the transducer; also the names and addresses of acceptable customer service facilities.

The "shock" that the transducer can withstand and still meet the standards requirements.

The "volume displacement" of the transducer and attached accessories. Volume displacement is one of the most important determinants of dynamic response.

The warm-up drift one might expect.

The changes in zero and sensitivity with temperature change over the range of 15°C to 40°C.

The light sensitivity of the transducer, since some of the newer disposable transducers are also light sensitive (Fig. 4-7).

COMPLICATIONS OF INVASIVE PRESSURE MONITORING

The three most important risks associated with vascular cannulation and direct blood pressure monitoring are air embolism, thrombosis, and infection.

Figure 4-7 Photograph of a disposable transducer shows its small size and rugged construction characteristics.

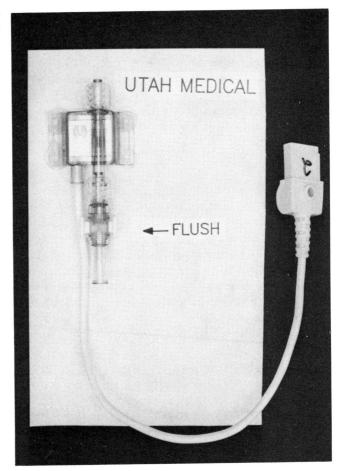

AIR EMBOLISM

Air embolism is the introduction of air into the circulatory system. Air insufflation can occur in a variety of ways into either the venous or arterial portion of the circulation. Venous air embolism may reduce or stop the flow of blood through the heart or may cause neurologic complications. The exact amount of venous air which is fatal to adults is not known, but it is estimated to be between 300 and 1600 ml.[22] The rate of air injection into the venous circulation is of primary importance. Death appears to be due to the right ventricle compressing the air rather than pumping blood.

The mechanism for arterial air embolism is different. Air entering the left side of the heart passes quickly into the aorta. Then, depending on the position of the patient, the air may flow into the coronary and/or the cerebral arteries.[22] Air entering these vessels then obstructs the flow of blood to areas supplied by these vessels. In dogs, small amounts of air in the range of 0.05 to 1 ml injected into the coronary circulation have been fatal.[22] Air embolism is best prevented by using continuous flush systems and keeping the plumbing systems closed.[22,25]

THROMBOSIS

Thrombosis can be caused by an invasive catheter, but it is an infrequent complication of arterial or pulmonary artery catheterization. Embolization of clots formed on a catheter can be flushed retrograde into the central circulation from radial arterial cannulation sites. To minimize thrombus formation, continuous flush systems have been developed to keep catheters patent and prevent the need to use syringes to flush catheters.[25,26] In recent years pulmonary artery catheters have had heparin-bonding added to their surface in an attempt to minimize thrombus formation, although no long-term data are available to demonstrate an effect.[27]

INFECTION

Although invasive pressure monitoring provides valuable monitoring information, it can also result in bacteremia due to contamination of catheters, stopcocks, pressure transducers, and flush solutions.[28-32] Early pressure transducers were reusable, and when they were not properly sterilized, they caused epidemics of bacteremia.[28] As a result, sterile diaphragm disposable domes were developed. These diaphragm domes did not eliminate the bacteremias and resulted in poor system dynamic response. The Centers for Disease Control now recommends changing domes and other disposable components every 48 hours.[31] Several recent studies, however, have supported extended use of the disposable components.[29,30,32] To prevent contamination of pressure monitoring systems and the patients to whom they are attached, the sterility of the monitoring plumbing system must be maintained.

SIGNAL AMPLIFICATION, PROCESSING, AND DISPLAY

Once the pressure signal has been transmitted to the transducer, the bedside monitor operates on that signal. Most monitors display the heart rate and systolic, diastolic, and mean pressure with a digital display. During a recent evaluation of bedside monitors it was found that applying the same pressure waveforms to each of three monitors gave different results.[33] In addition none of the monitors recognized and rejected the following artifact conditions: zeroing the transducer, fast-flushing of the system, and drawing blood from the patient.

These conditions occur several times a day during normal patient care and result in false alarms and erroneous trend data logging.[33]

To help eliminate these problems, new algorithms are being developed for bedside pressure monitors. Preliminary testing has shown that these enhanced algorithms produce dramatic improvements in the bedside monitor's ability to evaluate pressure waveforms in the clinical setting.[34] According to the study,

> Present monitoring systems allow far too much artifactual data to reach the monitor's display, trend buffer, and alarm logic.

> The enhanced pressure artifact rejection algorithm eliminates most of the false alarms caused by zeroing, flushing, and blood drawing.

> The trend displays of the new algorithm are more representative of actual patient conditions.

> Data sent from the bedside monitor to the computerized patient data management system is more valid and thus patient data management computer systems can be programmed to automatically acquire patient data.

Algorithms for enhancing the quality of data derived from pulmonary artery pressure waveforms have recently been developed and applied.[35]

REFERENCES

1. Gardner RM, Hollingsworth KW: Optimizing ECG and pressure monitoring. *Crit Care Med* 1986; 14:651
2. Gardner RM: Hemodynamic monitoring: From catheter to display. *Acute Care* (in press)
3. Gardner RM, Kutik M (co-chairmen): American national standard for blood pressure transducers. General. Association for the Advancement of Medical Instrumentation/American National Standards Institute 1986, Arlington, VA
4. Gardner RM, Kutik M (co-chairmen): American national standard for interchangeability and performance of resistive bridge type blood pressure transducers. Association for the Advancement of Medical Instrumentation/American National Standards Institute 1986, Arlington, VA
5. Disposable pressure transducers. *Health Devices*, September 1984; 13:268. ECRI, Plymouth Meeting, PA
6. Geddes LA: The significance of a reference in the direct measurement of blood pressure. *Med Instrum* 1986; 20:331
7. Gardner RM: Direct blood pressure measurement—Dynamic response requirements. *Anesthesiology* 1981; 54:227
8. Geddes LA: The direct and indirect measurement of blood pressure. Chicago, Year Book Medical Publishers, 1970
9. Hansen AT: Pressure Measurement in the Human Organism. *Acta Physiol Scand* 1949; 19(Suppl 68): 1
10. Hansen AT, Warburg E: The theory for elastic liquid containing membrane manometers. *Acta Physiol Scand* 1949; 19(Suppl 65): 306
11. Fry DL: Physiologic recording by modern instruments with particular reference to pressure recording. *Physiol Rev* 1960; 40:753
12. Wood EH, Sutterer WF: Strain-gauge manometers: Application to recording of intravascular and intracardiac pressures. In Glasser O (ed): *Medical Physics*, Vol 3, p 641. Chicago, Year Book Medical Publishers, 1960
13. Crul JF: Measurement of arterial pressure. *Acta Anaesthesiol Scand* 1962; 6(Suppl XI): 135
14. Shapiro G, Krovetz LJ: Damped and undamped frequency responses of underdamped catheter-manometer systems. *Am Heart J* 1970; 80:226
15. McCutcheon EP, Evans JM, Stanifer RR: Direct blood pressure measurement: Gadgets versus progress. *Anesth Analg* 1972; 51:746
16. Fox F, Morrow DH, Kacher EJ, Gilleland TH II: Laboratory evaluation of pressure transducer domes containing a diaphragm. *Anesth Analg* 1978; 57:67
17. Shinozaki T, Deane RS, Mazuzan JE: The dynamic response of liquid-filled catheter system for direct measurement of blood pressure. *Anesthesiology* 1980; 53:498
18. Gardner RM: Blood pressure monitoring: Sharing common elements, problems. *IEEE-EMB Magazine* 1982; 1:28
19. Boutros A, Albert S: Effect of the dynamic response of transducer tubing system on accuracy of direct pressure measurement in patients. *Crit Care Med* 1983; 11:124
20. Yeomanson CW, Evans DH: The frequency response of external transducer blood pressure measurement systems: A theoretical and experimental study. *Clin Phys Physiol Meas* 1983; 4:435
21. Soule DT, Powner DJ: Air entrapment in pressure monitoring lines. *Crit Care Med* 1984; 12:520

22. Toll MO: Direct blood-pressure measurements: Risks, technology evolution and some current problems. *Med Biol Eng Comput* 1984; 22:2

23. Taylor BC, Ellis DM, Drew JM: Quantification and simulation of fluid-filled catheter/transducers systems. *Med Instrum* 1986; 20:123

24. Gibbs NC, Gardner RM: Dynamics of invasive pressure monitoring systems: Clinical and laboratory evaluation (unpublished manuscript)

25. Gardner RM, Bond EL, Clark JS: Safety and efficacy of continuous flush systems for arterial and pulmonary artery catheters. *Ann Thorac Surg* 1977; 23:534

26. Gardner RM, Warner HR, Toronto AF, Gaisford WD: Catheter-flush system for continuous monitoring of central arterial pulse waveform. *J Appl Physiol* 1970; 29:911

27. Hoar PF, Wilson RM, Mangano DT, et al: Heparin bonding reduces thrombogenicity of pulmonary-artery catheters. *N Engl J Med* 1981; 305:993

28. Weinstein RA, Stam WE, Kramer L, et al: Pressure monitoring devices: Overlooked source of nosocomial infection. *JAMA* 1976; 236:936

29. Thomas F, Burke JP, Parker J, et al: The risk of infection related to radial vs. femoral sites for arterial catheterization. *Crit Care Med* 1983; 11:807

30. Sommers MS, Baas LS: Nosocomial infections related to four methods of hemodynamic monitoring. *Heart Lung* 1987; 16:13

31. Simmons BP: Centers for Disease Control: Guidelines for prevention of infections related to intravascular pressure-monitoring systems. *Infect Control* 1982; 3:68

32. Luskin RL, Weinstein RA, Nathan C, et al: Extended use of disposable pressure transducers: A bacteriologic evaluation. *JAMA* 1986; 255:916

33. Maloy L, Gardner RM: Monitoring systemic arterial blood pressure: Strip recording versus digital display. *Heart Lung* 1986; 15:627

34. Gardner RM, Monis SM, Oehler P: Monitoring direct blood pressure: Algorithm enhancements. *IEEE Computers in Cardiology*, Boston, MA, October 1986

35. Ellis DM: Interpretation of beat-to-beat blood pressure values in the presence of ventilatory changes. *J Clin Monit* 1985; 1:65

CHAPTER FIVE

CARDIAC OUTPUT MEASUREMENT TECHNOLOGY

Tina Banner
Michael J. Banner

Measurement of cardiac output (CO) in the intensive care setting has become an integral part of the assessment and management of critically ill patients. Due to technological advances over the past two decades, CO data are now easily obtainable at the bedside. Although the thermodilution technique still predominates, newer, noninvasive techniques are emerging and becoming popular for certain situations. This chapter will describe the rationale, theory, equipment, and procedures of CO measurement techniques, both invasive and noninvasive. An understanding of the theory of each technique is necessary to avoid the various sources of technical error, which are also included in the discussion.

INVASIVE TECHNIQUES

THERMODILUTION

CO can be easily measured at the bedside by the thermodilution technique by using a multiple-lumen pulmonary artery (PA) catheter. The thermistor lumen of the catheter consists of two fine insulated wires extending the length of the catheter and terminating at a thermistor embedded in the catheter wall approximately 4 cm from the tip of the catheter. This lumen connects to a cable from a single-purpose CO computer. The thermistor continuously records PA blood temperature, and changes in temperature affect the electrical resistance of the thermistor. Injecting a known amount of solution, at a known (colder than body) temperature through the proximal or right atrial lumen of the catheter, lowers the temperature of the blood as it passes the thermistor downstream (Fig. 5-1). This lowered temperature decreases the electrical resistance of the thermistor and, electronically, a curve is described. The area under this thermodilution curve is integrated, calculated as CO, and displayed on the computer in liters per minute. In actuality, right ventricular output is being measured: in the absence of intracardiac shunting, right and left ventricular outputs are equivalent, so that cardiac output is assessed based on right ventricular performance. It must be emphasized that the accuracy of the measurement is highly dependent upon correct technique.

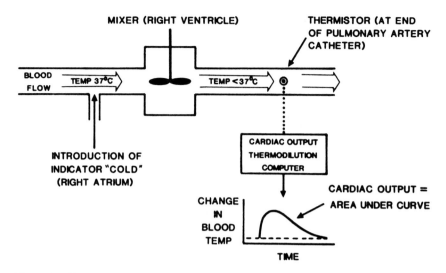

Figure 5-1 Thermodilution principle for measuring cardiac output. In this model, a change in the temperature of the blood is created at one point in the circulation (right atrium) by injecting a bolus of "cold" (lower than blood temperature) indicator. The resultant change in blood temperature is detected by the thermistor at a point "downstream" in the pulmonary artery (PA). As the "thermodiluted" (temperature-reduced) blood flows by the thermistor, a transient change in blood temperature with respect to time is detected by the thermistor altering its resistance and generating an appropriate curve. The area under this curve is integrated and cardiac output is calculated using the Stewart–Hamilton indicator dilution formula. (Modified from Banner MJ, Gallagher TJ: Respiratory failure in the adult: Ventilatory support. In Kirby RR, Smith RA, Desautels D (eds): *Mechanical Ventilation,* p 232. New York, Churchill Livingstone, 1985)

Preparation

Injectate. Either 5% dextrose in water or normal saline may be used for injection. Most currently available CO computers will accept room temperature or iced (0° C) injectate as a thermal indicator. An injectate reference probe from the CO computer is placed in the same temperature conditions as the injectate solution.

If a room temperature injectate is used, the probe may be placed in a nonsterile infusion bag (not to be used for patient injection, as the probe is not sterile) at room temperature in proximity (preferably side by side) to the sterile solution to be used as injectate. Neither solution should be placed on or near electrical equipment, which could warm these solutions. In commercially available systems, the injectate sensor is attached to the connecting tubing; the temperature is sensed as the solution enters the PA catheter.

If iced injectate is used, the probe should be placed in a nonsterile solution bag in the iced bath. It is essential that the temperature reference (probe) bag and injectate bag be the same temperature. Prefilled syringes may also be used as an alternate method for injectate preparation. Injectate temperature, measured by the reference probe, is displayed on the computer.

Computation Constant. Once the catheter model number and injectate temperature and volume are known, it is necessary to refer to the manufacturer's reference table to determine the appropriate computation constant. This information can be obtained from the computer manual or the pamphlet accompanying the catheter packaging. It is recommended that a copy of this table be permanently attached to the CO computer to provide quick reference. After determining the computation constant, the appropriate value is entered on the CO computer.

Catheter Position. Catheter position should be verified by observing the oscilloscope for a characteristic PA waveform that changes to a wedged or pulmonary artery occlusion waveform during balloon inflation and returns to a PA waveform after balloon deflation. For accurate CO values, the catheter tip should lie in a main branch of the PA (using radiographic verification).

Patient Position. The thermodilution technique should accurately reflect cardiac output in any position. However, it is recommended that CO be measured in the same position in which the other hemodynamic parameters are measured.

Computer Check. The thermistor lumen of the PA catheter is connected to the CO computer cable. Most computers have a self-test mechanism that will indicate if the integrity of the system is acceptable. This self-test may be performed to check the CO computer function. If the integrity of the system is inadequate, a fault message will appear on the display screen, after which all connections should be rechecked. If these are intact, the problem may be a defective thermistor.

Procedure

The procedure for measuring CO by thermodilution is easy; however, as stated, the accuracy of the method is highly dependent on adherence to proper technique. Once the described preparations are completed, the CO procedure may be initiated.

1 Check that the computer is in the measurement mode and is "ready."

2 Care should be·given to the withdrawal of injectate. If room temperature injectate is used, the bolus may be withdrawn at any time, providing the filled syringe remains at room temperature. (*Note:* Never lay filled syringe on electronic equipment.) In commercial systems, the syringe remains attached to the closed system, which includes the infusion bag, one-way valve, connecting tubing, and injectate probe.
   If iced injectate is used, the bolus for injection should be withdrawn from the solution source rapidly and injected immediately to prevent warming. The iced injectate bolus should be withdrawn and injected completely within 15 seconds.
   It is important that the exact amount of solution be injected, and that air bubbles or excess fluid are removed. Avoid holding the filled syringe, since heat transfer from the hand can warm the filled syringe (particularly iced solutions) and induce an error in the technique.

3 The bolus of indicator will be injected into the proximal (right atrial) lumen of the thermodilution PA catheter.

4 The computer is activated and the solution injected rapidly. The actual injection should be smooth and continuous without stopping or changing the injection rate. The injection should be completed within 2 to 4 seconds. These aspects of actual injection technique are crucial to the accuracy and reproducibility of the method.

5 CO will be displayed on the computer in liters per minute.

PRINCIPLE OF THERMODILUTION

The thermodilution method for measuring blood flow was first described by George Fegler in 1954.[1] Introduced into clinical medicine in 1971 by Ganz and co-workers,[2] this method for measuring cardiac output has been evaluated by investigators[2-7] over the past 15 years and is the most widely used technique for measuring CO in the clinical setting. The principle of thermodilution is an extension of indicator dilution, in which a known amount of indicator (*e.g.,* cold) is injected at a specified site "upstream" (*e.g.,* right atrium), and the resultant dilutional effect of the indicator as it mixes with blood at a "downstream" location (*e.g.,* PA thermistor) is measured (see Fig. 5-1). Using a thermal indicator (*e.g.,* cold), cardiac output can be calculated according to the Stewart-Hamilton indicator dilution formula:[8]

$$CO = \frac{V_I (T_B - T_I) \, K_1 \, K_2}{\int \Delta T_B \, dt}$$

where CO = cardiac output; V_I = injectate volume; T_B = blood (PA) temperature; T_I = injectate temperature; $\Delta T_B \, dt$ = change in blood temperature as a function of time; K_1 = density factor (injectate/blood); and K_2 = computation constant.

Familiarity with the components of this formula provides an understanding of the fundamental principles and technical aspects of thermodilution CO measurement and potential sources of errors.

The thermistor of the catheter represents one of four resistors in a Wheatstone bridge electrical circuit (Fig. 5-2). The catheter connected to the CO computer then functions as a complete Wheatstone bridge circuit.

Prior to injection, baseline blood temperature must be determined. In currently available CO computers and catheters, PA blood temperature (T_B) is measured at the PA thermistor, once this lumen is connected to the CO computer.

The temperature reference probe continuously measures and enters the injectate temperature (T_I). At baseline, before the injection, the Wheatstone bridge is said to be balanced, that is, there is no voltage difference across the bridge. The decreased blood temperature resulting from the injection of the cold indicator $(T_B - T_I)$ lowers the resistance of the thermistor, resulting in a voltage difference. This voltage differential describes a curve over time. The computer integrates the area under this curve $(\int \Delta T_B \, dt)$, and the resulting calculation is displayed on the monitor as CO in liters per minute. With this technique, CO varies inversely with the temperature–time integral change (and thus resistance change) created by the cold injection. Thus, the greater the blood flow over time, the smaller the temperature–time integral, the smaller the area under the curve, and the greater the CO, and *vice versa.*

Injectate Temperature. The current CO computers permit the selection of either room or iced temperature injectate. Several investigators have demonstrated the accuracy and reproducibility of both injectate temperatures.[6,9-12] In particular, Nelson and Anderson[9] and Shellock and colleagues[13] observed the same results in patient conditions once thought to be exceptions to the use of room temperature injectate: hypothermia, hypotension, and low-cardiac output. These studies showed that, despite the maximized signal-to-noise ratio (Fig. 5-3) associated with an iced injectate, in most cases it provides no particular advantage over room temperature injectate when 10-ml bolus volumes are used. However, when 5-, 3-, or

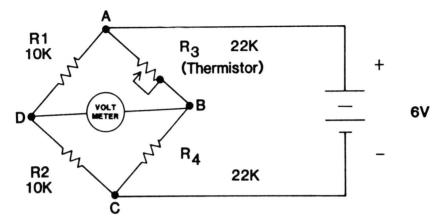

Figure 5-2 Wheatstone bridge electrical circuit in which R_1 and R_2 are resistors of 10 kilo-ohms (k) each and R_4 is a resistor of 22 k. Resistor R_3 is variable, that is, resistance is proportional to changes in temperature (lower the temperature, lower the resistance). The R_3 leg of the bridge represents the thermistor of the pulmonary artery catheter. At baseline, the resistance of R_3 is assumed to be 22 k.
When a driving voltage of, for example, 6 volts is placed across the bridge at points marked A and C, currents develop in the circuit with one current flowing through R_3 and R_4 and a second current flowing through R_1 and R_2. As long as the ratio of R_4/R_3 and R_2/R_1 are equal, (22/22 = 10/10), the voltage difference developed (measured by a voltmeter) between points B and D will be null. The bridge is then considered balanced. Any variation in the resistance of the thermistor causes the bridge to become unbalanced, resulting in a voltage difference across points B and D.

1-ml injectate volumes are used, iced temperature injectates may result in greater reproducibility than room temperature[12] due to the greater signal-to-noise ratio.

Room temperature injectate solutions offer several advantages:

There is less chance of obtaining spurious CO values, which can result when the injectate bolus is warmed as it is withdrawn through warm tubing, or from handling the syringe or injection delay.[8]

Cost is minimized because no special equipment is required to maintain iced temperature, and efficiency is improved because there is no need to wait for temperature equilibration. It takes about 45 to 60 minutes for syringes or infusion bags in an iced bath to reach equilibration at 0° to 4° C.

The chance of arrhythmias, which, although infrequent, have been reported to occur with iced temperature injectate,[14,15] is eliminated.

Injectate Solution and Volume. Either 5% dextrose in water (D_5W) or normal saline (NS) may be used as injectate. The density factor, (K_1: the ratio of the product of the specific heat and specific gravity of the injectate to that of blood) for each solution is similar,[3] allowing either to be used. The volume of injectate (V_I) used is determined by patient size and fluid status. In adult patients without fluid restrictions, 10-ml boluses are generally used. For pediatric or fluid-restricted patients requiring frequent cardiac output determinations, smaller volumes (5, 3, or 1 ml) may be used. The use of iced injectate volumes as small as 1 and 3 ml in pediatric patients was demonstrated by Freed and Keane,[16] and Wyse and

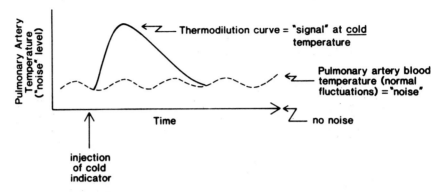

Figure 5-3 Diagrammatic representation of signal-to-noise ratio as related to the thermo-dilution cardiac output technique. Signal-to-noise ratio is the ratio of the amplitude of a signal after detection to the amplitude of the noise accompanying the signal. Relating this definition to thermodilution, signal-to-noise ratio could be described as the ratio of the thermistor resistance change created by the injection of cold indicator ("signal") and the temperature variations occurring in the PA ("noise"). The greater the difference between the temperature change resulting from the injection of cold indicator and the baseline PA temperature, the greater the signal-to-noise ratio and vice versa. Iced injectates result in a greater signal-to-noise ratio than room temperature injectates; larger injectate volumes produce a greater signal-to-noise ratio than smaller volumes.

associates[17] to produce accurate and reproducible results. However, the use of smaller volumes (5 ml or less) with room temperature injectate may reduce the signal-to-noise ratio sufficiently to result in less accurate CO measurements, as shown by Elkayam and co-workers[12] and Pearl and colleagues.[18] It would thus be advisable to consider iced injectate when smaller injectate volumes are indicated.

The volume of injectate used must be measured accurately to avoid spurious results. Moreover, the bolus volume must be injected in its entirety (*i.e.*, no leakage during injection). The injection of less indicator than specified produces falsely high CO values because this causes less cooling of the blood, interpreted as a higher flow than actual. Errors in delivered injectate volume are minimized with larger volumes (*e.g.*, an 0.1 ml error is 1% of 10 ml; the same error in volume is 3.3% of 3 ml). In addition, the catheter deadspace (injectate or proximal lumen volume) of various adult 7-French thermodilution catheters ranges from 0.71 ml to 0.94 ml and larger injectate volumes ensure a greater amount of indicator delivered into the circulation.

It is common in clinical practice to inject the indicator through a stopcock rather than directly into the proximal lumen port. Although direct injection into the catheter port would appear to be the ideal site, it "opens" the system to potential contamination and, because there is no stopcock, blood tends to back up through the catheter lumen. For these reasons, this method is less desirable. If injection is through a stopcock port and iced injectate is used, the injectate syringe should be connected to the stopcock port nearest the proximal lumen port in order to minimize stopcock deadspace, which is at room temperature. For example, 0.13 ml (with a Pharmaseal stopcock) to 0.2 ml (Luer-type stopcock) of injectate remains in the stopcock after injection. This is 1.3% to 2%, respectively, of a 10-ml injectate volume. Using smaller injectate volumes, the stopcock content percentage of the bolus volume is increased. However, with 5-ml volumes of iced injectate, there appears to be no significant difference when injection is via a stopcock or directly into the catheter port (personal observation). With less than 5-ml injectate volumes, it may be advisable to inject directly into the catheter port when using iced injectates. Minimization of errors in injectate temperature and volume is achieved through attention to accurate and reproducible technique.

Computation Constant. The computation constant (K_2) will be different for each manufacturer, computer, catheter model, injectate temperature (T_I) and injectate volume (V_I), and must be determined and adjusted prior to measurement. The constant is obtained by referring to the manufacturer's table, usually included in each catheter packaging, and in the CO computer operations manual. This constant takes into consideration a correction to the units of measurement (liters/min), injection or proximal lumen deadspace, heat transfer, injection rate, and volume and temperature of injectate.

The proximal lumen should be fluid-filled at all times while in a patient. That portion of lumen lying within the body contains fluid at body temperature, while the portion of lumen lying outside the body will contain fluid near room temperature. During injection, these two segments of fluid will be injected as a part of the indicator, while an equivalent amount of indicator will remain in this deadspace at the completion of injection. There is also an exchange of temperature during and after injection between the catheter wall and the surrounding blood. This "indicator loss" at both room or iced injectate temperature and various bolus volumes is considered in deriving this constant.

Thermodilution Curve. Referring to the Stewart–Hamilton formula for calculating cardiac output, it should be clear that the "numerator" variables are largely predetermined before the actual injection: the volume (V_I), temperature (T_I), and type of injectate solution (K_1) have been selected; the computation constant (K_2) has been entered into the computer, and once connected to the computer, the catheter thermistor should monitor the patient's PA blood temperature (T_B). The remaining determination is predominantly the denominator of the equation, or the integration of the thermodilution curve produced by the injection of the cold indicator, which will determine the CO. (*Note*: Faults in the actual injection technique can alter numerator variables, thus yielding possible erroneous CO values.)

Most currently available CO computers actually terminate the processing of the descending portion of the curve when it reaches a point equivalent to 30% of the upstroke. The decay of the curve from this point is assumed to be exponential, and the total area, using this assumption, is then integrated. This feature was designed to eliminate potential artifact (*e.g.*, "noise"), which may occur during this portion of the curve as a result of PA temperature changes related to other factors.

The shape of the curve is of vital importance, because it is the area under the curve that is integrated. A normal curve is smooth and typically consists of a rapid upstroke or peak, followed by a slower decay and return to baseline (Fig. 5-4A). Grossly irregular curves are not reliable and are frequently associated with inadequate mixing of the indicator with total blood flow (Fig. 5-4B). However, small irregularities are common and are the result of normal variations in pulmonary artery blood temperature. Many authors recommend using a strip-chart recorder in order to evaluate thermodilution curves for accuracy. Some computers now depict the curve on a liquid crystal display.

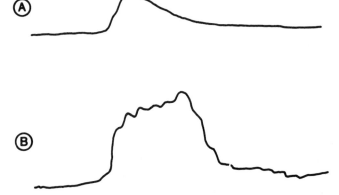

Figure 5-4 Examples of thermodilution curves.[8] The curve results from the thermistor resistance change created by the injection of "cold" indicator in the right atrium. Characteristically, the curve should be smooth and consist of a steep upstroke, followed by a slower decline toward baseline. **A.** Normal curve. **B.** Irregular curve.

Injection Technique

Accurate and reproducible thermodilution curves are produced by manual injections, which are rapid, smooth, and continuous. Ganz and Swan[3] demonstrated that when the injectate is delivered within a 2- to 4-second period, CO measurements are accurate and reproducible. (Injection rates that are too slow can influence K_2 in the indicator-dilution formula). Smooth and continuous curves are more commonly and easily obtained when pressure to the syringe plunger during injection is applied with the thenar eminence, as opposed to the thumb itself. Room temperature injectate does not warm to any significant extent from the time of filling the syringe to injection. However, Levett and Replogle[8] showed that the temperature of iced injectate does increase during this period but is minimal if injection is completed in less than 30 seconds (from initial withdrawal to completion of injection).

Nelson and Houtchens[19] reported that automatic injector devices show improved injection time, rate, and consistency in comparison to manual injection. These devices may serve to control variations between and within individuals performing manual injections. However, CO values were not statistically different when automatic injection was compared to manual injection performed by experienced personnel.

Injectate Systems

Three types of injectate systems are generally used in clinical practice for the maintenance and delivery of injectate: prefilled syringes, open two-bottle/bag, and closed injectate systems.

Prefilled Syringes. Barcelona and associates[20] showed that CO measurements obtained with 10-ml prefilled iced syringes and 10-ml prefilled room temperature syringes are comparable. Syringes can be prefilled and stored in an iced temperature environment or at room temperature. The major disadvantage of this type of system is the potential for contamination of the syringe contents. When syringes are chilled directly in ice baths, syringe hubs can become contaminated once the needle and cover or Luer-tip cap is removed; contamination of the catheter or stopcock port may then result.[21] In addition, bacterial growth was reported by Mattea, Paruta, and Worthen[21] to occur in an iced water bath after 3 hours. Syringes wrapped in plastic bags before immersion in the iced bath to prevent direct contamination of the syringe, cap, or hub may be less subject to possible contamination.

Burke and co-workers[22] demonstrated that when prefilled syringes are maintained at room temperature, 16% become contaminated within the first 24 hours and 45% become contaminated when stored more than 72 hours. The higher "incubation" temperature (room) may predispose this system to increased bacterial growth.

Open Systems. For iced temperature injectate, two intravenous infusion bottles or bags (D_5W or NS) are generally stored in an iced bath. One bottle/bag is maintained as a sterile source from which injectate is aspirated immediately before performing a CO measurement; the temperature reference probe is placed in the second (nonsterile) bottle/bag. Maintained in the same iced environment, the temperature of each bottle/bag, despite removal of fluid from the injectate bag, should not vary more than 0.5° C.[23]

The injectate may be aspirated either by a needle introduced into the bottle/bag or by some type of intravenous extension tubing. Two sources of injectate temperature error can occur with this set-up. First, if extension tubing is used, the tubing must also be immersed in the iced bath; otherwise, warmer (room temperature) fluid will comprise part of the injectate bolus. For example, one commonly used type of tubing (Novex Three-Way Stopcock with extension tube) has an approximate capacity of 3.6 ml. If all the tubing were in contact with room temperature rather than iced temperature, 36% of a 10-ml bolus would be at room temperature, which would create a rather significant injectate temperature error. Second, the syringe itself should be precooled by aspirating cold solution back and forth several times. Aspirating the cold solution directly into a room temperature syringe allows for some amount of cold transfer to the syringe material and thus another source of "warming" of the injectate.

Microbial growth was demonstrated by Nelson, Martinez, and Anderson[24] to occur in 35% of injectate bottles/bags within 48 hours using an open system for iced injectate. Moreover, greater numbers of CO measurements increase the likelihood of contamination because each measurement represents a "break" in the system.

The incidence of microbial growth in open room temperature systems has not been demonstrated. However, given the higher "incubation" of room temperature, the incidence reported with open iced systems, and the incidence with room temperature prefilled syringes, it would appear that this incidence could be significant.

Closed Systems. Commercially available closed systems for the maintenance and delivery of injectate are available (Fig. 5-5). These systems provide a sterile conduit from the injectate source to the catheter and are ideal for iced temperature injectate solutions. In addition, an in-line thermistor located near the injection lumen port measures the injectate temperature as it is delivered into the catheter. This minimizes many of the temperature errors commonly associated with iced injectate. For room temperature injectates, closed systems can be easily assembled (Fig. 5-6) at minimal cost.

Microbiologic testing by Nelson, Martinez, and Anderson[24] with a commercially available closed system for iced injectate (CO-set, from American Edwards Laboratories, Santa Ana, CA) showed that only 1 patient in 20 (this patient had 61 CO determinations) yielded a positive culture within a 48-hour period. In another study, Burke and colleagues[22] dem-

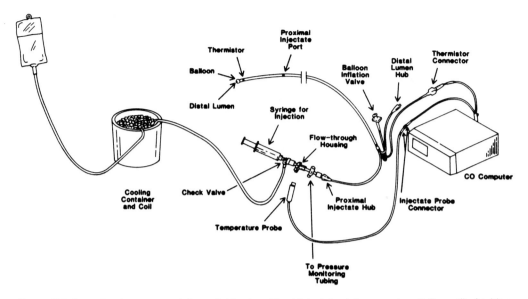

Figure 5-5 Example of a commercially available closed-iced injectate delivery system.* The coil of tubing filled with injectate is immersed in an ice bath. Injectate is withdrawn from the iced coiled tubing by the "check valve" and, when ready, is injected through the "flow-through housing" into the proximal lumen. Injectate temperature is monitored by an in-line temperature probe positioned proximal to the catheter port. (*Modified: Co-Set, American Edwards Laboratories, Santa Ana, CA)

onstrated microbial growth in only 1 of 81 samples (1.2%) within a 48-hour period using a closed system for room temperature injectate. These data indicate that closed systems can be maintained and changed every 48 hours without a significant incidence of bacterial growth.

Technique-Related Errors

Injectate Temperature Errors. Whenever the delivered injectate is warmer or cooler than the temperature selected and used in determining the computation constant, or than the fluid being monitored by the temperature reference probe, errors in CO measurement may occur. The most frequent temperature errors probably occur when iced temperature injectate is used, because the latter is predisposed to inadvertent warming of the injectate bolus prior to injection. Ten-milliliter iced injectate samples can warm from 0.6° C to 1.0° C within 30 seconds after removal from an iced bath and kept at room temperature and warmed 1° C every 13 seconds when clasped in a warm hand.[8,9] If all other factors are unchanged, a 10-ml bolus of iced injectate, which has warmed prior to delivery into circulation, can yield a 2% to 3% error per degree warmed, (e.g., injectate delivered at 7° C: the error would be almost 20%). Thus, meticulous attention to technique, specifically syringe handling and time lapse after withdrawal, is essential when using iced injectate solutions.

The use of room temperature injectate solutions minimize some of the potential temperature errors previously described with iced temperature. Warming of room temperature injectate is not affected by time lapse from solution withdrawal to injection. Holding

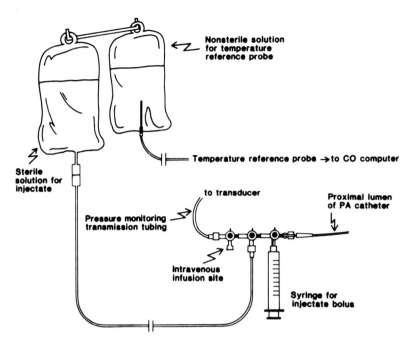

Figure 5-6 Example of a closed system for room temperature injectate delivery. The sterile solution bag for injectate is hung side-by-side with the nonsterile solution bag used for the injectate temperature reference probe (both bags are at the same temperature). Without "opening" the system, injectate can be withdrawn from the sterile source through stopcocks and injected into the proximal lumen. A third stopcock can be added for intravenous infusions. It is important that the syringe/injection port be that closest to the proximal lumen port to minimize catheter–stopcock dead space.

a room temperature syringe in a warm hand results in a temperature increase of 1° C per minute, an unlikely period of delay in clinical practice. In general, injected boluses that are warmer than the reference temperature tend to yield spuriously high CO values and *vice versa*.

Injectate Volume Errors. As previously mentioned, the selected injectate volumes should be accurately measured. If the delivered bolus volume (irrespective of temperature) is less than that chosen, falsely high CO values may result (the thermistor detects less cold and interprets it as higher flow).

A frequent source of volume error occurs when the injected bolus leaks from the site of connection to the catheter or stopcock during the forceful injection. If this occurs, these values should be disregarded and the measurements repeated. Another potential error may occur when intravenous infusions are passing through the proximal (right atrial) lumen or the distal lumen immediately before or after injection. Regardless of the injectate bolus temperature, the intravenous infusions are generally at room temperature (approximately 20° C), which is still a cold solution relative to body temperature. This additive effect of a cold indicator may compound both blood and injectate temperature errors and yield erroneous values. In this situation, fluids should not be infused for a few seconds before injection until the CO computer has completed the computation and displayed the CO value. (*Note*: In patients receiving vasoactive agents by the proximal lumen of a PA catheter and who do not tolerate the cessation of this infusion for approximately 45 to 60 seconds, it may be necessary to infuse these agents through a separate catheter. In addition, before injecting the indicator, the proximal lumen should be aspirated so that a bolus of vasoactive infusion will not be injected during CO measurement.)

Another source of operator error is entering an incorrect computation constant. A constant that is set too high will yield falsely high COs. Measurements already performed with an incorrect constant can be adjusted once the correct constant is determined, as follows:[25]

$$CO_{correct} = \frac{\text{computation constant}_{correct}}{\text{computation constant}_{incorrect}} \times CO_{incorrect}$$

It may be easier to enter the correct constant and repeat the measurement.

Catheter-Related Errors

Catheter Position. Accurate CO measurements are obtained when the catheter tip and thermistor are in proper position. Proper catheter position should be verified following catheter insertion. However, because catheters can migrate to some extent, position should be verified prior to CO measurement. In addition to radiographic verification, proper position is ascertained by observing both the pulmonary artery and pulmonary arterial occlusion waveforms. If the catheter tip becomes wedged without inflating the balloon, (*i.e.*, advanced too far in the PA), the thermistor may not be exposed to the entire indicator volume after injection, yielding erroneously high CO measurements. Ellis and colleagues[26] found that thermistor contact with the vessel wall may result in irregular curves and thus erroneous values.

Proximal lumen orifice (exit port) location in the right atrium is also an important factor for accuracy of the technique. Location of the proximal orifice below the right atrium (*e.g.*, right ventricle) may result in incomplete mixing of the indicator with total blood flow past the thermistor and thus yield spurious CO values. Location of the proximal orifice above the atrium (*e.g.*, superior vena cava or higher) may result in indicator loss prior to PA thermistor detection, again yielding false values. Verification of proximal lumen orifice position is obtained by observing a right atrial waveform on the oscilloscope. (*Note*: As mentioned, catheters are available with various proximal lumen orifice locations. This is an important consideration in selecting catheters for very small adults and children.)

Catheter Introducers. In recent years, the use of side-arm percutaneous central venous pressure introducer sets for inserting pulmonary artery catheters has become increasingly popular. Possible thermodilution measurement errors may result if intravenous fluids are infused through the side ports during CO measurement. The magnitude of the error depends on the volume and temperature of the infusing solution.

Another possible source of error associated with the use of side port extensions can occur if the *in vivo* portion of the introducer sheath covers the proximal (right atrial) exit port or orifice. Bears, Yonutas, and Allen[27] reported that if this occurs, the indicator may not be delivered rapidly or entirely into the circulation. The resulting error would be a falsely high CO value because less indicator would be detected. This is more likely to occur when PA catheters are inserted in the subclavian or internal jugular veins, in which case there is a shorter *in vivo* catheter distance. Most introducer sheaths are approximately 15 cm in length. By examining the PA catheter marking at the skin level and knowing the proximal lumen exit port location, one can determine the *in vivo* length and anticipate this problem. For example, if the PA catheter skin level is less than 45 cm in a catheter with the proximal exit port at 30 cm from the tip (*in vivo* catheter distance to the proximal exit port is then less than 15 cm), and 15 cm of introducer sheath is inserted into the patient, then it is likely that the sheath will cover the proximal exit port.

Patient-Related Factors

Effects of Ventilation. Fegler[28] in 1957 described a large error which could be introduced into the thermodilution calculations when respiratory movement was significant. Ganz and Swan[3] described cyclic changes with respiration in PA blood temperature which were negligible during quiet spontaneous breathing but which could be greatly amplified in the presence of abnormal respiratory patterns. Snyder and Powner[29] have identified unstable PA blood temperatures in patients receiving mechanical ventilation and undergoing coronary artery bypass surgery. Alterations in intrathoracic pressures and venous return were demonstrated by Armengol and associates[30] to change baseline PA blood temperature. These fluctuations in PA blood temperature, probably related to variations in thoracic venous inflow, represent a physiologic "noise" that lowers the signal-to-noise ratio and results in baseline (PA) temperature (T_B) drifts that may affect the reproducibility of CO measurements.[3,31] Most currently available CO computers moderate the potential baseline temperature drift problems by electronically averaging these values over a short period prior to indicator injection.[25]

Minimization of errors and variations due to respiratory-induced fluctuations in PA blood temperature may be accomplished by injecting the indicator at a consistent point in the ventilatory cycle, preferably at end-exhalation.[29,30] Unlike intracardiac pressure readings, which are more easily synchronized with end-exhalation, the thermodilution technique requires approximately 8 to 12 seconds of transit time for the injectate bolus to flow past the thermistor.[25] During this time, several cycles of ventilation may occur, making it impossible to obtain an instantaneous end-exhalation value. Jansen and co-workers[32] could not determine any satisfactory moment during the ventilatory cycle for injection during mechanical ventilation. However, Snyder and Powner[29] and Armengol and colleagues[30] concluded that reproducibility was best accomplished by averaging CO values obtained at regularly spaced intervals during the ventilatory cycle, especially when mechanical ventilation was employed.

Fegler[28] also noted that when distortion by respiratory movement was large, especially when it affected the steepest part of the thermodilution curve, a large error was introduced into the calculation. Hence, the actual injections should coincide with a period without mechanical ventilation, if possible. The injection should begin at the onset of exhalation from a mechanical ventilation, particularly with higher mechanical ventilatory rates. In this manner, the greatest amount of temperature change (*i.e.*, the steepest part of the curve) would be integrated during the end-exhalation phase of the ventilatory cycle.

An additional source of error reported by Wetzel and Latson[33] is the effect on baseline temperature fluctuations when rapid volume infusions are administered concurrently with CO determinations. In such situations, as previously mentioned, infusions should either be maintained at a constant rate or temporarily reduced before and during CO determinations.

Dysrhythmias. Dysrhythmias may result in variability in the CO measurement, because values reflect the cardiac rhythm and resulting right ventricular output during the computation time only. Although extremely rare, bradycardia[14] and atrial fibrillation[15] have been reported to develop following the right atrial injection of iced injectate solutions. The exact mechanisms are unclear; however, the alternative choice of a room temperature injectate might be considered in such situations.

Hypothermia. Merrick, Hessel, and Dillard[34] demonstrated accuracy in thermodilution cardiac output measurements during hypothermia when pulmonary artery blood temperature is continuously monitored. In hypothermic adult patients, both 10- and 5-ml injectate volumes at either iced or room temperature correlate well, even at core temperatures between 30.3°C and 34.8°C.[9,10] However, when fluid restriction is not a concern, 10-ml injectate volumes are recommended to maximize the signal-to-noise ratio.

High and Low Flow States. Few reports have clinically evaluated the accuracy of thermodilution using iced or room temperature injectate when CO was less than 3 liters/min. Above 3 liters/min, Pearl and co-workers[18] showed no difference in reproducibility and accuracy using 10-ml iced or 10-ml room temperature injectate. Variability in measurements increases when smaller volumes (5 ml, and especially 3 ml) of injectate are used, and even more so if smaller volumes of room temperature injectate are used.[18]

A study by Keen[35] showed a strong correlation between iced and room temperature injectate volumes when measuring CO in hyperdynamic cirrhotics with CO ranging from 6.4 to 11.2 liters/min.

Patient Position. Grose, Woods, and Laurent[36] compared CO measurements obtained in supine and semierect positions and demonstrated no significant differences in mean values. However, this study did show significant intrapatient changes in some individuals. The thermodilution technique will reflect cardiac output in any position. For consistency and comparison, CO determinations should be obtained in the same position in which the other hemodynamic parameters were obtained.

Intracardiac Shunts. Caution should be observed in performing thermodilution CO procedures in patients with intracardiac shunting. If this situation presents and thermodilution CO measurements are indicated, errors may occur. In the presence of right-to-left shunting, indicator injected into the right atrium may be "lost" to the left side of the heart and never pass the thermistor, resulting in falsely high CO values. In the presence of left-to-right shunting, recirculation of cold may occur, as "cooled" blood flowing through the right heart and pulmonary artery reaches the left side of the heart, passes back to the right side, and is then recirculated through the pulmonary artery past the thermistor. This can produce a second peak in the thermodilution curve, which becomes uninterpretable by the computer. In most situations, injections into central circulation would be contraindicated in the presence of intracardiac shunting. In a patient who might have an undiagnosed septal defect, the previously described findings after thermodilution injections might alert clinicians to this possibility.

Right Heart Valvular Dysfunction. Tricuspid or pulmonic valvular regurgitation may prevent accurate CO measurements due to indicator loss resulting from retrograde flow. In situations associated with significant right heart valvular regurgitation flow, the thermodilution technique may not be accurate.

Pediatric Considerations

Freed and Keane[16] and Wyse and colleagues[17] compared thermodilution to Fick CO measurements in critically ill children and infants, and demonstrated that thermodilution is an accurate and reproducible technique for measuring CO ($r = 0.93$ and 0.91, respectively). For intensive care management, 4- and 5-French thermodilution catheters with lumina for hemodynamic monitoring and indicator injection are available. These catheters may also be procured with proximal or right atrial orifice (exit port) locations at 10 or 15 cm from the catheter tip, enabling appropriate catheter selection for different body sizes (7-French catheters are also available with proximal orifice locations of 15 and 20 cm for large children or small adults). As mentioned previously, proximal lumen orifice position in the right atrium is an important factor in the accuracy of thermodilution. Location of the proximal orifice in the right ventricle may result in incomplete mixing of the indicator with total blood flow and yield erroneous CO values. Proximal orifice location above the right atrium might result in the loss of indicator before sampling (*i.e.*, detection by the thermistor).

The volume of injectate should be determined by the weight of the child or infant and fluid requirements. The potential for fluid overload in small infants can be minimized by using 1-ml injectate volumes. The use of excessive injectate volumes in small children and infants may result in CO errors due to recirculation.

Because of the small volumes used, most studies in children have employed iced injectate temperatures. Room temperature injectate, however, has yielded accurate thermodilution values when compared to Fick CO determinations.[17] In selecting the appropriate injectate temperature, it is recommended to consider the previously described signal-to-noise ratio factors to ensure or enhance the accuracy of the technique.

OTHER INVASIVE TECHNIQUES

Fick Technique

In 1870, Adolph Fick expounded a theory for quantitating blood flow that he never used in the laboratory: "The total uptake or release of a substance by an organ is the product of the blood flow to the organ and the arteriovenous concentration of the substance."[37] The Fick technique is a form of indicator dilution. In this method, oxygen entering the pulmonary circulation is the indicator that is measured in the pulmonary blood flow. According to the Fick principle, CO, in liters per minute, is equal to the oxygen consumption ($\dot{V}O_2$) divided by the arteriovenous oxygen content difference (($a - \bar{v}$)DO_2), multiplied by 100. If $\dot{V}O_2$ consumption = 250 ml/min, arterial blood O_2 content = 20 ml/dl, and mixed venous blood O_2 content = 15 ml/dl, then

$$CO = \frac{\dot{V}O_2}{(a-\bar{v})DO_2} \times 100$$

$$CO = \frac{250 \text{ ml/min}}{5 \text{ ml}} \times 100$$

$$= 5000 \text{ ml/min, or 5 liters/min}$$

The normal basal oxygen consumption index ($\dot{V}O_2$ in ml/min divided by body surface area) is between 110 to 150 ml O_2/min/m^2. The average error in $\dot{V}O_2$ measurement is approximately 6%, and the error for $(a-\bar{v})DO_2$ measurement is approximately 5%, making the total error in measurement of CO by this technique about 10%. This technique is generally used in the cardiac catheterization laboratory. The Fick technique is most accurate in low cardiac output states in which the $(a-\bar{v})DO_2$ is wide.[38]

Dye Dilution

In the indicator dye dilution technique, indocyanine green dye (the indicator) is injected rapidly as a bolus into the right atrium or pulmonary artery. Its appearance and concentration in a peripheral artery is detected by a cuvette densitometer. The result is a time–concentration curve resulting from the appearance and gradual disappearance of the dye. Due to recirculation, the curve characteristically consists of a second rise. The true "first-pass" (of the dye) curve is considered for CO calculations. CO is then calculated as

$$CO = \frac{\text{quantity of indicator}}{(\bar{c})\,(t)}$$

where $\bar{c}$ is the average concentration of the indicator during its first pass, and t is the total duration of the curve ($[\bar{c}][t]$ equals the area under the first pass curve). As with other indicator-dilution techniques, CO values are falsely high if the indicator is lost. Recirculation, which is unaccounted for, results in the indicator concentration being detected twice, yielding falsely low CO values.[37]

Errors with this technique are more common in patients with extremely low CO, severe mitral or aortic regurgitation, or intracardiac shunting.[38] This technique is generally limited clinically to cardiac catheterization laboratories.

This method is associated with the risk of allergic reactions to the dye and possible blood contamination during analysis. Repetitive injections may also result in accumulation of dye in the blood which may affect the accuracy of later measurements.

NONINVASIVE TECHNIQUES

Noninvasive technology for measuring CO has gained interest in the past few years and the potential advantages of lessened risk and cost to patients continue to generate enthusiasm. These techniques, which are currently available and are still being developed, have yet to achieve the confidence and reliability of the previously described invasive methods. However, the evolving noninvasive technology appears promising and, with further refinements, should overcome the present limitations and achieve widespread acceptance.

DOPPLER TECHNIQUE

Principles of Ultrasound

Ultrasound is defined as sound vibrations with frequencies (cycles per second or Hertz [Hz]) above the range of human hearing (20,000 Hz or 20 kHz). Ultrasonic technology deals with the transmission of high-frequency sound waves. The transducers used for clinical measurements have a piezoelectric element (crystal) that vibrates very rapidly and, in so doing, creates high-frequency sound waves, or ultrasound, which are directed through the body in the direction of the transducer aim.[39] (A piezoelectric element is a piece of crystal, which, when subjected to voltage, will undergo a change in shape, *i.e.*, vibrate). The ultrasound transducer functions both as a transmitter and as a receiver. The ultrasound technique used clinically for measuring CO is transcutaneous Doppler.

Doppler Principle. In the early 19th century, an Austrian physicist named Christian Doppler first described the principle now known as the "Doppler effect." He noted that the sound reflected or generated from a moving object shifted in frequency relative to the speed of that moving object[40] (Fig. 5-7). According to the Doppler principle, when an emitted ultrasonic wave is reflected from a moving object, the frequency of the reflected or returning wave is altered; the difference in frequency between the ultrasound emitted and that received will depend on the velocity of the reflecting (moving) interface and the angle at which the ultrasonic beam strikes the object. This change or shift in frequency is commonly referred to as the "Doppler shift." Doppler ultrasound is generally used to evaluate blood flow velocity, in which case it is the red blood cells that reflect the ultrasonic energy. As the ultrasound strikes the red blood cells and is reflected, a shift in frequency occurs which is proportional to the velocity of the reflecting blood cells. This "shift" results in a high-pitched sound. The faster the flow, the greater the shift, the higher-pitched the sound, and the greater the returning signal's amplitude. The measurement of blood flow velocity is then determined by the Doppler equation:[42]

$$f\Delta = \frac{2v\ f\emptyset\ \cos\ominus}{c}$$

where $F\Delta$ = Doppler shift frequency; v = velocity of erythrocytes; $f\emptyset$ = transmitted frequency (generally 2.5 to 3.5 MHz); $\ominus$ = angle between the ultrasound beam and the blood flow vector (ideally $\emptyset°$); and c = velocity of sound in blood (assumed to be 1570 ml/sec).

Measurement of Blood Flow Velocity. Two types of Doppler systems are available for obtaining CO measurements: continuous-wave and pulsed. (*Note:* Specific detailed descriptions of the actual measurement techniques will not be presented because each manufacturer's instrumentation varies to some extent.) The Doppler principle applies to both systems, in that measurement of aortic blood velocity through a known aortic diameter enables a quantification of CO. Measurement of ascending aortic blood flow velocity is usually obtained by placing a Doppler transducer in the suprasternal notch and aiming the ultrasound beam inferiorly toward the expected region of the ascending aorta and aortic root until blood flow velocity is detected (Fig. 5-8). (In some units, velocity can be measured at the aortic arch or other cardiac locations.) The aim is adjusted until the audio output of the Doppler

MOVING SOUND SOURCE

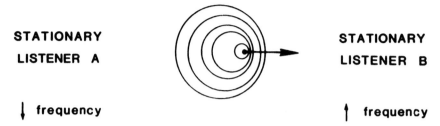

STATIONARY
LISTENER A

↓ frequency

STATIONARY
LISTENER B

↑ frequency

Figure 5-7 The Doppler effect. A higher frequency is heard when a moving sound source moves toward the stationary listener B than when it moves away from the stationary listener A.

shift frequencies yields the highest pitched sound (representing the highest velocity), concomitant with a perception of rapid onset and cessation of flow, and minimal diastolic flow,[42] characteristic of ascending aortic blood flow. In addition, the signal level output by visual display (digital or oscilloscopic representation) is also simultaneously assessed for optimal values.

The returning signals corresponding to blood flow velocity are processed into Doppler shift signals, which are then converted to velocities using the Doppler equation. Systolic

Figure 5-8 Diagrammatic representation of measurement of ascending aortic blood velocity. The Doppler transducer is placed in the suprasternal notch and aimed toward the expected region of the ascending aorta and aortic root. The aim is adjusted to yield the highest Doppler signal concomitant with the highest pitched audio output (see text).

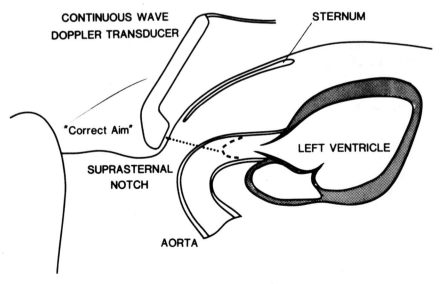

CONTINUOUS WAVE
DOPPLER TRANSDUCER

STERNUM

"Correct Aim"

LEFT VENTRICLE

SUPRASTERNAL
NOTCH

AORTA

velocity is then integrated (systolic velocity integral or SVI, (Fig. 5-9). CO is calculated as the product of SVI, the cross-sectional area (stroke volume), and the heart rate:[42]

$$CO = SVI \times \text{aortic cross-sectional area} \times \text{heart rate}$$

Aortic Cross-Sectional Area. Aortic diameter (from which cross-sectional area is calculated) may be determined in several ways: by measurement, using A-mode, cross-sectional (or M-mode), or two-dimensional echocardiography; or by estimation, using a table or a nomogram. Some commercially available Doppler units incorporate one of these techniques, in addition to the Doppler instrumentation. Whether measured or estimated, a value for aortic diameter is generally entered into the Doppler CO computer enabling calculation of cross-sectional area so that quantification of cardiac output can be obtained. (*Note*: If accurate measurements of aortic diameter cannot be obtained, arbitrary or estimated values can be entered allowing for monitoring of Doppler CO trend rather than volumetric flow.)

Continuous Wave Doppler

Continuous wave Doppler instruments use a two-crystal transducer. Ultrasound is continuously emitted from one crystal and continuously received by the other crystal. Blood flow velocity is measured all along the Doppler signal pathway. With the transducer placed in the suprasternal notch and aimed toward the expected location of the aortic root, the maximum frequency shift detected is assumed to correspond to the maximum velocity of blood flow within the ascending aorta.[41] Maximum velocity (or systolic velocity) is determined from both the audible and visual outputs of the Doppler device.

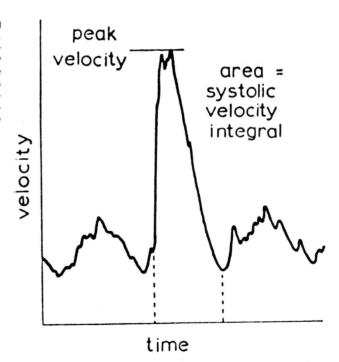

Figure 5-9 Aortic blood velocity from the ascending aorta in a dog. Velocity is zero at the abscissa. Moving blood and tissue interfaces cause the non-zero velocity during diastole. Peak systolic velocity and the area for systolic velocity integration are indicated. The "systolic velocity integral" (SVI) is equivalent to the area under the time course velocity curve during systole. (Colocousis JS, Huntsman LL, Curreri PW: Estimation of stroke volume changes by ultrasonic Doppler. Circulation 1977; 56:915)

The following studies in adults used a continuous-wave Doppler instrument (UltraCOM, from Lawrence Medical Systems, Inc., Seattle, WA) and compared the values to thermodilution CO measurements. Unless stated, aortic diameter was measured by the A-mode technique, which is incorporated into this instrument. A-mode measurements were not obtainable in all patients; the following reports reflect the patients in whom aortic diameter could be measured.

Huntsman and colleagues[42] using a prototype of the UltraCOM, demonstrated a correlation coefficient of 0.94. In this study, measurements were achieved in 45 of 53 adult patients (85%). Chandraratna and associates[41] showed a correlation coefficient of 0.97 in 36 of 39 (92%) patients studied. (This study also reported correlations for interobserver measurement variability of 0.98 and intraobserver variability of 0.97.) In a report by Rose and co-workers[43] the correlation of baseline Doppler and thermodilution in 16 patients was 0.919, yet in some patients the two techniques differed by as much as 1 liter/min. Various interventions, including pharmacologic vasodilatation (in 15) and pacing (in 1 patient), were used. After intervention, the correlation was 0.88. The closer correlation between the two techniques at baseline was postulated to be attributable to the vasodilator therapy. Nishimura and co-workers[44] found a correlation of 0.94 in 38 of 45 (84%) medical patients and 0.85 in 24 of 26 surgical patients (92%). The inability to obtain Doppler signals in all patients studied was due to either insufficient signal levels or prolonged ejection times (usually the result of signal detection from the innominate artery producing erroneously high CO values). Vandenbogaerde and colleagues[46] demonstrated a correlation coefficient of 0.97 in 28 of 41 patients (68%) but were, however, unable to obtain acceptable Doppler signals in 13 (32%) of the patients studied.

Rein and associates[45] compared thermodilution to Doppler CO measurements in children using another continuous-wave instrument (Sonacolor SC6310CD, Carolina Medical Electronics, Inc., King, NC). Aortic diameter was measured from a two-dimensional echocardiogram. Doppler measurements were obtainable in all 25 children and the correlation coefficient was 0.98.

Pulsed Doppler

Pulsed Doppler units use a single-crystal transducer which electronically alternates between a transmitter and a receiver mode. In contrast to the continuous-wave units, pulsed units measure the Doppler frequency shift at a selected depth from the transducer. Depending on the manufacturer and type of equipment, this sampling depth may be determined using either another echocardiographic ultrasound technique or by adjusting the depth selection until the velocity signals are maximized.[40] Systolic velocity is integrated and the average SVI over several heart beats is used for calculating CO as previously described. The primary advantage of this Doppler technique is that by selecting the sampling depth, the problem of ambiguity of the location of the detected flow is overcome. Hence, errors which might result from extraneous blood flow from other vessels are eliminated. The major limitation of the technique is the magnitude of frequency shifts that can be detected. At very high velocities, CO may be underestimated (such as might occur with aortic stenosis).[47]

Loeppky and co-workers[47] observed a correlation of 0.84 when comparing Doppler CO measurements to direct Fick measurements in adults using a pulsed Doppler echocardiograph (Advanced Technology Laboratories, Inc., Bellevue, WA). Alverson and associates[48] studied neonates and children and compared the same pulsed Doppler instrument with Fick CO measurements and found a correlation coefficient of 0.98.

Esophageal Doppler

In recent years, a Doppler ultrasound transducer has been incorporated into a standard esophageal stethoscope. This allows an essentially noninvasive method for monitoring CO continuously, by measuring descending aortic blood velocity. However, problems associated with calibration of descending volumetric flow relative to ascending flow and aortic diameter measurements are currently being evaluated. With further refinement and development, this technology should provide accurate, continuous monitoring of CO in patients who can tolerate the presence of an esophageal probe during anesthesia and operation.

Potential Errors and Limitations

There are several problems in measuring CO by the Doppler technique. First, the human aorta, unlike a rigid tube, is somewhat elastic and thus the cross-sectional area may change to some degree. Greenfield and Patel[49] demonstrated mean changes in cross-sectional area during the cardiac cycle of 11% of the diastolic value. In addition, aortic cross-sectional area can vary with changes in aortic pressure.[43,49] Because the currently available Doppler technology for quantifying CO assumes a constant aortic diameter, some measurement error may consequently occur if aortic diameter changes. Second, the velocity of the blood flow assumes a flat profile over most of the ascending aorta.[41,50] Although small regional differences may exist, Seed and Wood[50] demonstrated that measuring velocity in the ascending aorta through the center line gives an approximation of the mean velocity of the entire blood flow. Third, the amplitude of the velocity measurement is dependent on the angle between the direction of the Doppler signal aim and the direction of blood flow (angle of incidence). In the Doppler equation, this angle ($\cos \ominus$) is assumed to be 1°. However, for angles of more than 20°, the measurement error is less than 6%.[51] The specific limitations of continuous-wave and pulsed Doppler techniques have already been addressed.

An important aspect to this technique is the experience, skill, and knowledge of the operator. Loeppky and colleagues[47] stated that the technique requires an experienced operator with specialized training and knowledge of anatomy and flow characteristics of the aorta in order to obtain accurate and reliable measurements.

Noninvasive Doppler measurements of cardiac output cannot be obtained in all patients. The Doppler techniques for measuring CO previously described are not reliable in patients with aortic stenosis, due to high blood flow velocity through a narrowed orifice not representative of actual aortic diameter; aortic regurgitation/insufficiency, due to forward flow measurement only by this technique; or a prosthetic aortic valve, due to an altered flow channel size.[41] Inadequate Doppler signals are reported for unexplained reasons[41–46] and falsely elevated measurements (using continuous-wave) were observed by Nishimura and co-workers[44] and Vandenbogaerde and colleagues[46] in some patients in whom the inominate artery appeared to lie in the Doppler (continuous-wave) signal path. Difficulties in obtaining adequate Doppler signals were also reported in some mechanically ventilated patients.[46]

IMPEDANCE CARDIOGRAPHY

Principle and Theory of Measurement

Impedance cardiography (or thoracic electrical bioimpedance or transthoracic electrical impedance) is a noninvasive blood flow technology which provides real-time measurements of ventricular stroke volume.[52] Impedance cardiography utilizes four strip electrodes attached to the patient and connected to an impedance cardiograph. Two electrode strips are placed around the neck with approximately 3 to 4 cm distance between them. The third electrode strip is placed at the level of the xiphisternum and the fourth approximately 3 to 4 cm caudal to this location. To define the electrical field, a constant sinusoidal current is passed between the outer electrodes, and the rate of change in thoracic electrical impedance during systole is measured between the inner pair[53] (Fig. 5-10).

Kubicek Equation. Kubicek and associates[54] have posited an equation to assess ventilation stroke volume (SV):

$$SV = p(L/Zo) \, (LVET) \, (dZ/dt_{max})$$

Kubicek's method assumes that the adult thorax is, electrically speaking, a cylinder with a base circumference equal to the circumference of the thorax at the xiphoid level. This cylinder has an electrical length (L, in cm), which is the measured distance between the voltage-sensing circumferential band of electrode strips placed at the neck and at the xiphisternum. Moreover, this cylindrical thoracic volume conductor is homogeneously perfused with blood of a specific resistivity (p) in ohms per centimeter, which varies with the patient's hematocrit. Mohapatra and Hill[55] calculated the value of p as

$$(6.72 \, Hct + 75.176) - (0.104 \, Hct + 1.46) \, T \, °C$$

where Hct is the patient's hematocrit and T is body temperature in °C. The cylindrical thoracic volume conductor has a steady-state mean base impedance (Zo) in ohms. During systole, pulsatile variations in thoracic aortic blood flow cause a negative impedance change, and the maximum value of the rate of change in impedance during systole (dZ/dt_{max}) in ohms per second is proportional to peak ascending aortic blood flow. Multiplying these terms by left ventricular ejection time (*LVET*) in seconds yields stroke volume[52] (see Fig. 5-10).

Subsequent evaluations using Kubicek's method on groups of patients with varying illnesses produced poor correlations between the impedance cardiography method and other established methods of stroke volume measurement,[56] thus discouraging widespread clinical application of this technology in critically ill patients. Donovan and colleagues,[53] using Kubicek's empirical formula, found that cardiac output measurement was unsatisfactory in critically ill patients because of the technical difficulties associated with its use and the lack of precision when compared to the thermodilution method.

Figure 5-10 Diagrammatic representation of equipment used to measure cardiac output by impedance cardiography and the dZ/dt tracing used in calculating stroke volume. (See text; modified from references 52 and 53)

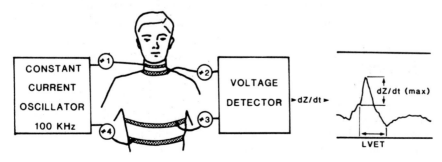

Sramek-Bernstein Equation. Sramek, Rose, and Miyaamoto[57] and Bernstein[52,58] proposed new equations which obviate the false assumptions of Kubicek's original equation. As Bernstein points out, the major problem in Kubicek's method is the quantitative importance of p. Specifically, no single p-Hct relationship has yielded good results when impedance stroke volume measurements were compared to reference standards.[52] Sramek determined that the actual electrical field distribution between the neck and lower thorax is that of a frustrum or truncated cone with the narrow end of the cone at the neck and divergent end at the lower thorax. The physical volume of this frustrum was determined to be 33% of the volume of the larger thoracic-encompassing cylinder.[57] Sramek and colleagues found that in adults, the measured linear distance is equal to 17% of body height (Ht) in centimeters.[57] It has been noted that in mammalian species, cardiac output is directly proportional to body weight,[59] and that ideal weight is a linear function of overall height.[60] Thus, the Sramek stroke volume equation is

$$SV = \left[\frac{(0.17 \text{ Ht})^3}{4.2} \right] (\text{LVET}) \left[\frac{dZ/dt_{max}}{Zo} \right]$$

where $(0.17 \text{ Ht})^3/4.2$ is the volume of the electrically participating thoracic tissue.

With the Sramek equation, systematic underestimations occur in patients who are 15% to 20% heavier than their ideal body weight.[52] Underestimations of stroke volume were also reported in morbid obesity using Kubicek's method.[61] It was reported that, as the lower thoracic circumference increases (as in obesity), the value of Zo decreases.[62] As a result of anthropometric considerations, Bernstein[52] subsequently appended Sramek's equation with a weight correction or scaling factor which represents the modified ratio of the patient's measured weight (Wt observed) to his or her ideal weight (Wt ideal) in kilograms:

$$SV = \beta \frac{(\text{Wt observed})}{(\text{Wt ideal})} \frac{(0.17 \text{ Ht})^3}{4.2} (\text{LVET}) \frac{dZ/dt_{max}}{Zo}$$

The symbol β represents the relative blood volume index, which equals the ratio of the average basal steady-state blood volume in ml/kg at any given deviation from ideal body weight to the average basal steady-state blood volume in ml/kg at ideal body weight. Blood volume in ml/kg may be derived from the data of Messerili and colleagues.[63]

Subsequently, the Sramek–Bernstein equation has been incorporated into the software of a microprocessor and is commercially available (NCCOM 3, from BoMed Medical Manufacturing, Ltd., Irvine, CA) for measurement of stroke volume and cardiac output. Using this instrument, Appel and associates[64] reported a correlation coefficient of 0.9 between the standard thermodilution method and the impedance cardiography method in 285 paired samples from 16 critically ill patients. It was pointed out that difficulties may arise with dysrhythmias, heart rates greater than 150/min, metal in the chest, sepsis, hypertension, and oily skin. Using the same impedance cardiography equipment and comparing it to the thermodilution of measuring cardiac output, Bernstein[58] found a correlation coefficient of 0.88 in 17 critically ill patients and Tremper and co-workers[65] reported a correlation of 0.84 in anesthetized dogs when blood pressure, blood volume, and blood flow were manipulated by hemorrhage and drug infusions.[65]

CONCLUSION

Schuster and Nanda[66] have addressed the problems of evaluating CO measurement techniques. In humans, we can only measure the reproducibility of a technique and its comparability to another technique which may also not be without limitations. Although accuracy may appear to be of primary importance, patient risk, cost, and technical limitations are also important practical considerations. The thermodilution technique is invasive; however, the pulmonary artery catheter provides additional hemodynamic information not available with the current noninvasive technology, which may justify the risk for certain patients. Certainly, noninvasive technology is attractive, but, as previously mentioned, still has limitations which should be overcome with further developments and refinements.

Ms. Hope Olivo provided editorial assistance; Mr. Jake Fuller, Ms. Barbara Brechler, and Ms. Joy Kuck provided the graphics.

REFERENCES

1. Fegler G: Measurement of cardiac output in anaesthetized animals by a thermo-dilution method. *Q J Exp Physiol* 1954; 39:153
2. Ganz W, Donoso R, Marcus HS, et al: A new technique for measurement of cardiac output by thermodilution in man. *Am J Cardiol* 1971; 27:392
3. Ganz W, Swan HJC: Measurement of blood flow by thermodilution. *Am J Cardiol* 1972; 29:241
4. Kohanna FH, Cunningham JN: Monitoring of cardiac output by thermodilution after open-heart surgery. *J Thorac Cardiovasc Surg* 1977; 73:451
5. Sorensen MB, Bille-Brahe NE, Engell HC: Cardiac output measurement by thermal dilution. *Ann Surg* 1976; 183:67
6. Stetz CW, Miller RG, Kelly GE, et al: Reliability of the thermodilution method in the determination of cardiac output in clinical practice. *Am Rev Respir Dis* 1982; 126:1001
7. Vandermoten P, Bernard R, De Hemptinne J, et al: Cardiac output monitoring during the acute phase of myocardial infarction: Accuracy and precision of the thermodilution method. *Cardiology* 1971; 62:291
8. Levett JM, Replogle RL: Thermodilution cardiac output: A critical analysis and review of the literature. *J Surg Res* 1979; 27:392
9. Nelson LD, Anderson HB: Patient selection for iced versus room temperature injectate for thermodilution cardiac output determinations. *Crit Care Med* 1985; 13:182
10. Shellock FG, Riedinger MS: Reproducibility and accuracy of using room-temperature vs. ice-temperature injectate for thermodilution cardiac output determinations. *Heart Lung* 1983; 12:175
11. Vennix CV, Nelson DH, Pierpont GL: Thermodilution cardiac output in critically ill patients: Comparison of room-temperature and iced injectate. *Heart Lung* 1984; 13:574
12. Elkayam U, Berkley R, Azen S, et al: Cardiac output by thermodilution technique: Effect of injectate's volume and temperature on accuracy and reproducibility in the critically ill patient. *Chest* 1983; 84:418
13. Shellock FG, Riedinger MS, Bateman TM, et al: Thermodilution cardiac output determination in hypothermic postcardiac surgery patients: Room vs. ice temperature injectate. *Crit Care Med* 1983; 11:668
14. Nishikawa T, Dohi S: Slowing of heart rate during cardiac output measurement by thermodilution. *Anesthesiology* 1982; 57:538
15. Todd MM: Atrial fibrillation induced by the right atrial injection of cold fluids during thermodilution cardiac output determination: A case report. *Anesthesiology* 1983; 59:253
16. Freed MD, Keane JF: Cardiac output measured by thermodilution in infants and children. *J Pediatr* 1978; 92:39
17. Wyse SD, Pfitzner J, Rees A, et al: Measurement of cardiac output by thermal dilution in infants and children. *Thorax* 1975; 30:262
18. Pearl RG, Rosenthal MH, Nielson L, et al: Effect of injectate volume and temperature on thermodilution cardiac output determination. *Anesthesiology* 1986; 64:798
19. Nelson LD, Houtchens BA: Automatic vs. manual injections for thermodilution cardiac output determinations. *Crit Care Med* 1982; 10:190
20. Barcelona M, Patague L, Bunoy M, et al: Cardiac output determination by the thermodilution method: Comparison of ice-temperature injectate versus room-temperature injectate contained in prefilled syringes or a closed injectate delivery system. *Heart Lung* 1985; 14:232

21. Mattea EJ, Paruta AN, Worthen LR: Sterility of prefilled syringes for thermal dilution cardiac output measurements. *Am J Hosp Pharm* 1979; 36:1156

22. Burke KG, Larson E, Maciorowski L, et al: Evaluation of the sterility of thermodilution room-temperature injectate preparations. *Crit Care Med* 1986; 14:503

23. Ray C, Carlon GC, Campfield PB, et al: Multiple determinations of cardiac output using a two-bottle technique. *Crit Care Med* 1979; 7:33

24. Nelson LD, Martinez OV, Anderson HB: Incidence of microbial colonization in open versus closed delivery systems for thermodilution injectate. *Crit Care Med* 1986; 14:291

25. American Edwards Laboratories—Models 9520 and 9520A. *Cardiac Output Computer Operations and Trouble-shooting Manual*, 1983

26. Ellis RJ, Gold J, Rees JR, et al: Computerized monitoring of cardiac output by thermal dilution. *JAMA* 1972; 220:507

27. Bearss MG, Yonutas DN, Allen WT: A complication with thermodilution cardiac outputs in centrally-placed pulmonary artery catheter. (lett). *Chest* 1982; 81:527

28. Fegler G: The reliability of the thermodilution method for determination of the cardiac output and the blood flow in central veins. *Q J Exp Physiol* 1957; 42:254

29. Snyder JV, Powner DJ: Effects of mechanical ventilation on the measurement of cardiac output by thermodilution. *Crit Care Med* 1982; 10:677

30. Armengol J, Man GCW, Balsys AJ, et al: Effects of the respiratory cycle on cardiac output measurements: Reproducibility of data enhanced by timing the thermodilution injections in dogs. *Crit Care Med* 1981; 9:852

31. Wessel HU, Paul MH, James GW, et al: Limitations of thermal dilution curves for cardiac output determinations. *J Appl Physiol* 1971; 30:643

32. Jansen JRC, Schreuder JJ, Bogaard JM, et al: Thermodilution technique for measurement of cardiac output during artificial ventilation. *J Appl Physiol* 1981; 51:584

33. Wetzel RC, Latson TW: Major errors in thermodilution cardiac output measurement during rapid volume infusion. *Anesthesiology* 1985; 62:684

34. Merrick SH, Hessel EA, Dillard DH: Determination of cardiac output by thermodilution during hypothermia. *Am J Cardiol* 1980; 46:419

35. Keen JH: The effect of injectate temperature on thermodilution cardiac output measurement in hyperdynamic cirrhotics (abstr). *Heart Lung* 1986; 15:312

36. Grose BL, Woods SL, Laurent DJ: Effect of backrest position on cardiac output measured by the thermodilution method in acutely ill patients. *Heart Lung* 1981; 10:661

37. Franch RH, King SB, Douglas JS: Techniques of cardiac catheterization including coronary arteriography. In Hurst JW (ed): *The Heart, Arteries, and Veins*, 5th ed, p 1851. New York, McGraw-Hill, 1982

38. Barry WH, Grossman W: Cardiac catheterization. In *Heart Disease: A Textbook of Cardiovascular Medicine*, p 289. Philadelphia, WB Saunders, 1983

39. Felner JM: Techniques of echocardiography. In Hurst JW (ed): *The Heart, Arteries, and Veins*, 5th ed, p 1773. New York, McGraw-Hill, 1982

40. Alverson DC: Neonatal cardiac output measurement using pulsed Doppler ultrasound. *Clin Perinatol* 1985; 12:101

41. Chandraratna PA, Nanna M, McKay C, et al: Determination of cardiac output by transcutaneous continuous-wave ultrasonic Doppler computer. *Am J Cardiol* 1984; 53:234

42. Huntsman LL, Stewart DK, Barnes SR, et al: Noninvasive Doppler determination of cardiac output in man: Clinical validation. *Circulation* 1983; 67:593

43. Rose JS, Nanna M, Rahimtoola SH, et al: Accuracy of determination of changes in cardiac output by transcutaneous continuous-wave Doppler computer. *Am J Cardiol* 1984; 54:1099

44. Nishimura PA, Callahan MJ, Schaff HV, et al: Noninvasive measurement of cardiac output by continuous-wave Doppler echocardiography: Initial experience and review of the literature. *Mayo Clin Proc* 1984; 59:484

45. Rein AJJT, Hsieh KS, Elixson M, et al: Cardiac output estimates in the pediatric intensive care unit using a continuous-wave Doppler computer: Validation and limitations of the technique. *Am Heart J* 1986; 112:97

46. Vandenbogaerde JF, Scheldewaert RG, Rijckaert DL, et al: Comparison between ultrasonic and thermodilution cardiac output measurements in intensive care patients. *Crit Care Med* 1986; 14:294

47. Loeppky JA, Hoekenga DE, Greene ER, et al: Comparison of noninvasive pulsed Doppler and Fick measurements of stroke volume in cardiac patients. *Am Heart J* 1984; 107:339

48. Alverson DC, Eldridge M, Dillon T, et al: Noninvasive pulsed Doppler determination of cardiac output in neonates and children. *J Pediatr* 1982; 101:46

49. Greenfield JC, Patel DJ: Relation between pressure and diameter in the ascending aorta of man. *Circ Res* 1962; 10:778

50. Seed WA, Wood NB: Velocity patterns in the aorta. *Cardiovasc Res* 1971; 5:319

51. Schuster AH, Nanda NC, Maulik D, et al: Doppler evaluation of cardiac output. In Nanda NC (ed): *Doppler Echocardiography*, p 144. New York, Igaku-Shoin, 1985

52. Bernstein DP: A new impedance stroke volume equation for thoracic electrical bioimpedance: Theory and rationale. *Crit Care Med* 1986; 14:904

53. Donovan KD, Dobb GJ, Woods WPD, et al: Comparison of transthoracic electrical impedance and thermodilution methods for measuring cardiac output. *Crit Care Med* 1986; 14:1038

54. Kubicek WG, Karegis JN, Patterson RP, et al: Development and evaluation of an impedance cardiac output system. *Aerospace Med* 1966; 37:1208

55. Mohapatra SN, Hill DW: The changes in blood resistivity with hematocrit and temperature. *Eur J Intens Care Med* 1975; 1:153

56. Keim HJ, Wallace JM, Thurston H, et al: Impedance cardiography for determination of stroke index. *J Appl Physiol* 1976; 41:797

57. Sramek BB, Rose DM, Miyaamoto A: A stroke volume equation with a linear base impedance model and its accuracy, as compared to thermodilution and magnetic flow meter techniques in humans and animals. *Proceedings of the Sixth International Conference in Electrical Bioimpedance*, p 88. Zadir, Yugoslavia, 1983

58. Bernstein DP: Continuous noninvasive real-time monitoring of stroke volume and cardiac output by thoracic electrical bioimpedance. *Crit Care Med* 1986; 14:898

59. Milnor WR: *Hemodynamics*, p 155. Baltimore, Williams & Wilkins, 1982

60. *Statistical Bulletin*, p 64. Metropolitan Life Foundation, Jan–June 1983

61. Rasmussen JP, Eriksen J, Andersen J: Evaluation of impedance cardiography during anesthesia in extremely obese patients. *Acta Anaesthesiol Scand* 1977; 21:342

62. Okutani H, Fujinami T, Nakayama K, et al: Studies on mean thoracic impedance (Zo). *Proceedings of the Fifth ICEBI*, p 31. Tokyo, August 1981

63. Messerili FH, Christie B, De Carvalho JGR, et al: Obesity and essential hypertension. Hemodynamics, intravascular volume, sodium excretion, and plasma renin activity. *Arch Intern Med* 1981; 81:141

64. Appel PL, Kram HB, Mackabee J, et al: Comparison of measurements of cardiac output by bioimpedance and thermodilution in severely ill surgical patients. *Crit Care Med* 1986; 14:933

65. Tremper KK, Hufstedler SM, Barker SJ, et al: Continuous noninvasive estimation of cardiac output by electrical bioimpedance: An experimental study in dogs. *Crit Care Med* 1986; 14:231

66. Schuster AH, Nanda NC: Editorial: Doppler echocardiographic measurement of cardiac output: Comparison with a non-golden standard. *Am J Cardiol* 1984; 53:257

CHAPTER SIX

PRACTICAL APPLICATION OF BLOOD GAS MEASUREMENTS

Philip G. Boysen
Robert R. Kirby

ATMOSPHERIC GASES

PARTIAL PRESSURE

The earth is enveloped by a layer of gas that has weight and exerts pressure. At altitudes above sea level, the density of gas (number of molecules per unit volume) decreases. Atmospheric (ambient) gas pressure at high altitude, therefore, is decreased relative to that at sea level (760 mm Hg or 14.7 lb/sq in). Each atmospheric gas exerts its own pressure (partial pressure) independent of other gases; although the partial pressures decrease with increasing altitude, their concentrations (percentage) remain constant.

COMPOSITION

For clinical purposes, we consider that atmospheric gas has only two components: oxygen (21%) and nitrogen (79%). When discussing the composition of the gas mixture within the lungs, however, we must also take into account carbon dioxide and water vapor, both of which change the partial pressures of oxygen and nitrogen from those of the inspired atmospheric gas (Table 6-1).

DETERMINANTS OF Pa_{CO_2}

The normal arterial partial pressure of carbon dioxide (Pa_{CO_2}) is 40 mm Hg (range, 36–44 mm Hg). Hypoventilation is defined as a Pa_{CO_2} above 44 mm Hg, and hyperventilation is a Pa_{CO_2} below 36 mm Hg.

Carbon Dioxide Production

Production of carbon dioxide is often ignored because it is relatively constant in most settings. However, in catabolic and hypermetabolic states, carbon dioxide production may increase significantly and affect Pa_{CO_2}. In the absence of shivering, production is decreased by hypothermia.

**TABLE 6-1   COMPOSITION AND PARTIAL PRESSURES OF
MAJOR ATMOSPHERIC AND ALVEOLAR GASES**

Atmospheric
Oxygen (21% of 760 = 159 mm Hg)
Nitrogen (79% of 760 = 600 mm Hg)

Alveolar	
Oxygen	100 mm Hg
Nitrogen	573 mm Hg
Carbon dioxide	40 mm Hg
Water vapor	47 mm Hg

Alveolar Ventilation

Total ventilation ($\dot{V}_E$) is partitioned between gas distributed to the alveoli and that passing to the non-gas-exchange (deadspace) areas of the lungs. Thus,

$$\dot{V}_E = \dot{V}_D + \dot{V}_A \tag{1}$$

where $\dot{V}_D$ is deadspace ventilation and $\dot{V}_A$ is alveolar ventilation. The conducting airways are termed anatomic deadspace. Alveoli that are ventilated but not perfused make up the alveolar deadspace.

If we relate volume to time, then

$$\dot{V}_E = V_T \times f/min \tag{2}$$

$$\dot{V}_A = V_A \times f/min \tag{3}$$

where V_T is tidal volume (including deadspace volume) and V_A is alveolar volume. The elimination of carbon dioxide is proportional to alveolar ventilation and the alveolar partial pressure of carbon dioxide (PA_{CO_2}):

$$\dot{V}_{CO_2} \, \alpha \, \dot{V}_A \times PA_{CO_2} \tag{4}$$

Because measurement of PA_{CO_2} is not always possible, we assume that $PA_{CO_2} = Pa_{CO_2}$. This relationship holds reasonably well in normal situations but can be quite aberrant in some clinical settings (*i.e.*, pulmonary embolism, profound pulmonary hypotension). Everything else being equal, however, increased $\dot{V}_A$ should be associated with decreased Pa_{CO_2}, whereas a decrease of $\dot{V}_A$ is associated with an elevation of Pa_{CO_2}.

DETERMINANTS OF Pa$_{O_2}$

When you measure the Pa_{O_2} from a sample of arterial blood, you need information on the alveolar gas composition to which the blood was exposed. First, estimate the alveolar P_{O_2} (PA_{O_2}); next, assume that both alveolar and arterial gas equilibration have occurred; finally, compare the estimated PA_{O_2} and the measured Pa_{O_2}. The initial step entails calculation of the partial pressure of humidified, inspired oxygen (PI_{O_2}):

$$PI_{O_2} = (P_B - P_{H_2O}) \times FI_{O_2} \tag{5}$$

At sea level, P_B = 760 mm Hg, PH_2O = 47 mm Hg (37°C body temperature and, in this example, $F_{I_{O_2}}$ = 0.21. Thus,

$$P_{I_{O_2}} = (760 - 47) \times 0.21 = 150 \text{ mm Hg}$$

Dead space gas maintains the same partial pressure. At the alveolar level, however, oxygen is removed and carbon dioxide added to the gas mixture. Total alveolar and atmospheric pressures are equal, but the composition and partial pressures of gases in the two phases differ. As we mentioned previously, the total pressure in each phase is equal to the sum of its partial pressures:

$$P_A = P_{A_{O_2}} + P_{A_{CO_2}} + P_{A_{N_2}} + P_{A_{H_2O}} \tag{6}$$

where P_A = the total alveolar gas pressure (equal to P_B).

Since $P_{A_{N_2}}$ and $P_{A_{H_2O}}$ remain essentially constant when ambient air is breathed, an *increase* in $P_{A_{CO_2}}$ implies a *decrease* in $P_{A_{O_2}}$. Thus, pulmonary capillary blood exposed to a lower $P_{A_{O_2}}$ enters the systemic circulation with a lower than normal $P_{A_{O_2}}$. The overall relationship defining these variables is described by the ideal alveolar air equation:

$$P_{A_{O_2}} = P_{I_{O_2}} - \frac{P_{A_{CO_2}}}{R} + [P_{A_{CO_2}} \times F_{I_{O_2}} \times \frac{1-R}{R}] \tag{7}$$

where R = the respiratory quotient, $\dot{V}_{CO_2}/\dot{V}_{O_2}$ (normally 0.8). This expression can be simplified to

$$P_{A_{O_2}} = P_{I_{O_2}} - (Pa_{CO_2} \times 1.25) \tag{8}$$

ABNORMALITIES OF OXYGENATION

P(A-a) Gradient

If the lung functioned as a perfect gas exchange organ, $P_{A_{O_2}}$ and Pa_{O_2} would be equal. To the extent that perfect ventilation and perfusion matching ($\dot{V}/\dot{Q}$) do not occur, a gradient between $P_{A_{O_2}}$ and Pa_{O_2} (P(A-a)O_2 is established. An increase of P(A-a)O_2 implies a deterioration in lung function. Alveolar hypoventilation also results in hypoxemia when *air* is breathed but is *not* associated with an increase of P(A-a)O_2 (Table 6-2). A number of abnormalities increase this gradient and produce hypoxemia (Table 6-3).

TABLE 6-2   CAUSES OF ALVEOLAR HYPOVENTILATION

Respiratory center depression	Myoneural junction
Drugs—narcotics, barbiturates, anesthesia	Myasthenia gravis
Medulla	Respiratory muscles
Encephalitis, trauma, neoplasm, hemorrhage	Muscular dystrophy
Spinal nerves	Thoracic cage
Cervical dislocation	Flail chest
Anterior horn cell disease	Upper airway
Poliomyelitis	Neoplasm, thymoma, aneurysm
Nerves to respiratory muscles	
Diphtheria, Guillain-Barré	

TABLE 6-3 CAUSES OF INCREASED P(A-a)O$_2$ GRADIENT

Post-traumatic pulmonary insufficiency	Near-drowning
Aspiration of gastric contents	Fat embolism
Sepsis	Uremia
Viral pneumonia	Pancreatitis
Smoke inhalation/respiratory burns	Neurogenic pulmonary edema
Inhalation of toxic chemicals	Altitude pulmonary edema
Oxygen toxicity	

Diffusion Block (Alveolocapillary Block)

Although it is theoretically possible that substances lie between the alveoli and the pulmonary capillaries and inhibit oxygen diffusion, this abnormality is of little clinical importance in the etiology of *acute* hypoxemia.

Relative Shunt (Decreased V̇/Q̇, "Shunt-like Effect")

A relative shunt results from reduced but finite ventilation that is less than the corresponding perfusion. Thus, some oxygenation of mixed venous blood occurs, but to a level far less than normal. This abnormality is the most common cause of hypoxemia in acute and chronic respiratory insufficiency. Diffusion block and relative shunt are corrected when patients inspire 100% oxygen.

Absolute Shunt

When mixed venous blood passing through the lungs does not come into contact with the alveoli, it is "shunted" past the gas-exchange surface. Venous admixture results when this shunted blood mixes with oxygenated blood from other normal lung areas. Absolute shunt is minimally improved by the administration of 100% oxygen.

Cardiac Output

A decrease in arterial oxygenation usually is thought to reflect increases of absolute or relative shunt and an overall deterioration of lung function. However, changes in cardiac output, by virtue of their effect on the content of oxygen in mixed venous blood, also ultimately affect Pa$_{O_2}$. Increases in cardiac output tend to minimize hypoxemia and the P(A-a)O$_2$ gradient that results from any right-to-left absolute and relative shunting. Conversely, decreases in cardiac output tend to accentuate this hypoxemia and to increase the P(A-a)O$_2$. Mechanical ventilation and positive end-expiratory pressure (PEEP) are used to improve lung function. However, by virtue of their potentially adverse effects on cardiac output, such therapy can be associated with a decreased Pa$_{O_2}$. Thus, pulmonary *and* cardiac function must be assessed to evaluate any given set of arterial blood gases accurately.

CLINICAL APPLICATION

TISSUE OXYGENATION

Tissue oxygen delivery depends on oxygen content of the blood and the cardiac output. Oxygen content of arterial blood (Ca$_{O_2}$) is determined by the Pa$_{O_2}$, hemoglobin content, and percentage of hemoglobin saturated with oxygen (Sa_{O_2}). The amount of dissolved oxygen is dependent on the Pa_{O_2}. Total content is expressed as milliliters of oxygen/100 ml blood (ml/dl). Calculation of Ca_{O_2} is as follows:

$$Ca_{O_2} = \text{oxyhemoglobin} + O_2 \text{ dissolved} = \text{Hgb} \times 1.34$$
$$\times \text{ } Sa_{O_2} + Pa_{O_2} \times 0.0031 \tag{9}$$

Normally, 25% of the Ca_{O_2} is extracted by the tissues. In general, an increased Ca_{O_2} in blood delivered to the tissues ensures a greater potential for maintenance of adequate tissue oxygenation. Thus oxygen content should be thought of not only in terms of the amount of oxygen that *is* delivered to the tissues, but also in terms of the amount that *can* be delivered in times of stress. This oxygen reserve of the blood is a major determinant of whether the tissues are oxygenated under such conditions.

Oxygen requirements usually remain constant over short periods of time. The amount of oxygen extracted from a given volume of blood depends on how much blood is presented to the tissues per unit of time. Of clinical importance is a knowledge of the Ca_{O_2} (amount of oxygen available to the tissues) and the mixed venous oxygen content ($C\bar{v}_{O_2}$) (amount of oxygen remaining in the blood after it has perfused the tissues and returned to the heart). You can then assess not only tissue oxygen use, but also the adequacy of the cardiopulmonary response to systemic oxygen demand. The concept is embodied within the Fick principle, which states that the amount of oxygen use by the tissues per unit time is equal to the amount of oxygen extracted from the circulated blood during the same time. Thus,

$$\dot{Q} = \frac{\dot{V}_{O_2}}{Ca_{O_2} - C\bar{v}_{O_2}} \tag{10}$$

where $\dot{V}_{O_2}$ = oxygen consumption (ml/min), $\dot{Q}$ = cardiac output (liters/min), and $Ca_{O_2} - C\bar{v}_{O_2}$ = ml/liter (ml/dl $\times$ 10).

PULMONARY ARTERY CATHETERIZATION

Systemic arterial blood represents a mixture of blood from the pulmonary capillary circulation that is "homogenized" in the left ventricle. Gas partial pressures and Sa_{O_2} normally are interpreted to reflect cardiopulmonary homeostasis because they represent the patient's capability of oxygen delivery necessary for tissue metabolism. Blood returned from the systemic tissues is mixed in the right ventricle and then pumped into the pulmonary artery. It is a homogenous mixture of systemic venous blood and reflects the patient's oxygen use. Flow-directed, balloon flotation pulmonary artery catheters allow direct sampling of this blood. Major indications for the use of these catheters are [1] hemodynamic assessment of left ventricular function and [2] measurement of gas partial pressures and oxygen saturation of pulmonary artery blood.

Arteriovenous Oxygen Content Difference

The arteriovenous oxygen content difference ($Ca_{O_2} - C\bar{v}_{O_2}$) represents the average amount of oxygen extracted per unit of volume of blood. It is sometimes used as a reflection of changes in cardiac output because it is inversely related to this parameter when oxygen consumption remains stable (see Equation 10).

Intrapulmonary Shunts

Right-to-left intrapulmonary shunt earlier was defined as that portion of the right ventricular cardiac output that does not participate in alveolar gas exchange ("wasted" perfusion). The *total* (physiologic) shunt is divided into *anatomic* and *capillary* components. The anatomic portion is composed of blood that does not enter the pulmonary capillaries, including [1] 2% to 4% of cardiac output that returns to the left side of the heart through bronchial, pleural, and thebesian veins (normal anatomic shunt); [2] congenital cardiac abnormalities with pulmonary to systemic blood flow (ASD, VSD, PDA); [3] highly vascular lung tumors; and [4] abnormal arteriovenous anastomoses.

Capillary shunt is represented by blood flow that has a *potential* for gas exchange with ventilated alveoli, but this exchange does not occur for some pathophysiologic reason. It is further divided into true capillary shunt and venous admixture. True capillary shunt exists when ventilation is absent but perfusion to the nonventilated regions continues at some finite value. Venous admixture (low $\dot{V}/\dot{Q}$, shunt-like effect) is best thought of as an abnormality in which ventilation is markedly reduced (but nevertheless present at some finite level) compared to perfusion. Even though the capillary shunt is composed of blood that *physically* traverses the pulmonary capillary bed, the net *physiologic* effect is that it is not oxygenated. True capillary shunt is commonly associated with atelectasis. Venous admixture also is commonly found in pulmonary edema, COPD, and partial airway obstruction from any cause.·

Cardiac Output

Cardiac output and its measurement are of major importance in the assessment of tissue oxygen utilization. Body tissues require a minimal amount of oxygen in order to maintain normal metabolic function. Whether the oxygen comes from a large or small quantity of blood makes no difference as long as the absolute amount is sufficient. When oxygen consumption remains constant, the amount of oxygen removed from a given quantity of blood is determined by the blood flow during the period of extraction. Thus, if 25 ml of oxygen is used by an organ every minute, and this requirement is constant, 25 ml will be removed whether the blood supply is 1 liter or 5 liters. As blood flow per unit time increases, less oxygen is extracted from any given quantity of blood and $C\bar{v}_{O_2}$ increases. Thus, cardiac output has a significant impact on the $C\bar{v}_{O_2}$ and on total oxygen availability.

THE SHUNT EQUATION

The classic shunt equation (see Appendix) expresses the total amount of right-to-left intrapulmonary shunted blood (anatomic and capillary) as a fraction of the cardiac output:

$$\frac{\dot{Q}s}{\dot{Q}t} = \frac{Cc'_{O_2}\ Ca_{O_2}}{Cc'_{O_2} - C\bar{v}_{O_2}} = Cv_{O_2} \tag{11}$$

where $\dot{Q}s$ = volume of shunted blood, $\dot{Q}t$ = cardiac output, and Cc'_{O_2} = end-capillary oxygen content (calculated from Pa_{O_2}, Equation 7).

In a broad sense, the numerator of this expression $(Cc'_{O_2} - Ca_{O_2})$ reflects the overall adequacy of respiratory function (*i.e.*, if perfect $\dot{V}/\dot{Q}$ matching is present, the numerator is 0, and no shunt is present). The denominator ($Cc'_{O_2} - C\bar{v}_{O_2}$), as has been indicated, reflects the overall adequacy of cardiovascular function (*i.e.*, oxygen uptake, which is cardiac output dependent). This single expression brings together all of the concepts we have discussed and allows you to dissect the various abnormalities that culminate in abnormalities of Pa_{O_2}. Important points to remember follow.

1 Shunt flow is 0 when Cc'_{O_2} and Ca_{O_2} are equal (hypothetical possibility only).

2 As increasing numbers of alveoli are collapsed or have their ventilation decreased, Ca_{O_2} is increasingly "diluted" by venous admixture, and $\dot{Q}s/\dot{Q}t$ increases.

3 In the face of a specific amount of lung damage and intrapulmonary shunt, an absolute increase in $\dot{Q}$ helps to maintain Pa_{O_2} at a higher level.

APPENDIX

Refer to Figure 6-1, where

$\dot{Q}t$ = total cardiac output

$\dot{Q}s$ = shunted portion of cardiac output

$\dot{Q}c$ = capillary flow

Ca_{O_2} = arterial oxygen content

$C\bar{v}_{O_2}$ = mixed venous oxygen content

Cc'_{O_2} = end-capillary blood oxygen content (after equilibration at alveolocapillary units with ideal $\dot{V}/\dot{Q}$)

PA_{O_2} = alveolar P_{O_2} in "ideal" alveoli

and

$\dot{Q}t$ = $\dot{Q}c + \dot{Q}s$

O_2 delivery = $\dot{Q}t \cdot Ca_{O_2}$

O_2 returned = $\dot{Q}t \cdot C\bar{v}_{O_2}$

O_2 consumption ($\dot{V}_{O_2}$) = O_2 delivered − O_2 returned

$= \dot{Q}t \, (Ca_{O_2} - C\bar{v}_{O_2})$

This is the previously described (Equation 10) Fick equation, commonly written as

$$\dot{Q}t = \frac{\dot{V}_{O_2}}{Ca_{O_2} - C\bar{v}_{O_2}}$$

and, rearranging

$$\dot{V}_{O_2} = \dot{Q}t \, (Ca_{O_2} - C\bar{v}_{O_2})$$

But, in terms of gas exchange, the same relationship can be represented as

$$\dot{V}_{O_2} = \dot{Q}c \, (Cc'_{O_2} - C\bar{v}_{O_2})$$

since only the capillary flow ($\dot{Q}c$), and not shunted flow ($\dot{Q}s$), participates in gas exchange.

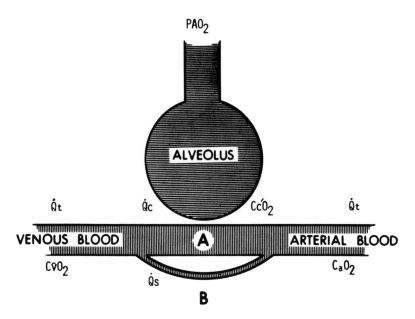

Figure 6-1 Venous blood in the pulmonary circulation may pass through areas that are well ventilated *(A)* or hypoventilated or nonventilated *(B)*. If the cardiac output decreases and systemic extraction of oxygen increases, the venous oxygen content will be less than normal. Any portion of the reduced cardiac output passing through B will cause a greater decrease in the resultant Ca_{O_2} and Pa_{O_2} than if cardiac output in normal $\dot{Q}t$ = total cardiac output; $\dot{Q}s$ = shunted portion of cardiac output; $\dot{Q}c$ = capillary flow; Ca_{O_2} = arterial oxygen content; $C\bar{v}_{O_2}$ = mixed venous oxygen content; Cc'_{O_2} = end-capillary oxygen content (after equilibrating with ideal alveolus); PA_{O_2} = alveolar P_{O_2} in "ideal" alveoli.

Therefore,

$$\dot{Q}t\,(Ca_{O_2} - C\bar{v}_{O_2}) = \dot{Q}c\,(Cc'_{O_2} - C\bar{v}_{O_2})$$
$$= (\dot{Q}t - \dot{Q}s)\,(Cc'_{O_2} - C\bar{v}_{O_2})$$

rearranging and solving for $\dot{Q}s/\dot{Q}t$

$$\dot{Q}s/\dot{Q}t = \frac{Cc'_{O_2} - Ca_{O_2}}{Cc'_{O_2} - C\bar{v}_{O_2}}$$

BIBLIOGRAPHY

Bendixen HH, Egbert LD, Hedley–Whyte J, et al: *Respiratory Care.* St. Louis, CV Mosby, 1965

Comroe JH: *Physiology of Respiration.* Chicago, Year Book Medical Publishers, 1962

Comroe JH, Forster RE, Dubois AB, et al: *The Lung,* 2nd ed. Chicago, Year Book Medical Publishers, 1962

Egan DF: *Fundamentals of Inhalation Therapy.* St. Louis, CV Mosby, 1969

Hodgkin JE, Collier CA: Blood gas analysis and acid–base physiology. In Burton GG, Hodgkin JE (eds): *Respiratory Care: A Guide to Clinical Practice,* 2nd ed, pp 258–266. Philadelphia, JB Lippincott, 1984

Nunn JF: *Applied Respiratory Physiology,* pp 178–245. London, Butterworths, 1977

CHAPTER SEVEN

ACID–BASE PROBLEM SOLVING

Philip G. Boysen
Robert R. Kirby

Systemic diseases are often accompanied by alterations in acid–base regulation. Occasionally, the abnormalities that result may become life-threatening, and the clinician must be able to differentiate and treat them. Failure to do so may result in morbidity or mortality that is preventable by the application of a few basic principles. This chapter does not discuss the various pathophysiological mechanisms by which alterations of acid–base occur, but rather focuses on simple, effective methods of diagnosis and treatment.

Historically, the subject of acid–base regulation has been made unnecessarily difficult by the use of terms such as "CO_2 combining power," "base excess," "buffer base," "standard bicarbonate," and "alkali reserve"—none of which has any readily apparent clinical meaning. When additional modifiers are added—for example, a "negative base excess"—these terms become almost incomprehensible. Regardless of the terminology used, however, acid–base disturbances involve one simple fact: the normal concentration or, more specifically, the activity, of the hydrogen ion (H^+) has been altered.

Part of the problem results from the traditional teaching that cations such as sodium are bases, and anions such as chloride are acids. Since most clinicians learn that acids are H^+ donors and bases are H^+ receptors, this confusion is understandable. We define acids as substances which, when in solution, dissociate to form H^+ and an anion (e.g., Cl^-, SO_4^{2-}, HPO_4^{2-}). Conversely, bases are substances which, when in solution, combine with (remove) H^+. The general reaction describing this relationship is

$$HA \leftrightarrows H^+ + A^-, \tag{1}$$

where HA represents an acid (H^+ donor) and A^- its conjugate base.

The presence or absence of an acid–base disturbance is commonly ascertained through an analysis of arterial blood pH and P_{CO_2}. With the exception of iatrogenic complications resulting from inappropriate mechanical ventilation, prolonged nasogastric suctioning, or the administration of sodium bicarbonate, most acid–base abnormalities originate intracellularly and are only secondarily manifested by extracellular compositional changes measured in arterial blood. Thus, although we can define the abnormality of H^+ in the extracellular fluid (ECF) compartment, we can only guess what disturbance is taking place intracellularly. Even when we are reasonably certain of the latter process, no specific therapy can be used to correct it.

BASIC PRINCIPLES

Another source of difficulty relates to quantitating the magnitude of acid–base derangements. The amount of H^+ is very small in comparison to the other common, physiologically important cations such as sodium and potassium. In normal plasma, sodium and potassium concentrations are 140 mmol/liter and 4.0 mmol/liter, respectively, whereas H^+ is only 0.000040 mmol/liter.[1,2] These small numbers commonly are expressed either as pH (the logarithm of the reciprocal of the activity or concentration of H^+) or in nanomoles (1 nmol $= 10^{-9}$ mole) per liter. The concentration of H^+ in normal arterial blood is 40 nmol, a considerably easier expression to write than 0.000000040 mol/liter.

Although pH is commonly used in acid–base chemistry, the concepts underlying its use are poorly understood by many clinicians. Quite apart from its definition, which is obscure to those who are not mathematically inclined, the use of pH tends to hide some facts that are of considerable importance. For example, the normal pH of arterial blood is 7.40 and the range is 7.36 to 7.44—a variation of only $\pm 0.54\%$. Actual H^+ is 40 nmol/liter ranging from 36 to 44 nmol/liter—a considerably greater numerical change of $\pm 10\%$. The apparent discrepancy results from the fact that pH is based upon a logarithmic scale. Thus small numerical changes in pH are associated with considerably larger absolute changes in H^+.

This fact can be further appreciated by comparing equivalent pH and nmol/liter H^+ values (Table 7-1). The pH range from 6.8 to 7.8 defines the extremes of H^+ that can be tolerated by human beings and represents a numerical variation of approximately 15%. The considerably larger change from 160 to 16 nmol/liter, over the corresponding pH range is evident in Table 7-1. Patients may have an H^+ concentration from 40% to 400% that which is normally present, a tenfold change in concentration that is not apparent when pH values alone are used. Thus, a change in pH from 7.0 to 7.2 represents a significantly greater improvement in acid–base status than does a change from 7.2 to 7.4; yet the absolute numerical change (0.2) is the same in both cases.

CLINICAL APPLICATIONS

RESPIRATORY DERANGEMENTS

Carbon dioxide alters H^+ according to the following reversible reaction:

$$CO_2 + H_2O \leftrightarrows H_2OCO_3 \leftrightarrows H^+ + HCO_3^-. \tag{2}$$

Respiratory derangements, by virtue of their effect on the partial pressure of arterial carbon dioxide (Pa_{CO_2}), may cause major changes in H^+ concentration within the body. For each acute 10 mm Hg deviation of Pa_{CO_2} above or below 40 mm Hg, the pH changes by approximately 0.07 units. In actuality, this change is not entirely linear, but with small acute changes in Pa_{CO_2}, the accuracy of the arterial blood gas values can be checked by knowing the approximate magnitude of change in pH that *should* occur for a given change in Pa_{CO_2}.

TABLE 7-1 H$^+$ EXPRESSED AS pH AND nmol/LITER

pH	nmol
6.8	160
7.0	100
7.2	63
7.4	40
7.6	25
7.8	16

Since there is a straightforward relationship between Pa_{CO_2} and alveolar ventilation, correction of the respiratory component in acid–base derangements is easy (at least in theory). If the pH is decreased and the Pa_{CO_2} levels are increased, an increase in alveolar ventilation will lower Pa_{CO_2} and return pH to normal. The opposite is also true. Remember that if *alveolar* ventilation is halved, Pa_{CO_2} is approximately doubled. Similarly, if *alveolar* ventilation is doubled, Pa_{CO_2} decreases by half. Respiratory disturbances and H$^+$ concentration can be easily assessed and corrected if the following relationship is appreciated:

$$\uparrow \dot{V}_A \rightarrow \downarrow CO_2 \rightarrow \uparrow pH. \tag{3}$$

METABOLIC DISTURBANCES

Hydrogen ion concentration also is affected by nonrespiratory ("metabolic") processes. Syndromes of metabolic acidosis fall into two patterns that can be separated by calculating the anion gap.

$$\text{Anion gap} = Na^+ - (Cl^- + HCO_3^-). \tag{4}$$

This "gap" represents unmeasured anions, most of which are offset by H$^+$. Thus an increased anion gap often implies the presence of a metabolic acidosis. Alternatively, Cl$^-$ may increase as H$^+$ concentration rises (Table 7-2). Causes of metabolic alkalosis can be categorized according to a pattern of anion (Cl$^-$) depletion into Cl$^-$ responsive or Cl$^-$ resistant types (Table 7-3).

Just as the change in Pa_{CO_2} from a normal value of 40 mm Hg is the prime indicator

TABLE 7-2   TYPES OF METABOLIC ACIDOSIS

Anion Gap	Hyperchloremic
Renal failure	Renal tubular acidosis
Diabetic ketoacidosis	Acetazolamide therapy
Salicylism	Diarrhea
Lactic acidosis (and starvation)	Ureteral diversions
Toxins	Addition of HCl (NH$_4$Cl, HCl, arginine, lysine)
Methanol	Early renal failure
Paraldehyde	
Ethylene glycol	

TABLE 7-3 TYPES OF METABOLIC ALKALOSIS

CL⁻ Responsive	CL⁻ Resistant
Vomiting or nasogastric suction	Adrenal disorders
Diuretic therapy	Hyperaldosteronism
Cl⁻ wasting diarrhea	Cushing's disease
Posthypercapnic alkalosis	Exogenous steroids
Carbenicillin or penicillin therapy	Bartter's syndrome
	Refeeding alkalosis
	Severe potassium depletion
	HCO_3^- therapy

of respiratory acid–base disturbance, a change in bicarbonate (HCO_3^-) concentration generally reflects disturbances that are metabolic in origin.

The normal value for plasma HCO_3^- is 24 mmol/liter. Bicarbonate is a "buffer." In the simplest terms, buffers, within their operational range, react with H^+ ions when these ions are present in excessive quantities, removing them from solution and thereby minimizing the increase in acidity that would otherwise occur. Conversely, if the milieu becomes too alkaline, the buffers release H^+ and, in so doing, tend to return the pH toward normal. Quantitatively, HCO_3^- is the more important ECF buffer, representing 75% to 80% of the total ECF against metabolically produced or exogenously administered acids. The other important buffers are hemoglobin, protein, and phosphates.

PROBLEM SOLVING

Determination of arterial pH by itself does not allow categorization of the H^+ excess or deficit. Arterial P_{CO_2} also must be known. For example, if a patient has an arterial pH of 7.0 and a Pa_{CO_2} of 40 mm Hg, metabolic acidosis is present, since ventilation, by definition, is normal. The magnitude of this disturbance is such that 60 excess nmol of H^+ per liter of ECF is present (see Table 7-1). However, if 60 nmol/liter of base (HCO_3^-) is administered in an attempt to correct this pH, no change results. The H^+ measured by the pH electrode is only a miniscule part of the patient's total H^+ load. As an example, if the arterial pH is reduced from 7.44 ($H^+ = 36$ nmol/liter) to 7.14 ($H^+ = 72$ nmol/liter) by an infusion of 0.1 M hydrochloric acid, approximately 14×10^6 nmol of H^+/liter ECF is added. Of this total, only 36 nmol/liter are responsible for the decrease of pH. The rest is buffered and thus rendered "harmless." If we can determine the change in body buffers, we can quantitate the H^+ that was added to or lost from the system. Since HCO_3^- is the major buffer, any change in its concentration can be interpreted as reflecting changes in H^+, with which it combines.

Extracellular fluid in a normal adult is composed of the interstitial fluid and plasma, and is equal to 20% of the body weight. If you know the amount of HCO_3^- change per liter from normal, and calculate the number of liters of ECF, a quantitative estimate of the HCO_3^- deficit (or excess) can be made. Consider the following example of a patient with a slight metabolic acidosis:

$$\text{Normal } HCO_3^- = 24 \text{ mmol/liter}$$
$$\text{Actual } HCO_3^- = 20 \text{ mmol/liter}$$
$$\text{Difference (normal } - \text{ actual)} = 4 \text{ mmol/liter}$$
$$\text{Body weight} = 70 \text{ kg}$$
$$\text{ECF (20\% body weight)} = 14 \text{ kg (14 liter)}.$$

Correction proceeds as follows:

$$
\begin{aligned}
HCO_3^- \text{ replacement} &= \text{Body weight} \times \%\,ECF \\
&\quad \times HCO_3^- \text{ deficit/liter} \\
&= 70 \text{ kg} \times 0.2 \times 4 \text{ mmol/} \\
&= \text{liter} \\
&\quad 56 \text{ mmol.}
\end{aligned}
\tag{5}
$$

In the absence of other abnormalities, the administration of 56 mmol of 8% $NaHCO_3$ (slightly more than one 50-ml vial) will correct the HCO_3^- deficit and restore plasma and interstitial fluid buffering capacity to within 75% to 80% of normal.

If changes in HCO_3^- always indicated only metabolic (nonrespiratory) acidosis or alkalosis, the presence and degree of the abnormality would be easily ascertained, as in the preceding example. However, this is not the case. Any process that changes Pa_{CO_2} (hyperventilation or hypoventilation, increased or decreased carbon dioxide production) also results in a change in HCO_3^- (see Equation 2).

The amount by which HCO_3^- is altered by different levels of Pa_{CO_2} depends on whether the change is acute or chronic. If you wish to determine how much of a decrease in HCO_3^- resulted from the buffering of acid (e.g., lactic, β-OH butyric,) you must first determine whether Pa_{CO_2} is normal. If it is, you can assume that all of the change noted is metabolic and that respiratory acidemia is not a factor in any HCO_3^- change. If Pa_{CO_2} is increased or decreased from a normal value of 40 mm Hg, however, you must first determine how much this change altered HCO_3^-. Only then can any additional change in HCO_3^-, over and above that resulting from Pa_{CO_2} change, be considered nonrespiratory in origin.

This differentiation is essential, since alterations in Pa_{CO_2} (respiratory acidemia or alkalemia) are corrected by correction of alveolar ventilation, as mentioned previously. Nonrespiratory abnormalities, if they are treated, require the administration of substances such as $NaHCO_3$ (acidosis) or HCl (alkalosis). Various techniques for separating respiratory and nonrespiratory changes in HCO_3^- have been introduced. One of the simplest and most effective is derived from studies in which experimental animals and healthy human subjects were allowed to reach acute and chronic "steady-state" conditions of Pa_{CO_2} between 15 and 100 mm Hg. Bicarbonate was measured at each level to define normal relationships between Pa_{CO_2} and HCO_3^- and 95% confidence limits were developed (Table 7-4).[3–8] If the actual HCO_3^- lies outside these limits for any given Pa_{CO_2}, the additional aberration is caused by a metabolic component. Specifically, HCO_3^- higher than the values in the table is caused by metabolic alkalosis, whereas lower HCO_3^- results from metabolic acidosis.

During acute and chronic hypocapnia and hypercapnia, changes in HCO_3^- are almost linear over the range of Pa_{CO_2} (20–100 mm Hg) encountered in altered pathologic states (Fig. 7-1).[3–8] Thus, you can predict what HCO_3^- "should be" for any Pa_{CO_2}. This observation

TABLE 7-4 ACUTE AND CHRONIC CHANGES IN Pa_{CO_2}, ARTERIAL pH, AND HCO_3^-

P_{CO_2} (mm Hg)	Arterial pH		HCO_3^-	
	Acute	Chronic	Acute	Chronic
15	7.61–7.74		15–21	
20	7.55–7.66		18–23	10–14
25	7.49–7.59		20–24	13–16
30	7.45–7.53	7.38–7.51	21–26	17–23
35	7.40–7.48		22–27	
40	7.37–7.44	7.37–7.51	23–27	22–31
45	7.33–7.39		24–28	
50	7.31–7.36	7.35–7.47	24–28	27–35
60	7.24–7.29	7.33–7.44	25–28	31–40
70	7.19–7.23	7.30–7.42	26–29	33–44
80	7.14–7.18	7.28–7.39	26–29	
90	7.09–7.13		27–29	
100		7.24–7.35		42–54

leads to certain rules of thumb to characterize various acid–base abnormalities.[3] These are as follow:

1 During acute hypercapnia, HCO_3^- increases 1 mmol/liter for each 10 mm Hg increase in Pa_{CO_2} above 40 mm Hg.

2 During chronic hypercapnia, HCO_3^- increases 4 mmol/liter for each 10 mm Hg increase in Pa_{CO_2} above 40 mm Hg.

3 During acute hypocapnia, HCO_3^- decreases 2 mmol/liter for every 10 mm Hg decrease in Pa_{CO_2} below 40 mm Hg.

4 During chronic hypocapnia, HCO_3^- decreases 5 to 7 mmol/liter for every 10 mm Hg decrease in Pa_{CO_2} below 40 mm Hg.

The greater change in HCO_3^- for chronic changes in Pa_{CO_2} is a result of renal compensation (increased conservation of HCO_3^- during chronic hypercapnia and increased elimination during hypocapnia), which tends to restore pH toward normal (see Table 7-4).

The rules of thumb make the delineation of acid–base disorders relatively simple, as demonstrated by two clinical examples.

Case 1: An otherwise healthy, 35-year-old, 70-kg man sustains acute airway obstruction. Repeated attempts at tracheal intubation are unsuccessful and he regurgitates and aspirates liquid gastric contents. Finally, an endotracheal tube is inserted. An arterial blood sample is sent to the blood gas laboratory and the following values are reported: Pa_{CO_2} = 70 mm Hg; arterial pH = 7.10; HCO_3^- = 21 mmol/liter.

To determine what type of acid–base disturbance this patient has, a stepwise analysis might proceed in the following manner. By convention, arterial pH below 7.36 represents acidemia (above 7.44 is alkalemia). Thus, the patient is acidemic and, because the Pa_{CO_2} is 70 mm Hg, at least a portion of the acidemia is respiratory. Is there also a component of nonrespiratory or metabolic acidosis? Application of rule of thumb 1 suggests that HCO_3^- should be at least 3 mmol above the normal values of 24 mmol/liter if only Pa_{CO_2} is changed. The

Figure 7-1 Linearity change in bicarbonate concentration with changing Pa_{CO_2}.

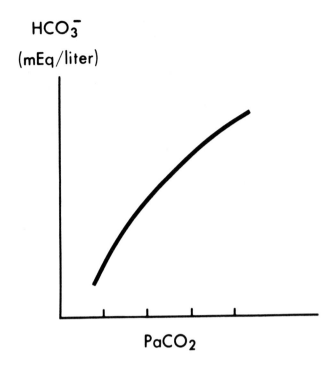

$$HCO_3^-$$

$$(mEq/liter)$$

$$PaCO_2$$

predicted HCO_3^- is 27 mmol//liter; hence a deficit of 6 mmol/liter exists. A combined respiratory acidemia and metabolic acidosis are present.

> Case 2: A 56-year-old, 70-kg man with chronic obstructive pulmonary disease and a resting Pa_{CO_2} of 70 mm Hg sustains an acute perioperative myocardial infarction. The blood pressure is 80/50 mm Hg, and he is diaphoretic, cool, and clammy. Arterial blood gas analysis shows the following: Pa_{CO_2} = 70 mm Hg: arterial pH = 7.10; HCO_3^- = 21 mmol/liter.

Here, the laboratory values are identical to those in case 1, but the clinical setting is considerably different. The arterial pH of 7.10 confirms acidemia and the Pa_{CO_2} of 70 mm Hg reveals that respiratory factors are present. However, in this instance, one is dealing with chronic hypercapnia, and the application of rule of thumb 3 predicts an HCO_3^- of 36 mmol/ liter. Actual HCO_3^- is only 21 mmol/liter, a deficit of 15 mmol/liter. The metabolic, or nonrespiratory, component of acidosis is much greater than in Case 1.

In both instances, ventilatory support is indicated to prevent worsening of the respiratory acidemia. If correction of the metabolic component is indicated, Equation 5 is used to determine the amount of HCO_3^- to be administered, as follows:

> For Case 1, 70 × 0.2 × 6 = 84 mmol HCO_3^-
> For Case 2, 70 × 0.2 × 15 = 210 mmol/HCO_3^-.

In practice, about three-fourths of the calculated amount of HCO_3^- would be administered initially. More can always be given; however, once the $NaHCO_3$ is "in," it cannot be taken out if too much was administered.

One might question whether the patient in Case 1 need be treated. This decision must be based on clinical judgment, not rule of thumb. The latter allows quantitation of the abnormality and represents the "science" of acid–base problem solving; the "art" is up to the physician. Although this approach is practical, we hasten to point out that major revisions in thought concerning the role of HCO_3^- therapy are taking place. The American Heart Association now urges restraint in the use of sodium bicarbonate during cardiopulmonary resuscitation (as opposed to their previous rather cavalier approach).[9] Experimentally, HCO_3^- administered to correct severe hypoxic lactic acidosis actually increases lactate production.[10] Part of the difficulty may be related to the fact that carbon dioxide elaborated by the reaction of H^+ and HCO_3^- (Equation 1) rapidly diffuses across cell membranes, creating intracellular acidosis even while the extracellular acidosis is decreased.

REFERENCES

1. Masoro EJ, Siegel PD: *Acid-Base Regulation: Its Physiology, Pathophysiology and the Interpretation of Blood Gas Analysis,* 2nd ed. Philadelphia, WB Saunders, 1977
2. Robinson JR: *Fundamentals of Acid-Base Regulation,* 5th ed. Philadelphia, Blackwell Scientific Publications, 1975
3. Bernards WC: *Interpretation of Clinical Acid-Base Data. Regional Refresher Courses in Anesthesiology,* pp 17-28. Philadelphia, JB Lippincott, 1973
4. Brackett NC Jr, Cohen JJ, Schwartz WB: Carbon dioxide titration curve of normal man. *N Engl J Med* 1965; 272:6
5. Brackett NC Jr, Wingo CF, Muren O, et al: Acid-base response to chronic hypercapnia in man. *N Engl J Med* 1969; 280:124
6. Cohen JJ, Brackett NC Jr, Schwartz WB: The nature of carbon dioxide titration curve in the normal dog. *J Clin Invest* 1964; 43:777
7. Schwartz WB, Relman AS: A critique of the parameters used in the evaluation of acid-base disorders. *N Engl J Med* 1963; 268:1382
8. Schwartz WB, Brackett NC Jr, Cohen JJ: The response of extracellular hydrogen ion concentration to graded degrees of chronic hypercapnia: The physiologic limits of the defense of pH. *J Clin Invest* 1965; 44:291
9. American Heart Association: Standards and guidelines for cardiopulmonary resuscitation and emergency cardiac care: Part III. Adult advanced cardiac life support. *JAMA* 1986; 255:2933
10. Graf H, Leach W, Arieff AI: Evidence for a detrimental effect of bicarbonate therapy in hypoxic lactic acidosis. *Science* 1985;227:754

CHAPTER EIGHT

PULMONARY FUNCTION TESTING IN THE CRITICAL CARE UNIT

Gregory R. Flick
Mark B. Berger

Measurement of pulmonary function in the intensive care unit (ICU) is quite different from testing performed in the pulmonary function laboratory. In the ICU, pulmonary function analysis may help determine the need for mechanical ventilation, or it may monitor ventilator safety, determine disease progression, or help decide when to wean the patient from mechanical ventilation. Test selection is important; some tests performed in the pulmonary function laboratory have little significance in the ventilated or acutely ill patient; a different set of normals is necessary (Table 8-1).

SPECIFIC DISEASE STATES: WHAT TO MONITOR

ACUTE ASTHMA

During an acute asthmatic event, resistance in the large and small airways progressively increases. Hyperinflation and air trapping occur, causing a reduction in vital capacity (VC). The diaphragm is placed at a mechanical disadvantage, decreasing respiratory muscle efficiency. As the respiratory muscles fatigue, ventilatory failure occurs; progressive respiratory acidosis and hypoxia result. Careful, repeated physical examination and arterial blood gases historically have been most useful in following asthma. Repeated determinations of peak expiratory flow rate (PEFR) and VC are less invasive and provide more objective measurements of disease progression. After four hours of treatment, improvement in PEFR greater than 50% of the admission peak flow rate predicts a rapid response to maximal therapy.[1] Carbon dioxide tension (P_{CO_2}), forced expiratory volume in 1 second (FEV_1), and VC differences do not always provide a reliable predictor to the speed of recovery. Those patients who have a 50% improvement in the presenting value of PEFR will obtain maximum improvement within 1 week of admission, whereas those who do not may take considerably longer.[1]

Patients with asthma and a PEFR 25% less than that predicted are particularly at risk for respiratory failure.[2] During treatment, bronchodilator response may be monitored with PEFR and VC; a comparison of the postbronchodilator value of the previous treatment with the prebronchodilator value of the current treatment may indicate the need for a shorter, more frequent treatment schedule.

TABLE 8-1 Selected Formulas to Calculate Pulmonary Function Variables

Variables	Formulas	Normal Values
Lung volumes		
Tidal volume	$V_T = \dot{V}insp \times T_I$	10–15 ml/kg (lean body weight)
Minute ventilation	$\dot{V}_E = V_T \times f$	6–10 liters/min
Alveolar ventilation	$\dot{V}_A = V_E - V_D \times f$	4.2–6.2 liters/min
Deadspace	$V_D = V_T(Pa_{CO_2} - PE_{CO_2}/Pa_{CO_2})$	$V_D/V_T = 0.30-0.40$
	$V_D = 150$ ml	
Mechanics		
Dynamic compliance	$Cdyn = V_T/Ppeak$	0.028 liters/ml H_2O ($V_T = 0.81$)*
Static compliance	$Cstat = V_T/Pplat$	0.045 liters ml H_2O ($V_T = 0.81$)*
Airway resistance	$Raw = (Ppeak - Pplat)/\dot{V}$	2.5 ml H_2O/(liters/sec)
Respiratory system resistance	$Rresp = Ppeak/\dot{V}$	10 ml H_2O/(liters/sec)†
Work		
Mechanical	$W = \int P \times dV_T$	0.85 kg-m/min or 0.08 kg-m/liter

* Bone RC: Diagnosis of causes for acute respiratory distress by pressure-volume curves. *Chest* 1976; 70:740.
† Peters RM, Hilberman M, Hogan JS, Crawford DA: Objective indications for respiratory therapy in post-trauma and postoperative patients. *Am J Surg* 1972; 124:262.

CHRONIC OBSTRUCTIVE PULMONARY DISEASE

Chronic obstructive pulmonary disease (COPD) is a broad disease category encompassing a number of distinct pathological processes, but in this discussion, it is limited to bronchitis and emphysema.

Bronchitis is characterized by mucus secretion, increased airways resistance, ventilation perfusion ($\dot{V}/\dot{Q}$) mismatch, and an increase in work of breathing. Hypoxemia and respiratory acidosis during exacerbation are common. For this reason, determination of arterial blood gases (ABGs) is important in the acute setting. PEFR and VC are useful for the same reasons as in asthma. Postoperatively, the bronchitic may experience increased secretions and decreased cough due to pain leading to atelectasis, increased $\dot{V}/\dot{Q}$ mismatch, and possibly, respiratory failure. Arterial blood gas determinations, serial physical examination, repeated PEFR, and VC facilitate management in these patients.

Emphysema is characterized by alveolar wall destruction and reduction in alveolar capillary units; an increase in compliance and deadspace ventilation results. Reduced airway compliance, airways collapse, and sputum production in some individuals result in air-flow obstruction. VC is often reduced because of air trapping, which produces an increased residual volume (RV). The reduced compliance promotes hyperinflation and places the diaphragm at a mechanical disadvantage, decreasing efficiency. ABGs are not markedly abnormal if there is good $\dot{V}/\dot{Q}$ matching in the remaining alveolar capillary units. ABGs also correlate poorly with the degree of dyspnea during an acute exacerbation. The deadspace to tidal volume ratio (V_D/V_T) increases slowly with disease progression and so is not particularly useful during an acute exacerbation. Some exacerbations are accompanied by increase in sputum production and $\dot{V}/\dot{Q}$ mismatching; there is considerable overlap between individuals with predominant emphysema or bronchitis. In this setting, initial determination of ABGs is important and measures of air flow (PEFR and VC) may be of help in determining treatment response.

RESTRICTIVE DISEASES

A reduction in respiratory system compliance due to increased lung or chest wall stiffness results in reduced total lung capacity (TLC) and VC. Expiratory flow rates are usually normal. Reduced TLC and lung compliance may be seen in several conditions, including diffuse pulmonary fibrosis, pulmonary parenchymal infiltrative diseases such as bronchopneumonia or extensive carcinoma, and conditions which increase lung water, including cardiogenic and noncardiogenic pulmonary edema. ABGs, lung compliance, and VD/VT are reasonable parameters to follow in the ventilated patient. A reduced chest wall compliance and relatively normal lung parenchyma characterize chest wall restriction. Resulting decreases in respiratory system compliance occur in high cord transection, scleroderma, burns, and kyphoscoliosis. Displacement or compression of the lungs by morbid obesity, effusion, large tumors, or ascites may also reduce TLC and produce restriction, usually without affecting lung compliance. If reducing TLC and VC leads to significant atelectasis, reduction in lung compliance may occur. With spinal cord transection, respiratory system compliance may be followed to determine when ventilator weaning may begin, as there is usually improvement with time.

Adult respiratory distress syndrome (ARDS), although defined by a clinical constellation of findings, is characterized by interstitial edema progressing to alveolar filling and destruction of alveolar capillary units with fibrosis. Increases in deadspace and VD/VT, reduction in VC, progressive hypoxemia, and a decrease in lung compliance result. Serial ABGs should be followed as the process worsens, and VD/VT, minute ventilation, and venous admixture (Q̇s/Q̇t) are very helpful during the recovery phase in determining when to wean from the ventilator.

NEUROMUSCULAR DISEASES

Myasthenia gravis, Guillain-Barré syndrome, motor neuron diseases, and spinal cord interruption may all lead to respiratory failure. In general, decreased muscular ability leads to reduced ventilation or an inability to respond to respiratory stress. Characteristically, VC is reduced and respiratory rate increased. Cough is weak, and thus the ability to clear secretions is compromised, leading to atelectasis, decreased compliance, V̇/Q̇ mismatch, and hypoxemia. Hypoventilation with respiratory acidosis may occur precipitously. In myasthenia gravis, the maximum minute ventilation (MVV) maneuver and peak inspiratory pressure (PIP) or VC may be helpful in diagnosis and following response to anticholinergic medication. Serial VC and PIP determinations predict respiratory failure better than serial ABGs in progressive neuromuscular diseases like Guillain Barré syndrome. A VC less than 1 liter or a PIP of less than -30 ml of water is a criterion for intubation. Difficulty with secretion clearance may become manifest when the mean maximal expiratory pressure is below $+40$ ml of water; this may also be an indicator for intubation.

REDUCED DRIVE

Reduced central ventilatory drive is responsible for hypoxemia and respiratory acidosis of varying degrees in several situations, including drug overdoses, central nervous system accidents, sleep apnea, the obesity hypoventilation syndrome, and central hypoventilation. Reduced minute ventilation, poor secretion clearance, atelectasis, and respiratory acidosis result. With extreme obesity, there may be an additional chest wall restrictive abnormality, reducing functional residual capacity FRC. Serial ABGs and specifically the arterial carbon dioxide tension (Pa_{CO_2}) must be followed in these patients. Spontaneous minute ventilation and VC during the recovery phase of drug overdose will help determine the time to wean. Actual measurement of respiratory drive is not commonly done in the intensive care setting.

WEANING CRITERIA USED IN THE INTENSIVE CARE UNIT

EXTUBATION VERSUS WEANING

Indications to discontinue mechanical ventilation must not be confused with indications to remove an artificial airway. Patients with altered states of consciousness, recurrent aspiration, or copious secretions may achieve ventilator independence, yet require continued airway protection.

There is little justification for pursuing tests of weaning readiness in unstable, critically ill patients. Withdrawal of ventilatory support (including mechanical inspiration and expiratory pressures) should not be considered until the underlying problem that necessitated support improves. Correction of nonpulmonary factors affecting the ability to breath spontaneously are important prior to weaning.

Various tests have been proposed to evaluate the need for continued ventilatory support. Such criteria seek to minimize premature weaning attempts, while decreasing unnecessary time spent on the ventilator. Generally, these tests can be separated into three areas of assessment: ability to oxygenate, resting ventilatory needs, and respiratory mechanical capability. They are based on three basic physiologic parameters: a $\dot{Q}s/\dot{Q}t$ of less than 15% to 20%, a V_D/V_T of less than 0.6, and an adequate "respiratory reserve" to enable a doubling of the resting work of breathing. Most other criteria listed are derivations of these three factors.

Oxygenation

Adequate blood oxygenation at an acceptably low inspired oxygen concentration is desirable before termination of ventilatory support. Once mechanical ventilation is withdrawn, the arterial oxygen tension (Pa_{O_2}) may decrease for a variety of reasons. Airway obstruction and atelectasis from secretions may reduce $\dot{V}/\dot{Q}$ matching and worsen intrapulmonary shunting. Respiratory frequency usually increases, increasing V_D/V_T and minute ventilation requirements. This, along with marginal cardiac output and extensive chest wall or parenchymal lung disease, increases the work of spontaneous breathing, which in turn increases oxygen consumption ($\dot{V}_{O_2}$) and depresses mixed venous oxygen saturations ($P\bar{v}_{O_2}$); Pa_{O_2} is lowered.

Several tests attempt to verify that an adequate Pa_{O_2} on an acceptably low fractional inspired oxygen concentration ($F_{I_{O_2}}$) is present before ventilatory support is discontinued.

Mixed Venous Blood Samples. Although a few patients with a high venous admixture ($\dot{Q}s/\dot{Q}t$) can be successfully weaned, in general it should be less than 20% before ventilatory support is discontinued.

$$\dot{Q}s/\dot{Q}t < 15\%\text{--}20\%$$

Usually patients who do not meet this criterion require a moderate to high $F_{I_{O_2}}$ or continuous positive airway pressure (CPAP) to maintain an adequate P_{O_2}. Subjects with low cardiac outputs may not successfully wean with a $\dot{Q}s/\dot{Q}t$ greater than 10%. Calculation of $\dot{Q}s/\dot{Q}t$ requires placement of a pulmonary artery catheter and sampling of mixed venous blood. Simpler tests of adequate oxygenation have, therefore, been proposed.

Alveolar-Arterial Oxygen Tension. Assuming a normal cardiac output, an alveolar-arterial oxygen tension difference below 350 mm Hg corresponds to a $\dot{Q}s/\dot{Q}t$ less than 15% to 20%.

$$P(A-a)O_2 < 300\text{--}350 \text{ mm Hg and } FI_{O_2} = 1$$

The test requires at least 20 minutes of ventilation with 100% oxygen, but a pulmonary artery catheter for sampling mixed venous blood is not necessary. Of course, the basic assumption (a normal cardiac output) must be a reasonable one. However, if the patient is considered for weaning, cardiovascular instability must not be present.

ABGs Determinations. This test requires only ABG determinations and is a frequently used criterion to assess adequacy of gas exchange prior to weaning.

$$Pa_{O_2} > 55 \text{ mm Hg and } FI_{O_2} < 0.4 \text{ and CPAP} < 5 \text{ ml } H_2O$$

Pa_{O_2} above 55 mm Hg on a FI_{O_2} less than 0.4 correlates well with a $\dot{Q}s/\dot{Q}t$ less than 20%. While this level may be used to initiate weaning, many would prefer a $Pa_{O_2} > 55$ on room air ($FI_{O_2} = .21$) before disconnecting ventilatory support entirely to avoid periods of hypoxia and desaturation which might occur if supplemental oxygen is not administered continuously. This is of practical significance because patients remove oxygen masks frequently.

Oximetry Measurements. Ear or finger oximetry measurements may occasionally be substituted for Pa_{O_2} values, since a Pa_{O_2} greater than 55 to 60 mm Hg should provide an oxyhemoglobin saturation (Sa_{O_2}) of at least 90%.

$$Sa_{O_2} > 90\% \text{ and } FI_{O_2} < 0.4 \text{ and CPAP} < 5 \text{ ml } H_2O$$

Oximeter calibration for each patient with spectrophotometric arterial blood oxygen saturations is recommended.

Ventilation Needs

Carbon dioxide tension and blood pH are dependent on alveolar ventilation. Increased carbon dioxide production must be matched with increased alveolar ventilation to maintain a steady-state Pa_{CO_2} and pH. Fever, sepsis, shivering, and excessive glucose loads during total parenteral nutrition may increase carbon dioxide production and ventilatory demands.

The amount of deadspace ventilation (VD) and central respiratory drive influence minute ventilatory needs and respiratory muscle demands. Assuming carbon dioxide production is stable, the various ventilatory criteria assess the relative proportion of VD present.

VD/VT Ratio. Patients whose VD/VT exceeds 0.6 are usually not weanable from ventilatory support. Small increases in VD/VT above 0.6 require large increases in minute ventilation ($\dot{V}E$) in order to maintain a given Pa_{CO_2}. Such increases in spontaneous $\dot{V}E$ may be difficult for many critically ill patients to achieve, ultimately resulting in hypercapnia and respiratory muscle fatigue.

Minute Ventilation. $\dot{V}E$ is determined by carbon dioxide production and the V_D/V_T. A patient whose V_D/V_T ratio is 0.3 to 0.4 will maintain a near normal Pa_{CO_2} with a $\dot{V}E$ of less than 10 liters/ min, providing less ventilatory reserve for stress situations. The $\dot{V}E$ limit may also be expressed as a function of body weight ($\dot{V}E$ less than 180 ml/kg/min), since carbon dioxide production is proportional to size. A V_T greater than 5 to 7 ml/kg with a RR of less than 30 breaths/min represents a limiting component of $\dot{V}E$ and may be used during a test of spontaneous ventilation ability.

Both V_D/V_T and $\dot{V}E$ offer an easy estimation of spontaneous resting ventilatory needs. Anxiety, pain, sedatives, or metabolic factors may alter $\dot{V}E$ and result in erroneous assessments of weaning readiness when $\dot{V}E$ is used as the sole criterion. Patients with advanced COPD may maintain an adequate pH through metabolic compensation despite V_D/V_T ratios exceeding 0.6. Regardless of the criterion selected, measurements of arterial pH and P_{CO_2} after a period of spontaneous ventilation are necessary to confirm acceptable ventilation.

Mechanical Capability

Extubated patients must generate adequate respiratory function at rest, while possessing sufficient ventilatory reserve for potential stress situations. The mechanical capability of the respiratory system may be impaired by neuromuscular weakness or factors which increase the work of breathing. Weaning criteria have therefore been proposed to assess the mechanical capability to sustain spontaneous ventilation during stress conditions.

Vital Capacity. Vital capacity (VC) is dependent on neuromuscular strength, motivation, and respiratory system compliance. A VC exceeding 1 to 1.5 liters or 10 to 15 ml/kg indicates that weaning may take place. A borderline VC achieved predominantly through accessory muscle use is not as predictive of successful weaning as similar values obtained when the diaphragm is working.

Maximum Voluntary Ventilation. If most of the mechanical ventilatory reserve is used to sustain resting V_T, a minimal stress could lead to exhaustion, resulting in a return to ventilatory support. If normal subjects can maintain a $\dot{V}E$ equal to 60% of their maximum voluntary ventilation (MVV) indefinitely, it follows that the ability to double resting $\dot{V}E$ predicts an adequate ventilatory reserve. Measurement of MVV is technically simple and reflects overall muscle strength and respiratory system compliance. Patient effort can greatly influence the results.

Peak Inspiratory Pressure. PIP reflects inspiratory strength but does not assess muscle endurance or lung compliance. A PIP below -30 ml H_2O correlates well with the ability to be weaned.[3] PIP determinations require less patient cooperation than VC or MVV measurements.

Work of Breathing. Using work of breathing as a weaning criterion is attractive because mechanical and ventilatory factors are assessed together and determinations are independent of patient effort. Normal work of breathing ranges from 0.4 to 0.8 kg-m/min (or 0.05 kg-m/liter) of ventilation. Patients are usually ventilator dependent if their resting work of breathing exceeds 1.8 kg-m/min.[4] Clinically useful data are otherwise scarce. Patients with COPD have a rate of approximately 1.5 kg-m/min.[5] Further investigation of this weaning criteria is needed in large groups of mechanically ventilated patients before it can be clinically useful.

NEGATIVE CLINICAL SIGNS FOR WEANING

Three physical findings seen during spontaneous ventilation tests may predict weaning failure: rapid shallow respirations, respiratory alternans (alternating between abdominal and rib cage breathing), and abdominal paradox (the inward movement of the abdominal wall during inspiration in the supine position).[6] These clinical signs, if present, may predict those patients still in need of ventilatory support; prospective confirmation is pending.

SHORT-TERM VENTILATOR PATIENTS

Patients requiring mechanical ventilation may be classified as either short- or long-term ventilator dependent. Classification is useful for choosing which, if any, weaning criteria should be applied. Short-term ventilator dependents require ventilatory support for less than 1 week and represent the majority of intubated patients, including most postoperative subjects, those suffering severe exacerbations of asthma, bronchitis, or heart failure, and those obtunded from drug overdoses. Most published studies assessing weaning criteria are of patients intubated for mean durations of only 3 to 55 hours and address only short-term ventilator dependence.[3,7]

In an early prospective study assessing multiple bedside weaning criteria, all subjects demonstrating a resting $\dot{V}E$ less than 10 liters/min, a MVV greater than double their $\dot{V}E$, and a PIP less than -30 ml H_2O were successfully weaned.[3] Although there were no false-positive results, a false-negative rate of 29% for the three criteria was noted. Although adequate performance on these weaning tests predicts a successful removal of assisted ventilation, many patients failing these criteria may have mechanical ventilation unnecessarily prolonged.

Subsequent prospective studies of postoperative patients have confirmed that no single or combination of criteria measuring mechanical ability can predict, with any degree of reliability, patients who can not be weaned. However, when gas exchange criteria (minimal Sa_{O_2} greater than 90% on a low FI_{O_2}) are used in addition, predictive weaning accuracy increases to 94%.[7]

Most short-term mechanically ventilated patients can be weaned, if, after 30 to 60 minutes of breathing through the ventilator without assistance, they are hemodynamically stable, have a normal body temperature, a low respiratory rate, a normal VT (10 ml/kg), and an adequate Pa_{O_2} with an FI_{O_2} of less than 0.4.[8] Evaluation of respiratory mechanics may not be applicable to patients requiring only brief ventilatory assistance, as mechanical ventilation may be unnecessarily prolonged. Specific criteria for deciding when to wean nonsurgical short-term ventilator dependent patients remain to be defined by prospective investigations.

LONG-TERM VENTILATOR PATIENTS

Fewer than 5% of mechanically ventilated patients require ventilatory support beyond 1 week. Most have COPD, pneumonia, sepsis, ARDS, restrictive lung diseases, refractory heart failure, or neuromuscular disease as causes for their prolonged ventilator dependence. Apart from those with neuromuscular disorders, very little has been written regarding appropriate weaning criteria for long-term ventilator dependent patients.

Sivak[9] reported on 15 patients with prolonged respiratory failure and suggested a VC of between 12 and 15 ml/kg and a PIP of less than -25 ml H_2O as appropriate guidelines for weaning. Attention to the underlying cause of respiratory failure and correction of nonpulmonary factors did result in successful weaning in 12 of 15 patients. The recommendations were not, however, prospectively tested.

Morganroth and co-workers[10] retrospectively studied 10 subjects with 11 instances of prolonged mechanical ventilation. Spontaneous ventilatory measurements did not predict ability to wean; mean values for V_T, FVC, $\dot{V}_E$, respiratory rate, and PIP were not significantly different between successful and failed weaning periods. Interestingly, withdrawal of ventilator assistance was accomplished despite deterioration of spontaneous ventilator measurements in a few patients. What discriminated successful from aborted weaning trials was a reduction in "adverse factor" and "ventilator scores." Adverse factors generally assessed cardiac performance, presence of infection, mental status, nutritional status, bronchial hygiene, and psychologic factors. Reduction of these "adverse factors" highlights the contention that successful correction of underlying pulmonary and nonpulmonary complications will best predict whether long-term mechanical ventilation may be terminated.[9] The lowest ventilator scores were achieved with an F_{IO_2} equal to or less than 40%, CPAP of 0 ml H_2O, effective static compliance of greater than 60 ml/ml H_2O, dynamic compliance of greater than 40 ml/ml H_2O, ventilator $\dot{V}_E$ of less than 10 liters/min, and a triggered ventilatory rate of less than 20/min. The fall in ventilator score before successful weaning suggests that an improving gas exchange is an important indication for beginning weaning trials in these patients. All of these parameters, however, await prospective evaluation. Until such investigations are available, the most dependable criteria for successful weaning remains the correction of underlying pulmonary and nonpulmonary factors.

Today, modes of ventilatory support often blend contributions of the patient with mechanically supplied work from the ventilator. Intermittent mandatory ventilation, pressure support ventilation, mandated minute ventilation, and continuous positive airway pressure supply, incrementally, work that the patient is unable to perform. Weaning, using these modes, is possible independent of specific objective instantaneous criteria. Once ventilatory support has produced a clinically acceptable breathing pattern and satisfactory blood gases and the disease process has been controlled, the clinical setting for withdrawal of ventilatory support has been satisfied. Decrements in mechanically supplied work must then be followed by augmentation of the patient's efforts. As long as the clinical breathing pattern remains satisfactory and blood gases continue within acceptable limits, decrementations may proceed. A spontaneous ventilatory rate of less than 30 is a simple, sensitive but nonspecific parameter to document progress.

SPECIFIC TESTS AND APPLICATIONS

MEASUREMENT OF RESPIRATORY FREQUENCY AND LUNG VOLUME

Measurement of respiratory frequency is primarily for monitoring ventilation. Ideally, both apneas and hypopneas (shallow breaths) must be detected. To do this, it is usually necessary to detect flow or a change in lung volume. Serial observation may miss significant events. Nasal thermistors measure air flow by the change in temperature, and they are sensitive but uncomfortable and often fall off. Magnetometers measure displacement: a magnet on one side of the chest induces a current in a coil placed on the other, which varies with the distance of separation. The magnetometer detects thoracic motion but does not detect obstructive apneas characterized by continued thoracic motion and cessation of air flow. The pressure pneumograph measures displacement of volume by encircling the chest with an expandable tube or a mercury strain gauge. These devices miss obstructive apneas as well, and are somewhat uncomfortable to wear. Impedance pneumographs rely on the changing impedance of the expanding chest wall to detect chest wall motion. They are convenient and fairly sensitive but suffer from movement artifact and therefore may produce an inordinant number of false alarms. The inductive plethysmograph relies on a series of coils placed around the chest and abdomen, usually incorporated in a close-fitting, vestlike garment. Although the inductive plethysmograph is relatively stable over time and has less movement artifact than other methods, it is tedious to calibrate and fairly expensive. It does, however, detect obstructive apneas and provide quantitative measurement of V_T when properly calibrated.

Intubated patients are easier to monitor because their airway is cannulated. Frequently, ventilators provide a display of V_T, respiratory frequency, and inspiratory flow rate. Newer ventilators and monitoring systems often display, in addition, respiratory system compliance and resistance, oxygen consumption, carbon dioxide production, and, recently, some measure of mechanical work. Unless careful calibrations are performed and artifacts are sought and eliminated, these values are accurate enough to be used for decision making.

Alveolar ventilation ($\dot{V}_A$) is physiologically most important to follow and cannot be accurately monitored. It is a function of frequency (f), V_T, and V_D.

$$\dot{V}_A = (V_T - V_D) \times f \text{ (liters)}$$

Vital Capacity (VC)

VC is the volume difference between functional residual capacity (FRC) and TLC and is determined by lung elasticity, airway resistance, airway wall compliance, gas density, and patient effort. It is a function of height, age, sex, and race.

VC is measured with a spirometer, with the water seal and rolling seal spirometers the standards by which others are judged. The Wright spirometer is a vaned instrument which produces accurate volume determinations so long as flow rates are high enough to overcome friction inherent in the device and no sputum is introduced into the instrument. Electronic spirometry uses a pneumotachograph to measure flow which is integrated to provide volume. Common pneumotachographs include the Fleisch-type pneumotachograph, which measures the pressure drip when air flows across a screen; the vortex pneumotachograph, which counts eddy air flow currents around a small obstruction using an ultrasonic mechanism; and the heated wire or heated bead pneumotachograph, which employs a thermocouple and detects air flow by measuring changes in resistance, proportional to cooling.

Minute Ventilation ($\dot{V}_E$)

$\dot{V}_E$ is the product of V_T and f; it is determined by the alveolar ventilation, deadspace ventilation, and central drive.

$$\dot{V}_E = V_T \times f \text{ (liters/min)}$$
$$\dot{V}_E = (V_A + V_D) \times f$$

Many ventilators display V_E or it can be measured with a Wright spirometer or a large Tissot bell–type spirometer.

If patients have decreased compliance and are ventilated with high peak inspiratory pressure (PIP) and distensible disposable ventilator circuits are used, the ventilator display will overestimate the amount received by the patient. Many circuits have a compliance of 3 to 4 ml/cm. If PIP is 50 cm H_2O, approximately 200 ml of gas will be compressed in the tubing during inhalation, reexpand during exhalation, and be measured as minute ventilation. Accurate measurements can be made only if the measuring device is connected directly to the patient's endotrachial tube, thus measuring only exhaled gas.

Deadspace Ventilation (V_D)

V_D is important in illness and its determination should accompany all measurements of $\dot{V}_E$. The anatomic deadspace includes the volume of the airways to the level of the respiratory bronchiole; the physiologic deadspace includes, in addition, alveolar volume that is well ventilated but poorly perfused. Calculation of V_D/V_T requires measurement of end-tidal carbon dioxide tension (PE_{CO_2}) and Pa_{CO_2}. Several assumptions simplify the equation.

$$V_D/V_T = Pa_{CO_2} - PE_{CO_2}/Pa_{CO_2}$$

Expired Pa_{CO_2} may be determined by collecting a large quantity of exhaled gas in a Douglas bag or Tissot spirometer and measuring the mixed carbon dioxide concentration. Alternatively, PE_{CO_2} may be measured, since it theoretically approaches mixed carbon dioxide concentration. The latter method, although not as accurate, is much easier.

A convenient nomogram developed by Seleky and associates[11] allows rapid determination of V_D/V_T once the $\dot{V}_E$ and Pa_{CO_2} are known. A carbon dioxide production of 200 ml/min is assumed to make the calculation possible. Once the V_D/V_T is known, the nomogram may be used further to predict changes in Pa_{CO_2} induced by alterations in ventilator imposed minute ventilation. This nomogram should be used with caution because of the basic assumption. Critically ill patients have large variations in oxygen consumption, which at a constant respiratory quotient will produce large variations in CO_2 production. Additionally, respiratory quotient varies significantly. The assumption would be valid only for stable patients with normal O_2 consumption (250 ml/min) and respiratory quotient (0.8).

Increases in V_D/V_T can be seen with pulmonary emboli, vascular obliteration in emphysema or ARDS, pleuropulmonary air leaks, and shock with low cardiac output state (Fig. 8-1).

Functional Residual Capacity (FRC)

FRC is the lung volume when the ventilatory system is at rest (end-expiration) and is not usually determined in the ICU. Measurement is difficult as high oxygen concentrations make gas dilution determinations inaccurate. FRC is reduced most commonly in diseases with increased pulmonary elastic forces, such as interstitial lung disease and ARDS. Mechanical ventilation with CPAP is used to increase the FRC and improve $V/\dot{Q}$ matching.

Forced Expiratory Volume in One Second (FEV_1)

The volume exhaled in the first second of a forced expiration (FEV_1) from TLC is determined by lung recoil pressure at a given volume, airway resistance and compliance, and patient effort. An FEV_1 determination is difficult to perform in ventilated patients, and bedside

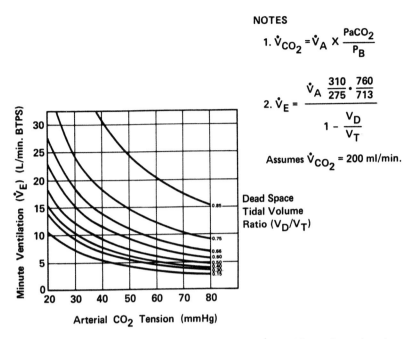

NOTES

1. $\dot{V}_{CO_2} = \dot{V}_A \times \dfrac{PaCO_2}{P_B}$

2. $\dot{V}_E = \dfrac{\dot{V}_A \dfrac{310}{275} \cdot \dfrac{760}{713}}{1 - \dfrac{V_D}{V_T}}$

Assumes $\dot{V}_{CO_2}$ = 200 ml/min.

Dead Space
Tidal Volume
Ratio (V_D/V_T)

Figure 8-1 Relationship between minute ventilation ($\dot{V}_E$) and Pa_{CO_2} for various iso-pleths of V_D/V_T. Use to calculate V_D/V_T or, once this is known, affect of alterations in $\dot{V}_E$. (Selecky et al: *Am Rev Respir Dis* 1978; 117:181)

determination requires a spirometer. For this reason, other tests of air flow are employed more often.

Peak Expiratory Flow Rate (PEFR)

Peak expiratory flow rate is easy to determine at the bedside; inexpensive instrumentation and relative accuracy contribute to the value of the measurement. It is most commonly used in the spontaneously breathing patient. Repeated determinations correlate well within the same individual and compare favorably to values derived from a pneumotachograph. The patient is instructed to blow out through the instrument as hard and fast as possible; the best of three tries is used.

MEASUREMENT OF PULMONARY MECHANICS

Inflation Pressures

Airway pressure during inspiration is a test for a number of derived variables including resistance, conductance, and compliance. Most ventilators display airway pressure during lung inflation. Pressure measured at the airway opening at end-inspiration after subtracting applied CPAP is termed the *peak airway pressure*. If expiration is prevented following an inspiration, the respiratory muscles relax and pressure at the airway opening then equals alveolar pressure (after subtracting applied CPAP); this is termed the *plateau pressure*. Error is introduced if insufficient time is allowed for pressure equilibration, and some degree of volume compression occurs depending on the respiratory system recoil.

Several other derived pressures are commonly encountered. Transpulmonary pressure, the pressure across the lung, is the difference between alveolar and pleural pressure. Alveolar pressure equals the airway opening pressure when there is no flow (at end-inspiration or end-expiration and during occlusion with relaxed muscles). Esophageal pressure approximates pleural pressure and may be measured with an esophageal balloon. Transthoracic pressure is the difference between the pressure at the chest wall (barometric pressure) and alveolar pressure.

Airway Resistance and Conductance

Airway resistance and conductance can be determined in the ICU. Resistance in a tube is the amount of driving pressure divided by flow rate. The driving pressure is the drop in pressure along the airway and, thus, the difference between the alveolar pressure and mouth pressure.

Airway conductance is the reciprocal of resistance: airway resistance decreases as lung volume increases. The relationship of resistance to lung volume is nonlinear. However, conductance is a linear function of lung volume.

In the pulmonary function laboratory, airway resistance is measured using a body plethysmograph. This is not possible in the ICU, but information may be derived in the ventilated patient by examining the pressure and flow relationships. Respiratory system resistance is a measure of the elastic and viscous resistance of the lung tissue, chest cage, and airway. It is determined by relating airway opening pressure to inspiratory flow, and it increases with increasing lung volume because of the elastic component. Airway resistance may be approximated using peak and plateau airway pressures displayed on the ventilator. The plateau pressure (equals alveolar pressure), when subtracted from the peak airway pressure, gives the pressure drop down the airway at a given lung volume. Dividing this pressure drop by the inspiratory flow yields the inspiratory airway resistance at a particular lung volume. It follows that a large difference between peak and plateau airway pressure is due to increased airway resistance.[12]

Lung Compliance

Compliance is determined by the elastic properties of the lung and chest wall by measuring a change of volume and relating it to a change in recoil force or pressure. Several different components of compliance are commonly measured. In the ICU, total respiratory system compliance is usually measured, that is, the compliance of the lung and chest wall combined. To determine static, or effective, respiratory system compliance, inspiratory volume is divided by the plateau pressure at end-inspiration. Static effective compliance is useful to follow because the chest wall compliance component usually remains constant during the course of many acute disease processes. Changes in static effective compliance then reflect changes in lung compliance. Exceptions to this may be in cases of massive obesity, spinal cord transections, and ascites when the volume of ascitic fluid is changing.

The dynamic compliance characteristic[12] is obtained by dividing inspiratory volume by peak pressure. A curve may be constructed at various tidal volumes and peak pressures. It is not truly compliance (hence the term characteristic) but rather a sum of elastic and flow resistance properties of the lung, and as such, it can be quite useful. Comparison of the static compliance and dynamic compliance characteristic at a given lung volume or at several lung volumes can give information about acute events during mechanical ventilation.[12] Comparison with determinations done at the onset of mechanical ventilation may suggest the presence of pulmonary edema, bronchoconstriction, retained secretions, pneumothorax, atelectasis, and intubation of the main-stem bronchus. Once the clinician is familiar with the shapes of these curves, he or she can make quick evaluation of acute changes in patient status. The only equipment necessary is the mechanical ventilator. Changes in the dynamic compliance characteristic that are unaccompanied by changes in static compliance are in general due to changes in the flow resistive properties of the lung and suggest problems of increased resistance, such as bronchoconstriction (*e.g.,* asthma, pulmonary embolus, bronchitis), intubation of the main-stem bronchus, and pneumothorax. Alterations in both determinations of compliance suggest a change in lung stiffness, such as with pulmonary edema (*e.g.,* congestive heart failure or ARDS) or pneumonia.

Respiratory Timing

Respiratory timing is not routinely measured in the intensive care setting, but an understanding of the inspiratory (T_I) and expiratory (T_E) time intervals is necessary for proper ventilator adjustment. The total respiratory cycle time (T_{TOT}) is the sum of the inspiratory and expiratory times.

$$T_{TOT} = T_I + T_E$$

Changing T_I and T_E produces changes in ventilation. The inspiratory gas flow rate and V_T determine T_I while the inspiratory to expiratory (I:E) ratio determines T_E. The relation may be expressed as

$$V_E = V_T/T_I \times T_I/T_{TOT}$$
$$V_E = V_T \times frequency$$

V_T/T_I is the inspiratory flow rate and relates to drive; T_I/T_{TOT} is the duty cycle and relates to the frequency expression. Many patients with COPD require a prolonged T_E to avoid progressive hyperinflation. Alternatively, patients with interstitial disease producing restriction and increased elastic forces have a very short T_E and may be best ventilated with inverse ratio breathing. *Inverse ratio breathing* is breathing with T_I greater than 50% of T_{TOT}. The benefits of this are reduced airway pressures and better oxygenation.[13]

MEASUREMENT OF MUSCLE PERFORMANCE

Inspiratory and Expiratory Pressures

Peak inspiratory (PIP) and expiratory pressure (PEP) both are measures of the ability of the ventilatory muscles to generate a pressure against a closed orifice. Performance decreases when muscles are weak due to fatigue, malnutrition, deconditioning, or neuromuscular disease. The peak or maximal inspiratory pressure is dependent on lung volume and is greatest at residual volume. Conversely, the peak or maximal expiratory pressure is highest when performed at TLC. Measurement requires a pressure gauge with a measuring capacity of $+300$ to -160 ml/H_2O. The patient is asked to perform a maximal inspiratory maneuver from FRC and a maximal expiratory maneuver from TLC. The determination is effort-dependent, and some motivation on the part of the tester is necessary to obtain good results.

Leaks in the tubing and around the mouth, especially with weak facial muscles, may be a source of error. Alteration of TLC and FRC by pre-existing obstructive or restricting disease may also alter the results without clinically evident muscle weakness being present.

Some believe that the ability to generate a VC is a better determinant of muscle performance than PIP. Evidence cited to support this view is that performance of a VC maneuver measures not just muscular performance but also mechanical properties of the lung and chest wall. PIP, in contrast, measures only the muscle component. Those who favor measurement of PIP for determining muscle weakness cite the fact that VC may not decline until significant muscle weakness exists.

Work of Breathing

Ventilatory muscle work may be expressed as mechanical, metabolic, or tension–time work. For the most part determination has been an experimental procedure due to the complexity of measurement, but new microprocessor ventilators allow some components of work to be measured. At present, however, it does not seem that, without careful elimination of artifacts and calibration, these values can be considered accurate enough to use as validated objective measurement. In fact, there have been no reports validating these values as produced when the microprocessor ventilators are used in routine clinical situation. Mechanical work is performed against elastic, resistive, friction, and inertial forces during inspiration; the stored elastic work is then used to perform passive expiration. The elastic forces are derived from the lung parenchyma and chest wall; the resistive forces are provided by the airways and to some extent the tissues of the chest wall. Frictional, inertial forces, and work against gravity are usually regarded as relatively insignificant.

Mechanical work to move a gas is determined by multiplying pressure (P) by change in volume. This is the area under the inspiratory pressure–volume curve or the integral of the pressure–tidal volume product.

$$\text{Work} = \int P \times dV_T$$

A substitution of terms provides a more useful relationship:

$$\text{Work} = \int P \times \dot{V} dt$$

Integration is performed during the inspiratory time interval.

Work performed by the ventilatory muscles "on the lung," excluding work on the chest wall and abdominal contents, may be measured in spontaneously breathing patients. That pressure is the transpulmonary pressure. Work performed only on the lung underestimates the total respiratory system work in patients with obesity, kyphoscoliosis, ascites, or other chest wall restrictive processes.

In ventilated patients the total respiratory system work may be determined by measuring ventilator work during controlled ventilation. Ventilator work is equal to the product of airway pressure and inspiratory flow during the period of inspiration, both measurements that are available from the ventilator. When the patient is relaxed and the chest is inflated by the ventilator, all the mechanical work is performed by the ventilator. The work measured is the total work of inflating the lung, moving the chest wall, and displacing the abdomen. It is more representative of the actual burden on the respiratory muscles than work performed on the lung.

Work may also be described in metabolic terms. Oxygen consumption and carbon dioxide production are descriptive of metabolic work performed. Measurement of metabolic work perhaps is most useful in determining nutritional requirements of ill patients. Increased carbon dioxide production due to overfeeding of glucose may lead to an increase in the minute ventilation requirement. Mechanical ventilation, when appropriately applied, reduces oxygen consumption by the respiratory muscles and may be beneficial in patients with acute myocardial infarction and reduced cardiac output.

Measurement of tension–time work, although not a true measure of mechanical work, has been used to study diaphragm fatigue. Placing an esophageal and gastric balloon allows measurement of transdiaphragmatic pressure (Pdi) which is proportional to developed tension. The Pdi measurement must be equated to a standard maximal transdiaphragmatic pressure (Pdi_{max}) maneuver for comparison purposes. The time interval is the inspiratory time as a portion of the total respiratory cycle time (T_I/T_{TOT}). Fatigue has been shown to develop when the $(Pdi/Pdi_{max})(T_I/T_{TOT})$ product is greater than 0.15.[14]

REFERENCES

1. Petheram IS, Jones OA, Collins JV: Patterns of recovery of airflow obstruction in severe acute asthma. *Postgrad Med J* 1979; 55:877
2. Martin TG, Elenbass RM, Pingleton SH: Use of peak expiratory flow rates to eliminate unnecessary arterial blood gases in acute asthma. *Ann Emerg Med* 1982; 11:70
3. Sahn SA, Lakshminarayan MB: Bedside criteria for discontinuation of mechanical ventilation. *Chest* 1973; 63:1002
4. Peters RM, Hilberman M, Hogan JS, Crawford DA: Objective indications for respiratory therapy in post-trauma and postoperative patients. *Am J Surg* 1972; 124:262
5. Fleury B, Murciano D, Talamo C, et al: Work of breathing in patients with chronic obstructive disease in acute respiratory failure. *Am Rev Respir Dis* 1985; 131:822
6. Cohen CA, Zagelbaum G, Gross D, et al: Clinical manifestations of inspiratory muscle fatigue. *Am J Med* 1982; 73:308
7. DeHaven CB, Hurst JM, Branson RD: Evaluation of two different extubation criteria: Attributes contributing to success. *Crit Care Med* 1986; 14:92
8. Prakish O, Meij S, Borden B, Saxena PR: Cardiorespiratory monitoring during open heart surgery. *Crit Care Med* 1981; 9:530
9. Sivak ED: Prolonged mechanical ventilation, an approach to weaning. *Cleve Clin Q* 1980; 47:89
10. Morganroth ML, Morganroth JL, Nett LM, Petty TL: Criteria for weaning from prolonged mechanical ventilation. *Arch Intern Med* 1984; 144:1012
11. Seleky PA, Wasserman K, Klein M, Ziment: A graphic approach to assessing interrelationships among minute ventilation, arterial carbon dioxide tension, and ratio of physiologic dead space to tidal volume in patients on respirators. *Am Rev Respir Dis* 1978; 117:181
12. Bone RC: Diagnosis of causes for acute respiratory distress by pressure-volume curves. *Chest* 1976; 70:740
13. Cole AGH, Weller SF, Sikes MK: Inverse ratio of ventilation compared with PEEP and adult respiratory failure. *Intensive Care Med* 1984; 10:227
14. Bellamare F, Grassino A: Effect of pressure and timing of contraction on human diaphragm fatigue. *J Appl Physiol* 1982; 53:1190

CHAPTER NINE

OXYGEN THERAPY

Robert A. Smith

In 1775, Joseph Priestley and Carl Wilhelm Scheele published reports describing their respective discoveries of "dephlogisticated air" and "fire-air." Priestley noted,

> The feeling of it to my lungs was not sensibly different from that of common air; but I fancied that my breast felt peculiarly light and easy for some time afterwards. Who can tell but that in time, this pure air may become a fashionable article in luxury. Hitherto only two mice and myself have had the privilege of breathing it.[1]

Scheele observed,

> Hence it is the fire-air by means of which the circulation of the blood and of the juices in animals and plants is so fully maintained.[2]

Following its discovery, oxygen was employed in an empirical and frequently irresponsible manner to treat a variety of illnesses, and its limited clinical use shortly fell into disfavor. In 1915, John S. Haldane treated soldiers who had suffered phosgene gas poisoning and noted that oxygen administration improved their cyanosis and overall clinical situation.[3] This observation marked the beginning of modern oxygen therapy.

Atmospheric air contains 20.9% oxygen, corresponding to a partial pressure of 0.209 atmospheres absolute (ATA). A rise in the inspired partial pressure of oxygen ($P_{I_{O_2}}$) can be achieved by increasing the fraction of inspired oxygen ($F_{I_{O_2}}$) or the total atmospheric pressure. This presentation reviews techniques of administering supplemental oxygen at ambient pressure and briefly examines the potential complications of oxygen therapy.

OXYGEN THERAPY

Gas exchange between air and blood occurs by diffusion across the air–blood barrier, driven by the partial pressure gradient of oxygen between alveolar air ($P_{A_{O_2}}$) and pulmonary capillary ($P\acute{c}_{O_2}$) blood. Alveolar P_{O_2} never reaches $P_{I_{O_2}}$ because of the residual air that remains in alveoli at end-exhalation. At atmospheric pressure (760 mm Hg at sea level), $P_{I_{O_2}}$ is 160 mm Hg. Water vapor (47 mm Hg at 37°C) and carbon dioxide ($\simeq 40 \pm 5$ mm Hg) partial pressures reduce $P_{A_{O_2}}$ to approximately 100 to 105 mm Hg. Pulmonary capillary P_{O_2} varies from $\approx$ 40 mm Hg (pulmonary arterial) to a level similar to $P_{A_{O_2}}$ if the blood equilibrates completely with alveolar gas. However, an irreducible gradient exists between alveolar gas and arterial blood, resulting in a systemic $P_{a_{O_2}}$ of about 90 to 95 mm Hg. This $P(A - a)_{O_2}$ gradient is often used as an index of pulmonary function. When cardiac output is normal, a gradient of 20 mm Hg represents an intrapulmonary shunt of $\approx$ 1% if the patient breathes 100% oxygen.

The potential for oxygen transfer across the lungs is estimated by the pulmonary diffusing capacity for oxygen. It quantitates the oxygen flow rate resulting from the P_{O_2} gradient of 1 mm Hg, thus estimating global lung conductance for oxygen transfer to the blood via diffusion. When normal oxygen transfer is decreased by a functional "diffusion block" resulting from pulmonary injury or disease, this flow can be maintained by increasing $P_{A_{O_2}}$ with supplemental oxygen. Elevating the fraction of inspired oxygen $(F_{I_{O_2}})$ by 0.01% increases $P_{I_{O_2}}$ by $\sim$ 8 mm Hg and $P_{A_{O_2}}$ by $\sim$ 7 mm Hg.

PRINCIPLES OF AIR DILUTION

Various concentrations of inspired oxygen may be provided by oxygen-powered air-entrainment devices or the blending of compressed air and oxygen. Air entrainment is accomplished with either an injector (Venturi tube) or a jet-mixing device. Injectors are relatively uncommon in contemporary supplemental oxygen therapy; however, they are incorporated in some mechanical ventilators (Bird IPPB devices) and continuous positive airway pressure (CPAP) systems. The most frequently used air-entrainment mechanism employs jet-mixing. The jet exit is in or near the plane of the entrainment port; at this point and within the mixing chamber, pressure is ambient. Thus, air entrainment is not due to high-velocity jet flow (Venturi effect) but rather to viscous shearing between moving and static air layers. The dynamic gas (oxygen) transfers kinetic energy to the static air mass (ambient gas), "dragging" (entraining) ambient air into the moving stream. The amount of air dilution is regulated by selection of a jet orifice size (*e.g.* color-coded jet nozzles for air–oxygen mixing masks) or adjusting an air-entrainment orifice (*e.g.*, wall-mounted nebulizer).

Entrainment efficiency is affected by delivery circuit pressure. Whenever delivery circuit pressure increases above atmospheric pressure, the entrainment volume diminishes while jet flow (100% oxygen) remains unaltered, producing a higher $F_{I_{O_2}}$. To provide a consistent $F_{I_{O_2}}$, the gas flow from jet mixing devices must vent to ambient. A method of $F_{I_{O_2}}$ control virtually unaffected by circuit pressure fluctuations utilizes mechanical blending of compressed air and oxygen. Blenders are commonly powered by 40 to 50 psig (pounds per square inch gauge) air and oxygen sources (Fig. 9-1). Source gases are matched to the lowest source pressure by reducing valves, and air and oxygen at a common pressure are interfaced with a proportioning valve and mixed to a selected $F_{I_{O_2}}$. Blended gas is then directed to the outlet port for delivery by a metering device.

SUPPLEMENTAL OXYGEN ADMINISTRATION

Supplemental oxygen administration is facilitated by either fixed or variable performance modes. Fixed performance systems deliver a predictable and consistent $F_{I_{O_2}}$ independent of fluctuations in the patient's breathing pattern. These are functionally large capacitance systems providing gas flow that exceeds peak inspiratory flow $(\dot{V}_I)$ demand. Variable systems (*i.e.*, small or noncapacitance) are patient-dependent. A noncapacitance device, such as a

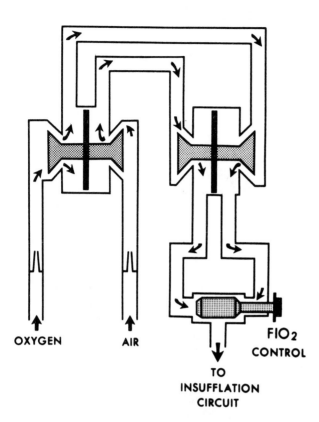

Figure 9-1 Schematic representation of an air-oxygen blender. High-pressure air and oxygen are equilibrated by pressure regulators; each is then interfaced with the F_{IO_2} control valve for delivery to the circuit.

OXYGEN AIR FIO$_2$ CONTROL

TO INSUFFLATION CIRCUIT

nasal catheter or cannula using a low flow rate ($\leq$ 4 liters/min), produces insufficient storage of oxygen during exhalation to affect the next inspiration substantially. Therefore, oxygen enrichment is a function of $\dot{V}_I$ and the oxygen flow rate. A nasal or pharyngeal oxygen delivery device may provide some capacitance at flow rates > 4 liters/min. An oxygen mask or face tent increases capacitance to a variable extent that is dependent on the presence of a reservoir.

NASAL CANNULA AND CATHETER

Supplemental oxygen may be administered with a cannula or catheter. An oxygen cannula consists of two prongs placed approximately 1.0 cm into the nares and held stationary by an elastic head strap. The catheter should be lubricated with water-soluble jelly and then inserted into a naris until its tip is just visible below the soft palate. It is secured to the upper lip or nose with tape. Cannulas and catheters should be changed at least every day, and more frequently if crusting of the outlet ports occurs. The F_{IO_2} administered with either device depends on oxygen flow rate, the patient's $\dot{V}_I$, respiratory rate (RR), duration of the expiratory phase, and the anatomic reservoir (*i.e.*, nasopharyngeal volume). A rule-of-thumb for cannula or catheter systems is that F_{IO_2} is increased by 0.03 to 0.04 for each liter per minute of oxygen flow rate. However, maximum tracheal F_{IO_2} is unlikely to exceed 0.50; therefore, flow rates > 8 liters/min are unlikely to increase delivered oxygen further and may prove uncomfortable.

FACE MASKS

Four types of face masks are used to supplement oxygen delivery: simple, partial rebreather, nonrebreather, and air entrainment (high-flow oxygen-enrichment masks).

Simple oxygen masks do not contain valves or a reservoir, and provide an $F_{I_{O_2}}$ of 0.35 to 0.50 when the oxygen flow rate is 6 to 10 liters/min. Oxygen flow should exceed the patient's minute ventilation to minimize expired gas rebreathing. The mask augments the anatomic reservoir volume by providing supplemental oxygen about the nose and mouth; however, variation in $\dot{V}_I$ and RR can alter $F_{I_{O_2}}$. Sellers and Haggs recently showed that a simple oxygen mask delivery of 2 to 4 liters/min offered no advantage over either a nasal cannula or catheter in providing a higher or more consistent tracheal $F_{I_{O_2}}$.[4]

Partial rebreathing and nonrebreathing masks facilitate delivery of a relatively high $F_{I_{O_2}}$. These masks incorporate an oxygen reservoir bag from which the patient breathes (Fig. 9-2). An advantage of the partial rebreather is that it provides a high $F_{I_{O_2}}$ while conserving the oxygen supply. Oxygen flow rate is regulated to permit the initial one third of the expired tidal volume (V_T) (anatomic dead space) to distend the reservoir maximally, thus preventing the entry of gas containing carbon dioxide, which instead exits through side ports in the mask. Theoretically, this mask reduces the oxygen requirement by approximately 30%, making it applicable to situations such as patient transport where the availability of oxygen is limited. A mean $F_{I_{O_2}}$ between 0.70 and 0.85 may be obtained with proper application of this device.

Nonrebreathing masks have unidirectional valves on each side of the mask that permit

Figure 9-2 Partial rebreathing reservoir and mask systems provide delivery of almost 100% oxygen.

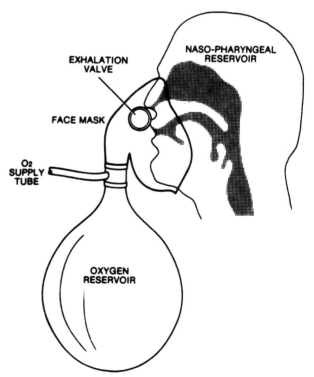

EXHALATION VALVE

NASO-PHARYNGEAL RESERVOIR

FACE MASK

O₂ SUPPLY TUBE

OXYGEN RESERVOIR

venting of exhaled VT while preventing inspiration of room air. Another one-way valve separates the reservoir bag from the mask to prevent retrograde flow of expired gas. Oxygen flow rate should be adequate to sustain the reservoir bag volume. When a disposable, bubble-through humidifier is employed, oxygen is vented to ambient through the pressure valve in the delivery unit at flow rates $\geq$ 15 liters/min; therefore, if a patient's minute ventilation exceeds that level, the humidifier must be bypassed or another one interfaced to provide sufficient gas flow. For short periods, the former solution is quick and generally proves innocuous for an hour or so. A mean $F_{I_{O_2}}$ of 0.80 to 0.95 is attainable with correct application of this system.

Oxygen-powered air-entrainment masks are designed to provide a high flow of gas at a known $F_{I_{O_2}}$ (Fig. 9-3). Oxygen is delivered to a small tube or jet-mixing device (previously discussed) that increases gas velocity. As the high-velocity stream exits from the jet nozzle, ambient air is entrained and dilutes the stream of pure oxygen. This high flow of mixed gas into the mask substantially exceeds the patient's minute ventilation; thus, no valving or reservoir is necessary to prevent rebreathing. The high flow also promotes consistent $F_{I_{O_2}}$ despite fluctuations in a patient's ventilatory pattern (*i.e.*, provides high capacitance of oxygen-enriched gas). Often, these masks are referred to as "venti-masks," implying that a Venturi tube is used, but the air-dilution mechanism actually occurs by jet-mixing.

Commercial air-entrainment masks facilitate the delivery of oxygen with an $F_{I_{O_2}}$ from 0.24 to 0.50. The level is controlled by graded adjustment of an entrainment port or by specific injector attachments. The latter masks are accompanied by a number of color-coded and labeled jets that produce a known $F_{I_{O_2}}$ at a given oxygen flow rate. The desired injector is connected to the inlet hose of the mask and powered by the designated oxygen flow. Most

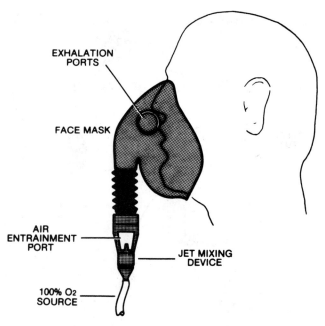

EXHALATION PORTS

FACE MASK

AIR ENTRAINMENT PORT

JET MIXING DEVICE

100% O₂ SOURCE

Figure 9-3 Air-entrainment masks are powered by 100% oxygen, which is diluted by air entrained through a jet-mixing device.

air-entrainment masks also have an adaptor that permits aerosol therapy at a lower $F_{I_{O_2}}$ than is possible with conventional oxygen-powered wall-mounted nebulizers.

NEBULIZERS

Wall-mounted nebulizers are often used to administer humidified oxygen to patients with artificial airways through a T-adaptor (Fig. 9-4) or tracheostomy collar. Oxygen is directed through a restricted orifice, creating a high-velocity jet stream, and then passes across one end of a small-diameter tube immersed in water, producing a subatmospheric pressure immediately adjacent to the tube. Because water surface pressure is atmospheric, liquid migrates up the tube; droplets are continuously fractured (aerosolized) by the jet stream and delivered to the inspiratory circuit.

Oxygen-powered nebulizers have an adjustable air-entrainment port providing $F_{I_{O_2}}$ from approximately 0.35 to 1.0. Two considerations are important. Because of inherent jet restriction, the maximum oxygen flow available to power most large-reservoir (wall-mounted) nebulizers is 14 to 16 liters/min at 50 psig. Normally, peak $\dot{V}_I$ is approximately three to four times resting minute ventilation (*i.e.*, 10–30 liters/min). When total flow to an aerosol circuit is less than the inspiratory demand, ambient air may be inhaled, thus decreasing the $F_{I_{O_2}}$. This problem often occurs when one treats a tachypneic patient with a high $F_{I_{O_2}}$ gas mixture because total gas flow is decreased. If a low-capacitance device (mask or tracheostomy collar) is used, two nebulizers may be interfaced in order to provide adequate gas flow. In T-tube circuits, the problem is solved by addition of sufficient reservoir tubing to the distal end of the T-adaptor.

HUMIDIFICATION

Humidity refers to moisture or water vapor in a gas. Completely saturated gas at 37°C contains 43.8 mg of water per liter, which generates a vapor pressure of 47 mm Hg. Alveolar gas has a relative humidity of 100% at 37°C. When the water content of inspired gas is

Figure 9-4 Jet nebulizer circuit with large water reservoir.

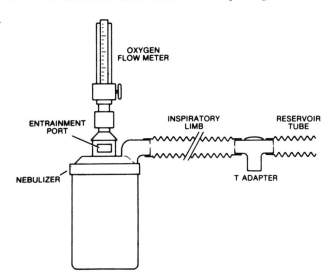

< 43.8 mg/liter at 37°C, vapor pressure is < 47 mm Hg, creating a "negative" pressure gradient (humidity deficit) between the inspired gas and respiratory mucosa. The amount of mucosal evaporation depends on this deficit. Mucosal dehydration increases mucus viscosity and reduces mucociliary clearance.

The humidification of oxygen delivered with a nasal cannula or catheter, partial rebreathing or nonrebreathing mask, or air-entrainment mask ("optional" since the gas mixture is partially humidified by entrained air) is often accomplished by passing gas through ambient temperature water. Usually it is directed into a submerged grid that fractionates the gas into tiny bubbles, thus increasing the gas–liquid interface area. Most commercially available bubble-through humidifiers increase the relative humidity of compressed oxygen from 0 to ~ 80% to 90% at 25°C.[5]

Warming, filtration, and humidification of inspired air occur in the upper respiratory tract. When this conditioning system is partially bypassed by an artificial airway, adequate humidification must be employed to minimize the humidity deficit. Under these conditions, a heated humidifier or an aerosol generator should be used. The Puritan-Bennett Cascade humidifier directs gas through a submerged grid causing small bubble formation (Fig. 9-5). The water reservoir is warmed by a heating element that was adjusted manually on the original model. A newer version employs a servo system in which water temperature is controlled by a thermistor at the proximal airway.

A recently manufactured wick humidifier is made by Bird Corporation (Fig. 9-6). Gas passes into a heated chamber containing a water-saturated wick. The water level is maintained uniformly by a reservoir feed system. A float mechanism periodically opens a valve, allowing water inflow to replace that which has evaporated from the wick. Wick chamber temperature is manually controlled, while the proximal airway temperature is measured by a thermistor and displayed on the control unit. Airway temperature is monitored to ensure

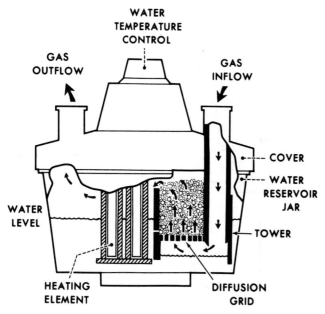

Figure 9-5 Schematic illustration of the Bennett Cascade humidifier. Dry gas flows through the tower and is fractionated by a submerged diffusion grid into small bubbles, which are dispersed through heated water.

Figure 9-6 The Bird humidifier.

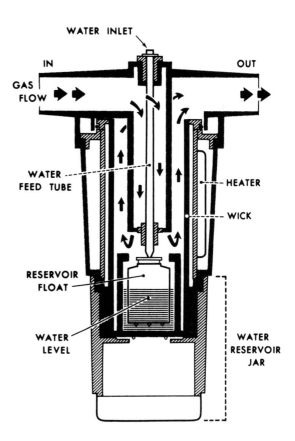

adequate moisture-carrying capacity (*i.e.*, almost 100% relative humidity at 37°C) and to avoid mucosal burns from hot inspired air.[6]

POTENTIAL COMPLICATIONS

HYPERCAPNIA

Patients with severe chronic obstructive pulmonary disease (COPD) develop progressive hypoxemia and hypercapnia. Despite these alterations, arterial and cerebrospinal fluid *p*H are normal because of increased bicarbonate levels. A few patients become "desensitized" to the respiratory stimulant effects of carbon dioxide, presumably maintaining ventilation by means of "hypoxemia receptor" drive originating in the carotid arteries and aortic arch. If this drive mechanism is ablated by administration of oxygen so that the Pa_{O_2} is above 55 to 60 mm Hg, ventilation is reduced significantly and carbon dioxide retention is exacerbated, possibly resulting in narcosis.[7]

Another cause of hypercapnia in chronically hypoxemic patients who receive supplemental oxygen is postulated to involve reduction of hypoxic pulmonary vasoconstriction in areas with low ventilation/perfusion ($\dot{V}/\dot{Q}$) ratios.[8] This vascular autoregulatory mechanism becomes inactive as a result of increased Pa_{O_2}, and the resulting failure to direct blood flow away from hypoventilated regions increases carbon dioxide retention. Nevertheless, potential ventilatory depression should never contraindicate oxygen therapy in severe hypoxemia. If hypoventilation is a major problem, other support measures, including mechanical ventilation, can be employed.

ABSORPTION ATELECTASIS

Alveoli in low $\dot{V}/\dot{Q}$ regions tend to remain patent because of the presence of nitrogen, which exhibits little tendency to volume change (nitrogen splinting). However, these lung units become unstable and collapse when high concentrations of oxygen rapidly "wash" nitrogen out of the alveoli. If oxygen uptake into the pulmonary capillary blood exceeds the amount supplied to low $\dot{V}/\dot{Q}$ units, alveolar collapse occurs.[9] This phenomenon has been reported in healthy individuals at an $F_{I_{O_2}} > 0.60$[9] and probably occurs at lower levels in patients with acute respiratory insufficiency.[10, 11]

PULMONARY OXYGEN TOXICITY

In 1775, Joseph Priestley recognized that

> though pure dephlogisticated air might be very useful as a medicine, it might not be so proper for use in the usually healthy state of the body; for, as a candle burns out much faster in dephlogistated than in common air, so we might live out too fast, and the animal powers be too soon exhausted in the pure king of air. A moralist may say that the air which nature has provided for us is as good as we deserve.[1]

In some respects, the dependence of living organisms on oxygen is paradoxic. Although it is essential for aerobic metabolism, too much oxygen or inappropriate oxygen metabolism can be toxic. Thus, survival in an oxygen environment involves a complex interaction between the biologic generation of very reactive chemical species called free radicals (atoms or molecules with one unpaired electron occupying an outer orbital) and the ability to harness these substances.

Mammals derive most of their cellular adenosine triphosphate by controlled, four-electron reduction of oxygen and the formation of hydrogen peroxide (H_2O_2, which is not a free radical) by the mitochondrial electron transport system. During the course of normal metabolism, oxygen can accept less than four electrons to form reactive species that may be cytotoxic to cells. These reactions include:

$$O_2 + e^- \longrightarrow O_2^{\cdot -} \text{ (superoxide)}$$
$$O_2 + 2\,e^- + 2\,H^+ \longrightarrow H_2O_2$$
$$O_2^{\cdot -} + H_2O_2 \longrightarrow {}_1O_2 + OH\cdot + OH^-$$
(singlet oxygen, hydroxyl radical, hydroxyl ion)
$$O_2 + 4\,e^- + 4\,H^+ \longrightarrow 2\,H_2O \text{ (water)}$$

The latter metabolites are thought to be particularly cytotoxic.[12]

The lone electron present in the outer orbital of a free radical endows it with very unusual chemical reactivity and physical characteristics. Free radical reactivity is accounted for by the strong tendency of this electron to pair with another, forming a chemical bond. These metabolites may be responsible for the inactivation of sulfhydral enzymes, the peroxidation of unsaturated membrane lipids and accompanying loss of membrane integrity, and the disruption of DNA syntheses.[13] Cells, however, contain protective antioxidants such as the enzymes superoxide dismutase (SOD), catalase, and glutathione reductase.[14]

Lung antioxidant enzyme levels are correlated with tolerance to hyperoxia, as shown by investigations with agents that induce production of these enzymes.[15,16] Pretreatment of rats with *Salmonella* endotoxin produces increased SOD and oxygen tolerance.[17] Laboratory animals pre-exposed to 0.80 ATA oxygen for several days increase SOD production and have increased survival rates when subsequently exposed to a near lethal dose treatment schedule of hyperoxia.[18] Other antioxidants, including alphatocopherol (the most active form of vitamin E), ascorbic acid (vitamin C), and β-carotene (vitamin A), also may play an important role in the scavenging and conversion of free radicals to less harmful forms.[14] During hyperoxia, increased free radical production presumably overwhelms intracellular scavenging and detoxification, precipitating cell damage and death.

Granular pneumocytes (type II cells) may be inherently resistant to hyperoxia.[16] Since ultrastructural changes appear relatively late, their response may be adaptive rather than toxic. They are thought by some to produce the majority of antioxidants available in the lungs. Thus, lungs with a high ratio of type II to type I pneumocytes (infants and patients recently exposed to hyperoxia or acute lung injury) appear to exhibit significant resistance to oxygen toxicity. Increases of lung enzyme activity in oxygen-tolerant and adapted animals apparently reflect alterations in the antioxidant capacity of individual cells or an increase in the number of cells exhibiting high antioxidant enzyme activity (*e.g.*, type II cells and alveolar macrophages). Further investigation of modalities that increase tolerance to hyperoxia may lead to significant improvement in our ability to administer oxygen therapeutically.

The $P_{I_{O_2}}$, rather than $F_{I_{O_2}}$, is the culprit in pulmonary oxygen toxicity. Overt histologic damage occurs at > 6 ATA oxygen, although individual susceptibility varies substantially, and more subtle alterations may occur at lower $P_{I_{O_2}}$.[16] The earliest manifestation of pulmonary hyperoxic toxicity is tracheobronchitis. Associated physiologic alterations include decreased mucociliary clearance, chest pain (usually substernal), cough, and reduced vital capacity. These changes develop within 24 hours at 1.0 ATA oxygen. Continued hyperoxic exposure between 48 and 72 hours produces progressive cellular changes, and areas of capillary endothelium and alveolar epithelium may become denuded. These histologic alterations are accompanied by interstitial fluid accumulation, decreased lung compliance and gas transfer, and polymorphonuclear leukocyte infiltration.[18–20] Death occurring at ≈ 72 hours of 1.0 ATA oxygen is attributed to pulmonary edema and respiratory failure.

Sublethal oxygen exposure is associated with repair and chronic pulmonary changes superimposed on the alterations induced by the underlying lung injury. Initial cytotoxicity and lung edema is followed by increased collagen formation and proliferation of interstitial fibroblasts and granular pneumocytes.[20] Hyperoxic breathing at 1.0 ATA oxygen for up to 24 hours is not associated with any significant risks. No clinically significant alterations in pulmonary function or gas exchange have been reported in subjects exposed to < 0.06 ATA oxygen for several weeks.

REFERENCE

1. Priestley J: Experiments and observations on different kinds of air. Reprinted in *The Discovey of Oxygen*, Part I, pp. 53–54. London, Gurney and Jackson, 1923

2. Scheele CW: Chemical treatise on air and fire. In *The Discovery of Oxygen*, Part II, p 41. London, Gurney and Jackson, 1923

3. Haldane JS, Priestley JG: *Respiration*, pp 8–26. Oxford, Clarendon Press, 1935

4. Sellers WFS, Huggs CMB: Comparison of tracheal oxygen concentrations using Hudson mask, nasal cannula and nasal catheter. *Anesth Analg* 1987; 66:S153

5. Klein EF Jr, Shah DA, Modell JH, et al: Performance characteristics of conventional and prototype humidifiers and nebulizers. *Chest* 1973; 64:690

6. Klein EF Jr, Graves SA: "Hot pot" tracheitis. *Chest* 1974; 65:225

7. Weil JV, Byrne-Quinn E, Sodal IE, et al: Hypoxic ventilatory drive in man. *J Clin Invest* 1970; 49:1061

8. Wagner PD, Dantzker DR, Dueck R, et al: Ventilation perfusion inequality in chronic obstructive lung disease. *J Clin Invest* 1977; 59:203

9. Nunn JF: *Applied Respiratory Physiology*, 2nd ed, p 367. London, Butterworths, 1979

10. Douglas ME, Downs JB, Dannemiller FJ, et al: Change in pulmonary venous admixture with varying inspired oxygen. *Anesth Analg* 1976; 55:688

11. Register SD, Downs JB, Stock MC, et al: Is 50% oxygen harmful? *Crit Care Med* 1987; 15:598.

12. Brigham KL: Role of free radicals in lung injury. *Chest* 1986; 89:6

13. Nickerson PA, Matalon S, Farhi LE: An ultrastructural study of alveolar permeability to cytochrome C in rabbit lung: Effect of exposure to 100% oxygen at one atmosphere. *Am J Pathol* 1981; 102:1

14. Beckman JS, Freeman BA: Antioxidant enzymes as mechanistic probes of oxygen-dependent toxicity. In Taylor AE, Matalon S, Ward PA (eds): *Physiology of Oxygen Radicals*, pp 39–53. Bethesda, MD, American Physiological Society, 1986

15. Massaro D, Massaro GD: Biochemical and anatomical adaptation of the lung to oxygen-induced injury. *Fed Proc* 1978; 37:26

16. Fisher AB, Forman HJ: Oxygen utilization and toxicity in the lungs. In Fishman AP, Fisher AB (eds): *The Respiratory System: Vol 1. Circulation and Nonrespiratory Functions*, pp 231–254 Bethesda, MD, American Physiological Society, 1985

17. Frank L, Summervile J, Massaro D: Protection from oxygen toxicity with endotoxin: The role of the endogenous antioxidant enzymes of the lung. *J Clin Invest* 1980; 65:1104

18. Kaplan HP, Robinson FR, Kapanci Y, et al: Pathogenesis and reversibility of the pulmonary lesions of oxygen toxicity in monkeys: I. Clinical and light microscopic studies. *Lab Invest* 1969; 20:94

19. Kapanci Y, Weibel ER, Kaplan HP, et al: Pathogenesis and reversibility of the pulmonary lesion of oxygen toxicity in monkeys: II. Ultrastructural and morphometric studies. *Lab Invest* 1969; 20:101

20. Pratt PC, Vollmer RT, Shelburne JD, et al: Pulmonary morphology in a multihospital collaborative extracorporeal membrane oxygenation project. I. Light microscopy. *Am J Pathol* 1979; 95:191

CHAPTER TEN

MECHANICAL VENTILATION

Michael J. Banner
Robert A. Smith

Mechanical ventilators are used to facilitate the movement of gas in and out of the lungs. The mechanisms of accomplishing this goal vary in design and performance. A comprehensive appreciation of the relationship between design and function is important not only in deciding which device to use in a particular situation but also in evaluating changes in the patient's ventilatory status. To understand the effects of mechanical ventilation on the lungs, it is necessary to be aware of pneumatic flow, pressure, and volume profiles.

CLASSIFICATION

All ventilator modes are divided into inspiratory and expiratory phases (Table 10-1). These phases allow a clinically oriented discussion of the design specifications and functional evaluation of mechanical ventilatory support mechanisms.

INSPIRATORY PHASE

Dynamic

Various mechanisms are used to facilitate positive-pressure inspiration (Table 10-2). Traditionally, such devices are grouped as flow or pressure generators, although no commonly employed ventilator functions entirely as one or the other. Indeed, some microprocessor-operated ventilators can be adjusted to function either way, depending on the selected mode. Nonetheless, the concept of flow and pressure generators is fundamental to understanding ventilator performance characteristics.

Flow generators produce a characteristic gas flow pattern despite changes in pulmonary mechanics. Ideal pneumatically powered flow generators must have a driving pressure at least 10 times the maximal encountered airway pressure. Structurally competent electromechanical flow generators are, in theory, not influenced by changes in airway pressure. In contrast, pressure generators develop consistent pressure waveforms, regardless of breath-to-breath patient changes. Almost all ICU ventilators are flow generators.

Flow generator output usually assumes one of four contours: constant (square wave),

TABLE 10-1 FUNCTIONAL CLASSIFICATION OF MECHANICAL VENTILATION

I. Inspiratory Phase
  A. Dynamic
    1. Flow generator
    2. Pressure generator
  B. Static
    1. End-inspiratory plateau
  C. Termination
    1. Volume-cycled
    2. Time-cycled
    3. Flow-cycled
    4. Pressure-cycled
	II. Expiratory Phase
	  A. Passive
	  B. Retardation
	  C. PEEP
	  D. Active
	  E. Termination
	    1. Time-cycled
	    2. Pressure-cycled
	    3. Flow-cycled

TABLE 10-2 MECHANISMS OF INSPIRATORY GAS FLOW

Injectors
  Bird Mark series ventilators, IMV Bird; Puritan-Bennett MA-1, MA-2; Engström Erica
Pistons
  Engström ER 300; Emerson 3PV, 3MV
	Solenoids
	  Bear-1, Bear-2; Puritan-Bennett 7200; Hamilton Veolar; Ohmeda CPU 1
	Stepper-Motors
	  Siemens Servo ventilators; Bear-5

sinusoidal, accelerating, or decelerating (Fig. 10-1). Some flow generators fail to maintain a uniform flow pattern in the face of increasing airway pressure; these devices actually have pressure generator characteristics. Flow generators incorporate injectors, pistons, on/off solenoid valves, servo-controlled solenoid valves, and servo-controlled stepper-motor valves. Pressure generators typically produce sigmoidol or constant, increasing rectilinear pressure curves.

Injectors. An injector is functionally based on the Bernoulli and Venturi principles. In 1738, Bernoulli observed that in tubes of varying caliber, the lateral pressure of a moving fluid is inversely proportional to velocity (Fig. 10-2). In 1797, Venturi demonstrated that to restore lateral wall pressure to a value similar to that proximal to a constriction, the tube distal to the constriction must gradually expand. If the widening angle exceeds 15°, pressure cannot be reestablished (Fig. 10-3).

As subatmospheric pressure is created by the accelerated gas flow velocity at the constriction, additional gas is entrained and the total flow output is delivered either directly to the lungs (Bird Mark series ventilators, IMV Bird) or to a chamber where a gas-filled bellows (Puritan-Bennett MA-1, MA-2) (Fig. 10-4) or bladder (Engström Erica) is compressed, delivering its contents to the patient. Injector performance is affected by the outlet pressure; as the latter increases during inspiration, entrained gas flow rate and total flow decline. Against zero back-pressure (*i.e.*, at the onset of inspiration), the flow rate is constant. As downstream pressure reduces injector efficiency, flow decelerates. When outlet pressure rises sufficiently to prevent further gas entrainment, the injector stall point is reached. Completion of tidal volume delivery necessitates that the duration of inspiration be increased (Fig. 10-5). Injector performance is nearly optimal when the stall pressure exceeds 100 cm H_2O.

Figure 10-1 Four common inspiratory flow ($\dot{V}$I) trajectories (patterns). The trajectory is determined by the location of the peak $\dot{V}$ point during inspiration and whether $\dot{V}$ is sustained (constant) or incrementally altered (decelerating, sinusoidal, accelerating).

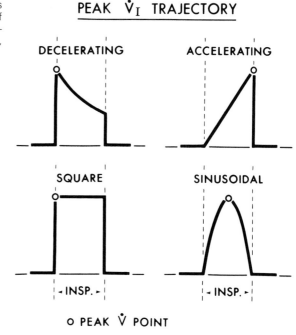

Piston Pumps. Positive–negative displacement devices (piston pumps) move a specific volume of gas with each stroke (Fig. 10-6). "Negative" displacement (*i.e.*, downward motion within the cylinder) entrains a preselected volume of gas. Positive (upward) piston motion displaces the gas volume into the breathing circuit (Emerson 3PV, 3 MV) or into a rigid canister to compress a gas-filled rubber bag (Engström ER 300). Gas within the bag is then delivered to the lungs. In most cases, the inspiratory stroke is guided by a linkage rod attached to the perimeter of a revolving wheel. This mechanical configuration provides a sinusoidal flow contour.

Figure 10-2 The Bernoulli principle. A laminar restriction tube is depicted at *B*. Bulk flow rate is equal at points *A, B,* and *C*; however, flow is more rapid through the restriction. Bernoulli observed that lateral wall pressure is inversely proportional to fluid velocity.

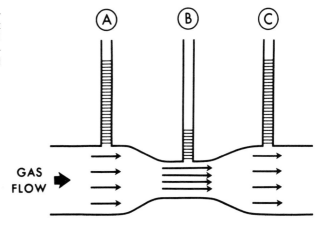

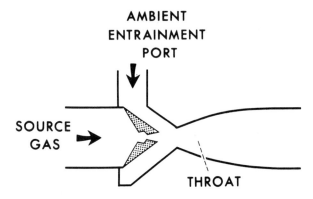

AMBIENT ENTRAINMENT PORT

SOURCE GAS

THROAT

Figure 10-3 An injector (Venturi tube) incorporates principles elucidated by Bernoulli and Venturi. Compressed source gas is directed through a restriction (jet) creating subatmospheric pressure which causes air entrainment. Total flow in the throat equals the sum of jet and entrained flows.

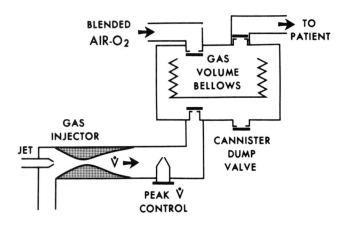

Figure 10-4 During mechanical inspiration, flow from a gas injector (Bennett MA-1, MA-2) is directed into a rigid canister to compress a bellows. The bellows content is delivered to the breathing circuit.

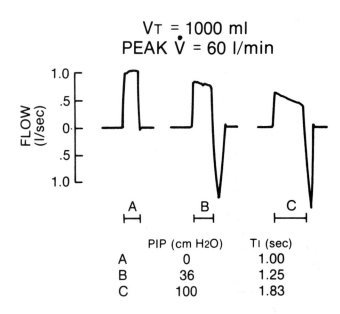

$V_T = 1000$ ml
PEAK $\dot{V} = 60$ l/min

	PIP (cm H2O)	TI (sec)
A	0	1.00
B	36	1.25
C	100	1.83

Figure 10-5 Flow curves during volume-cycled, injector-powered, mechanical insufflation (Bennett MA-2) at 0 (A), 36 (B), and 100 (C) cm H_2O PIP. Since injector flow decreases with increased PIP, inspiratory time (TI) must increase to maintain V_T.

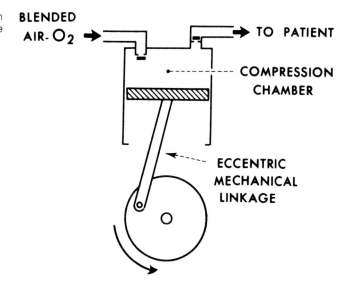

Figure 10-6 The mechanical inflation mechanism used by a piston ventilator (Emerson 3 MV; see text).

On/Off Solenoid Valves. These valves are used in conjunction with a high-pressure gas source to generate inspiratory flow. A solenoid valve insufflation mechanism is illustrated in Figure 10-7 (Bear-1). In this example, source gas is regulated to a driving pressure of 3.2 or 1.8 psig (225 cm H_2O and 127 cm H_2O, respectively). During inspiration, the solenoid opens, directing gas through the peak flow control and into the breathing circuit. When the driving pressure is 3.2 psig, gas flow into the circuit is constant at the selected peak flow rate. However, at 1.8 psig, as the gradient between driving pressure and breathing circuit pressure narrows, flow rate declines from the selected peak value.[1] Significant flow deceleration does not occur until the peak inspiratory (inflation) pressure (PIP) exceeds 70 cm H_2O.

Servo-Controlled Solenoid Valves. These mechanisms are used in some microprocessor operated ventilators (Puritan-Bennett 7200, Hamilton Veolar). The Hamilton flow valve (Fig. 10-8) is a representative microprocessor-controlled solenoid. Gas flows from a high-pressure reservoir through an isosceles-triangle-shaped orifice into the inspiratory limb of the breathing circuit. The orifice opening (height) is modulated by a motor through a shaft, which oscillates similarly to the high-speed positive–negative movement (vibration) of a loudspeaker. Electric current is passed through a coil connected to the triangular plunger by a

Figure 10-7 An On/Off electronic solenoid valve (Bear 2) used to facilitate positive-pressure inflation. A toggle switch is positioned to regulate the driving pressure of blended gas delivered to the peak flow control.

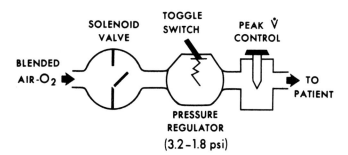

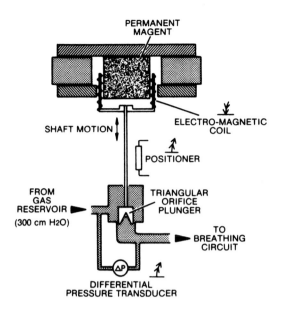

Figure 10-8 Microprocessor-controlled electromagnetic flow valve (Hamilton Veolar; see text).

shaft, producing a variable magnetic field at the apex of the valve housing. The magnitude of the electric current is altered by a microprocessor that compares (references) the preselected ventilatory parameters entered into its memory from the control panel to the actual gas flow traversing the valve. The height of the triangular orifice is a determinant of its area and is measured by a position sensor that generates a continuous signal to the microprocessor. When the differential pressure across the orifice is constant, the flow is proportional to the area. By sensing the height of the triangular orifice and continually correcting variations in differential pressure, the ventilator delivers flows from 20 to 3000 ml/sec in constant, sinusoidal, decelerating, or accelerating waveform patterns. This closed-loop, servo-controlled system functions almost instantaneously.[2]

A block diagram of the servo loop for mechanical inspiration with the Hamilton Veolar is depicted in Figure 10-9. Analog signals from the various inspiratory control knob potentiometers are converted to digital signals to allow microprocessing. A digital signal is generated for each parameter: tidal volume (V_T), inspiratory time (T_I), inspiratory flow ($\dot{V}_I$)

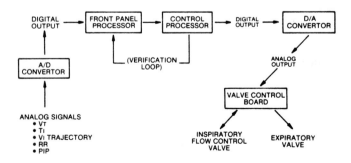

Figure 10-9 Electronic subsystem of a microprocessor-controlled mechanical inspiration (see text).

pattern or trajectory, respiratory rate (RR), and PIP. Once digitized, parameter-specific signals are sent (bused) to the front panel processor (FPP) and then to the control processor (CP). The FPP and CP operate in different areas of the ventilator but are linked with a verification loop to ensure that each digitized command is executed correctly. Digital output from the CP is converted to an analog signal and bused to the valve control board. Appropriate current is then passed to the electrodynamic motor of the insufflation valve to facilitate V_T delivery with the specified characteristics. During this phase, the exhalation valve is simultaneously closed.

Servo-Controlled Stepper Motors. A servo-controlled stepper motor insufflation valve is incorporated into the Bear-5 ventilator (Fig. 10-10). Blended gas from 10 to 18 psig (703 to 1265 cm H_2O) enters the flow control valve. Gas flow is controlled by a variable orifice. The valve shaft is attached to a stepper motor, the position of which is controlled by the central processing unit (CPU) through linear movement of the shaft. This motion determines the position of a ball, which creates a variable orifice. Two optical sensors detect zero and full flow positions of the valve. An optical disc mounted on the shaft interrupts the zero optical sensor light beam when the valve is closed. The same optical disc blocks the full-range optical sensor when the valve is maximally open. Nominal rotation is 189 steps (170°). The valve, in conjunction with the internal flow transducer and CPU, forms a servo gas control system capable of up to 150 liters/min peak flow rate in constant, sinusoidal, decelerating, or accelerating contours.

Once V_T, peak $\dot{V}_I$, waveform, and circuit compliance compensation (optional adjustment) are entered by the operator, the CPU monitors gas flow ($\dot{V}$) and sends instructions to the stepper motor. The internal transducer measures real time $\dot{V}$ output and transmits this value to the CPU. If actual $\dot{V}$ is different from that stipulated, adjustments are made accordingly. If during spontaneous breathing the selected peak $\dot{V}$ is exceeded, causing a

Figure 10-10 A microprocessor-controlled, stepper-motor actuated inspiratory flow valve system (Bear 5; see text).

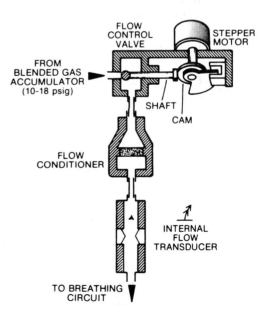

reduction in proximal airway pressure, the demand system provides supplemental $\dot{V}$ up to 170 liters/min for the duration of inspiration; thus, delivered V_T may exceed programmed V_T.[3]

Automatic flow supplementation illustrates the uniqueness of servo-controlled inspiration. This feature may be of particular importance in managing patients with labile ventilatory drive and inspiratory $\dot{V}$ demand during patient-triggered (assisted) mechanical ventilation. If peak $\dot{V}$ is adjusted improperly, significant patient–ventilator phasing problems can precipitate excessive work of breathing and/or a sensation of "air hunger," despite the fact that each breath is volume-augmented. Servo-controlled $\dot{V}$ supplementation helps to buffer the inadequacies of suboptimal mechanical breaths.

Static

During dynamic mechanical positive-pressure inspiration, gas flow into the lungs is facilitated by the pressure gradient developed between the proximal airway and alveoli. Proximal airway pressure generated for a given V_T depends primarily upon pulmonary (lung–thorax) resistance and compliance characteristics. This relationship can be expressed as follows:

$$PIP = V_T/Cdyn + (Raw \times \dot{V}_I),$$

where PIP = peak inspiratory pressure (cm H_2O); Cdyn = effective dynamic compliance (ml/cm H_2O); Raw = airway resistance (cm H_2O/liter/sec).

Resistive and elastic components of the PIP can be estimated by performing a 1.5- to 2.5-second postinflation hold or end-inspiratory plateau (EIP). This phase represents a no-flow component of mechanical inspiration (Fig. 10-11). After V_T delivery, exhalation valve opening is delayed for a selected time interval. The EIP can be used to distinguish between Cdyn and static compliance (Cst). Impedance to gas flow (airway resistance) and volume expansion (lung–chest wall elastance) determine Cdyn. It is equal to V_T divided by the PIP minus baseline pressure (PEEP or atmospheric). Static compliance quantitates the distensibility of the lung–chest wall and is equal to V_T divided by EIP minus baseline pressure. Compliance is commonly expressed as ml/cm H_2O. The disparity between Cdyn and Cst is a reflection of Raw.

Figure 10-11 Inspiratory and expiratory pressure components of mechanical ventilator cycles.

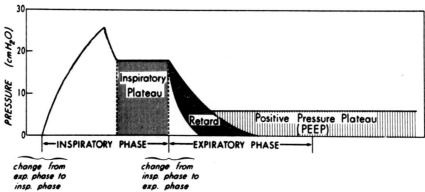

Calculation of Raw is problematic, since instantaneous $\dot{V}$ measurement is required along with simultaneous calculation of the pressure gradient between the proximal and distal ends of the resistor (*e.g.,* airway). Some microprocessor ventilators provide both inspiratory and expiratory Raw. However, inspiratory Raw can be estimated when VT is delivered by a constant flow generator:

$$Raw = PIP - EIP/\dot{V}_{peak.}$$

An EIP presumably facilitates more homogeneous distribution of inspired gas volume, particularly when lung compartments have dissimilar time constants (Raw × Cdyn). When adjacent lung units are ventilated, the gas volume delivered to each is dependent on its respective total impedance. Lung regions with high impedance fill slowly (slow spaces), whereas those with low impedance inflate more rapidly (fast spaces). Ventilation to slow spaces is adversely affected by high velocity and turbulent inspiratory flow.

Termination (Inspiratory to Expiratory Cycling)

Volume. Volume-cycled inspiration is terminated after delivery of a preselected VT to the ventilator circuit. A common misconception is that volume delivery to the patient is also constant despite alterations in pulmonary mechanics. However, a portion of the VT is lost by distention of and compression within the ventilator and breathing circuit and does not reach the lungs. The magnitude of this volume loss is determined primarily by breathing circuit compliance and PIP. Similar disparities in the preselected versus patient-delivered volumes occur with all conventional ventilators, regardless of their inspiratory cycling mechanisms. The Bear-5 microprocessor ventilator permits automatic circuit compliance compensation. A compliance factor, determined by the volume/pressure characteristic of the breathing circuit and humidifier, is entered into the CPU. The PIP is "read" by the CPU every fourth breath, and flow adjustments are made to add the necessary additional volume to compensate for that "lost" in the circuit.

Time. Time-cycled inspiration is terminated after a preselected interval. Ventilatory cycling phases are programmed by manipulating one of the following: inspiratory and expiratory time (Emerson 3PV, IMV Bird); inspiratory time (Emerson 3MV, Bear-5); or inspiratory and EIP times as a percentage of total cycle time (Siemens Servo 900C, Hamilton Veolar). The VT delivered by time-cycled ventilators is either selected (Emerson, Servo 900C, Hamilton Veolar) or is a function of inspiratory time and $\dot{V}_I$ (IMV Bird).

Pressure-controlled ventilation with the Servo 900C is a time-cycled mode in which the ventilator functions as a constant pressure generator. Gas flow to the breathing circuit is adjusted automatically to maintain a constant pressure for a selected time interval, even in the face of moderate air leaks. Since the exhalation valve remains closed throughout inspiration, this technique effectively provides an inspiratory pressure plateau (the so-called reverse I:E ratio) only in patients whose breathing patterns are well phased with the ventilator (*i.e.,* those who are not attempting to breathe spontaneously during the mechanical inspiratory phase).

A time-cycled, pressure-limited inspiratory plateau can also be administered with the Bear-5 ventilator. In this case, a continuous fresh gas flow is provided to the breathing circuit. The exhalation valve pilot tube pressure equals the selected inspiratory pressure, thereby allowing effective spontaneous ventilation to occur during the plateau phase (in essence, spontaneous continuous positive airway pressure, or CPAP). This feature should reduce rebreathing by tachypneic patients during a plateau phase exceeding 1.5 seconds.

In the pressure-controlled mode, ventilators function as flow-servoed, time-cycled, constant pressure generators. Tidal volume is principally dependent on effective Cdyn. Also, since additional $\dot{V}i$ is available, this is a dynamic rather than a static inspiratory plateau mode.

Flow. Flow-cycled inspiration is terminated when the gas flow rate decreases to a predetermined level. This mechanism is employed by microprocessor-based ventilators offering inspiratory pressure support (PS) modes. When PS is activated, inspiration continues until the flow rate decays to 25% (Servo 900C, Hamilton Veolar, Bear-5) of the initial peak value. This technique is discussed in detail later.

Pressure. Pressure-cycled inspiration is terminated when a preselected pressure is achieved within the ventilator circuit. At this point, inspiratory gas flow ceases and the exhalation valve opens. Tidal volume and Ti are related directly to pulmonary compliance and inversely to airway resistance and circuit impedance. Significant leaks in the circuit or at the airway prevent development of the requisite inspiratory cycling pressure. Many of the ventilators employed for intermittent positive pressure breathing (IPPB) therapy (Bird Mark series) are pressure-cycled. Nearly all time-, volume-, and flow-cycling ventilators can be adjusted to terminate inspiration at a preselected PIP. This feature is incorporated as a safety measure in case the primary cycling mechanism fails. Notable exceptions include the Emerson and IMV Bird ventilators, which employ an adjustable mechanical relief valve to limit circuit pressure. When this relief pressure threshold is reached, time-cycled gas flow continues but is vented to ambient.

EXPIRATORY PHASE

Mechanical expiration commences when the exhalation valve opens. As lung deflation occurs, pressure normally declines rapidly to the atmospheric (ambient) level. Alternatively, the valve may open gradually (or only partially) to provide resistance (retardation) to exhalation (see Fig. 10-11). Finally , it may open until the circuit pressure decreases to a preselected positive level, at which point it again closes to maintain this pressure (PEEP).

Exhalation valves are pneumatically or electronically seated. A pneumatic balloon valve is illustrated in Figure 10-12. The exhalation pilot control solenoid is a three-way valve that selects the pneumatic source for exhalation valve control. During all mechanical inspirations (spontaneous or controlled), pneumatic power is shunted from the main insufflation valve, pressurizes the exhalation valve pilot tube, and closes the balloon valve, preventing gas leakage out of the circuit. During exhalation, the valve is depressurized to ambient or PEEP levels.[4]

An electronic exhalation valve is incorporated by the Hamilton Veolar ventilator (Fig. 10-13). The exhalation valve consists of a metallic disc incorporated into a silicone rubber membrane enclosed in a plastic housing. It is closed with a linear motion electronic motor similar to the inspiratory flow control valve (see Fig. 10-8). During inspiration, electric current is passed through the coil, creating an electromagnetic field with the same polarity as the permanent magnet; thus, the silicone membrane is seated by the downward motion (repulsion) of the actuating shaft, which also compresses a spring. Expiration occurs when

Figure 10-12 Pneumatically actuated balloon exhalation/PEEP valve system (Bennett 7200; see text).

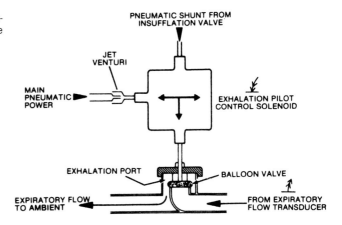

the electric current switches off, eliminating the electromagnetic field. The weight of the coil/actuating shaft is offset by the spring tension, thus minimizing valve resistance and allowing the exhalation valve to open.

Passive

Expiration usually is a passive event facilitated by a positive alveolar-to-ambient pressure gradient resulting from lung–chest-wall recoil. Expiration time depends on the magnitude of this pressure gradient and the airway resistance. Resistance to expiration also results from external sources (endotracheal tubes, ventilator circuitry).

Retardation

Expiratory flow retardation occasionally is employed to prevent premature airway closure and air trapping in patients with obstructive pulmonary lesions. Retardation of expiratory gas flow decreases the slope of the expiratory pressure curve (see Fig. 10-11), maintaining back pressure in the small airways and, in effect, splinting them open. Indications for this application are debatable but generally include conditions in which the inspired volume exceeds that which is expired. In such circumstances, if a circuit leak is not present, one can reasonably infer that pulmonary air trapping is occurring.

Figure 10-13 Electromagnetic exhalation/PEEP valve mechanism (Hamilton Veolar; see text).

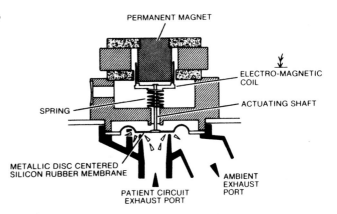

Apart from acute or chronic obstructive lung disease (asthma, emphysema), the most frequent causes of air trapping ("inadvertent" PEEP) are iatrogenic and involve an excessively high ventilator cycling frequency or VT. Persistent pulmonary hyperinflation is associated with hypercapnia, reduced venous return, increased pulmonary artery pressure, and parenchymal injury or barotrauma.

Positive End-Expiratory Pressure

Positive end-expiratory pressure is produced by maintaining a residual positive circuit pressure during expiration (see Fig. 10-11). Several mechanisms are employed to generate this pressure with the exhalation valve. In the Hamilton Veolar, an electric current is directed to the coil of the electromagnetic exhalation valve, producing the force required for the desired pressure (see Fig. 10-13). When the patient's expiratory force falls below the downward force of the silicone membrane, the valve seats, preventing further exhalation and loss of lung volume. Pneumatically actuated PEEP/CPAP mechanisms are discussed in detail later.

Active

Reduction of circuit pressure during the expiratory phase speeds up or actively facilitates expiration. The effect depends on the duration and magnitude of the reduction. If it is maintained only until ambient airway pressure is restored, expiration is accelerated, lung volume does not decrease below FRC, and intrapleural pressure does not fall below its resting level. However, if a subatmospheric circuit pressure develops (negative end-expiratory pressure, or NEEP), lung volume falls below FRC and intrapleural pressure decreases beyond its normal end-expiratory level. A significant reduction in FRC is associated with atelectasis and hypoxemia. If such a pressure is applied to the airway in patients with chronic obstructive pulmonary disease, premature airway collapse and air trapping can result.

Originally, NEEP was introduced to buffer the hemodynamic effects of positive-pressure ventilation. However, its use in adults was short-lived because the induced lung dysfunction outweighed any potential hemodynamic benefit.

Termination (Expiratory to Inspiratory Cycling)

Changeover from the expiratory to inspiratory phase can be time-, pressure-, or flow-cycled.

Time. During controlled mechanical ventilation (CMV), the duration between breaths is time dependent and is unaffected by patient effort. Direct selection of mechanical expiration time (TE) with a function-specific control is available on a limited number of adult ventilators (Emerson 3PV, IMV Bird). Indirect control results from interaction between the selected CMV rate (or total cycle time) and either TI (Emerson 3MV), I:E ratio or percent of total cycle time (Siemens 900C, Engström Erica, Hamilton Veolar), or peak $\dot{V}$, $\dot{V}_I$, $\dot{V}_I$ waveform, and VT (Puritan-Bennett 7200, Bear-5). In the latter case, $\dot{V}_I$ determines how rapidly VT is delivered (see Fig. 10-5). Thus, at a constant CMV rate and VT, TE is directly proportional to $\dot{V}_I$. Time-cycled controlled exhalation is used in intermittent mandatory ventilation (IMV) and high-frequency ventilation (HFV) techniques.

Pressure. Pressure-cycled termination of expiration results from a decrease in airway pressure caused by the patient's inspiratory effort. It is independent of time. A pressure transducer is interfaced with the breathing circuit, threshold (sensitivity) control, and cycling mechanism. The magnitude of airway pressure reduction necessary to terminate exhalation is adjusted with the sensitivity control. Spontaneous breaths (no driving pressure) are provided by demand-flow mechanisms or from reservoir bags (discussed later).

Flow. Exhalation can be terminated by flow-cycling (Engström Erica). A patient-triggered 0.1 liter/sec flow rate is sensed by a pneumotachometer, which is claimed (although not proven) to be more responsive than pressure-cycled mechanisms.

AIR–OXYGEN BLENDING

The fraction of inspired oxygen ($F_{I_{O_2}}$) must be adjustable and independent of circuit pressure fluctuations during prolonged mechanical ventilation. All modern ventilators incorporate either a compressed air and oxygen mixing mechanism or a system to dilute compressed oxygen with ambient air. The latter method is facilitated by ventilators with a bellows design (Puritan-Bennett MA-1, MA-2; Monaghan 225; Ohio 550). The compressed oxygen source gas is regulated to a low pressure (*e.g.*, 1 to 4 cm H_2O) and, along with ambient air, is combined to produce the selected $F_{I_{O_2}}$ as both gases are "pulled" into the descending bellows during exhalation (see Fig. 10-4).

Nonbellows ventilators blend compressed air and oxygen to the desired $F_{I_{O_2}}$. Air–oxygen blenders are commonly powered by 40 to 50 psig air and oxygen sources. One of the original designs, conceived by Forrest M. Bird, matches source gas pressures to the lowest value with a pair of reducing valves (Fig. 10-14), following which air and oxygen are interfaced with a proportioning valve and mixed to the selected $F_{I_{O_2}}$. The blended gas is then delivered through a needle valve to the inspiration circuitry.

Later air–oxygen blending mechanisms, such as that in the Hamilton Veolar, exhibit similar technical features (Fig. 10-15). A movable piston is located within a cylinder containing a series of radial orifices. Compressed air and oxygen enter the cylinder separately. Piston position is set with the $F_{I_{O_2}}$ control knob and determines the proportion of air and oxygen. Three to four liters (depending upon pressure) of mixed gas compressed at approximately 300 to 350 cm H_2O is accumulated as a reservoir for the inspiratory flow circuitry. Such reservoirs are also used in the Bear-5 and Siemens Servo 900C ventilators and tend to minimize fluctuations in $F_{I_{O_2}}$, particularly during conditions of high flow and frequent cycling.

CONTINUOUS POSITIVE AIRWAY PRESSURE AND SPONTANEOUS POSITIVE END-EXPIRATORY PRESSURE

Continuous positive airway pressure and spontaneous positive end-expiratory pressure (sPEEP) are positive pressure modes used with spontaneous breathing. They can be employed individually or in conjunction with mechanical ventilation (IMV). With CPAP, both inspiratory and expiratory pressures are positive, although the inspiratory level is less than is the expiratory. With sPEEP, airway pressure is zero or negative (subambient) during inspiration but increases at the end of expiration to a predetermined positive pressure (Fig. 10-16). The level of CPAP or sPEEP used is designated by the value measured at end-expiration. Both are designed to increase expiratory transpulmonary pressure and lung volume (functional

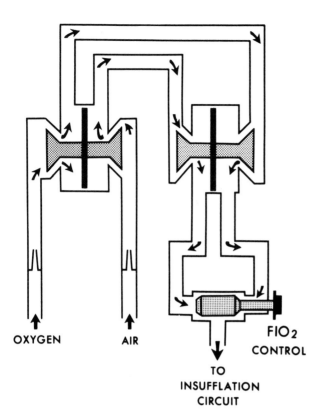

Figure 10-14 Air–oxygen blender uses staged pressure equilibration and a needle valve to provide the desired F_{IO_2} (see text).

OXYGEN

AIR

FIO_2
CONTROL

TO
INSUFFLATION
CIRCUIT

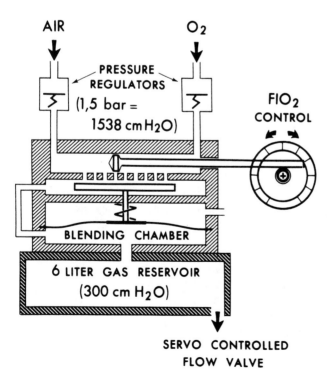

Figure 10-15 Air–oxygen blender system (Hamilton ventilator) that incorporates a mixed gas reservoir (see text).

AIR

O_2

PRESSURE
REGULATORS
(1,5 bar =
1538 cm H_2O)

FIO_2
CONTROL

BLENDING CHAMBER

6 LITER GAS RESERVOIR
(300 cm H_2O)

SERVO CONTROLLED
FLOW VALVE

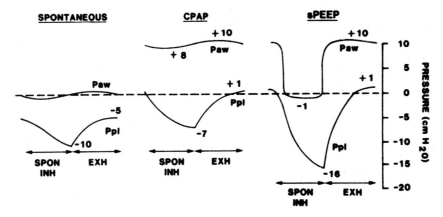

Figure 10-16 Paw and Ppl waveforms for spontaneous ventilation, CPAP, 10 cm H_2O, and sPEEP, 10 cm H_2O. The periods of spontaneous inspiration and expiration are indicated for all three forms of breathing. Transpulmonary pressure (Paw − Ppl) at end-inspiration increases normally from 5 to 10 cm H_2O for spontaneous ventilation, and in these examples from 9 to 15 cm H_2O for CPAP and sPEEP.

residual capacity). Inspiratory and mean airway pressures do not reflect the total alveolar distending pressure at end-expiration (Fig. 10-17).

EQUIPMENT

A variety of mechanical devices are used to deliver CPAP. A common and convenient method, with or without a ventilator, uses continuous gas flow (usually 10 to 20 liters/min

Figure 10-17 Pressure and volume changes in the lung during spontaneous ventilation with CPAP. *A,* With ARDS, the lung characteristically has reduced FRC; airway pressure is zero. *B,* CPAP increases the airway pressure to 10 cm H_2O and restores FRC to normal. *C,* During spontaneous inspiration, airway pressure decreases to 5 cm H_2O while inspiratory transpulmonary pressure (see Fig. 10-1) and lung volume increase. *D,* At end-expiration, airway pressure returns to 10 cm H_2O, and the lung volume to FRC.

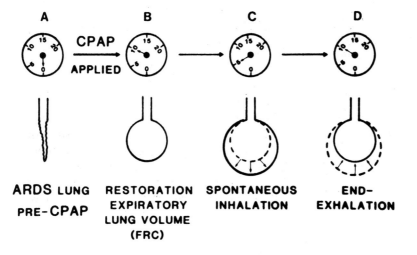

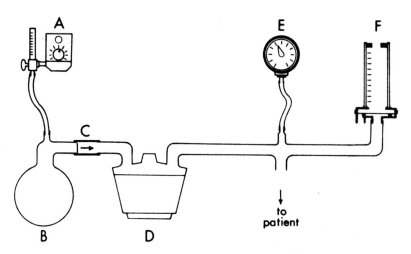

Figure 10-18 Reservoir bag CPAP system. *A,* Air/oxygen blender and flowmeter; *B,* 3-liter reservoir bag; *C,* one-way valve; *D,* humidifier; *E,* aneroid pressure manometer; and *F,* threshold resistor expiratory pressure valve (Emerson).

at a specified $F_{I_{O_2}}$), a reservoir bag, one-way valve, humidifier, and an expiratory pressure valve (Fig. 10-18). Both $F_{I_{O_2}}$ and gas flow rate are precisely regulated by an air–oxygen blender with a back-pressure-compensated flow meter. The gas is directed into a 3-liter bag that acts as a reservoir for the patient's breathing. It then passes through the one-way valve, which opens during spontaneous inspiration and closes during expiration. During expiration, when breathing circuit/airway pressure is greatest, a compliant reservoir bag will distend or "balloon" to a larger volume. Expiratory closure of the one-way valve precludes retrograde flow to the reservoir bag and maintains a fairly nondistensible breathing circuit, with only the expiratory valve influencing airway pressure.

Expiratory Pressure Valves

Expiratory pressure valves regulate the level of airway pressure during CPAP and sPEEP, as well as during mechanical ventilation with PEEP. They are characterized as threshold resistors and flow resistors.[5,6] In theory, threshold resistors generate pressure (P) without associated additional flow resistance.[7] Pressure from a threshold resistor results from a force (F), expressed in newtons (N), over a discrete surface area (SA), expressed in square meters (m^2):

$$P \propto F/SA$$

A loading F of 1000 N applied to an SA of 1 m^2 generates a P of 10 cm H_2O (100 $N/m^2 \simeq 1$ cm H_2O). Exhaled gas passes freely through the completely open threshold resistor orifice until the balance of forces on opposite sides of the valve mechanism comes into equilibrium at end-expiration.[6] At this point, the valve closes abruptly, preventing further gas loss from the airways and lungs (Fig. 10-19).

In contrast, flow resistors generate P by imposing resistance (R) to exhaled flow by means of an adjustable orifice (Fig. 10-20):

$$P \propto R\dot{V}$$

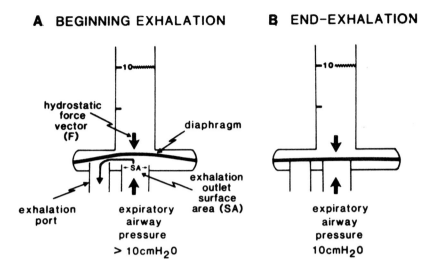

A BEGINNING EXHALATION   **B** END-EXHALATION

Figure 10-19 Emerson water column threshold resistor ($P\alpha^F/_{SA}$). Positive pressure (P) results from a force (F) applied to a surface area (SA). Opening and closing of the valve diaphragm is dependent on the balance of forces across it. *A,* At the beginning of exhalation, force resulting from the patient's airway pressure against the bottom side of the diaphragm is greater than the hydrostatic F vector, resulting from pressure of the water column against the upper surface. Consequently, the diaphragm rises, allowing exhalation. *B,* At end-expiration, the forces acting across the valve are in equilibrium and the diaphragm descends, occluding the exhalation outlet. (Banner MJ, Lampotang S, Boysen PG, et al: Flow resistance of expiratory positive pressure valve systems. *Chest* 1986; 90:212)

Assuming V is constant, P varies directly with R. This relationship holds true only under laminar flow conditions and within a given range of flow rates. For example, if R is 10 cm H₂O/liter/sec and exhaled V̇ is 1 liter/sec, so long as these conditions prevail, P ≈ 10 cm H₂O. A threshold resistor should maintain a set pressure regardless of variations in exhaled

Figure 10-20 A flow resistor (PαRV̇) screw-clamp variable orifice) generates expiratory positive pressure *(plus sign)* dependent on the product of resistance *(R)* and flow *(V)* directed through the valve. Resistance varies inversely with orifice size. A smaller exhalation orifice increases R and P (assuming constant flow) and vice versa. (Banner MJ, Lampotang S, Boysen PG, et al: Flow resistance of expiratory positive pressure valve systems. *Chest* 1986; 90:212)

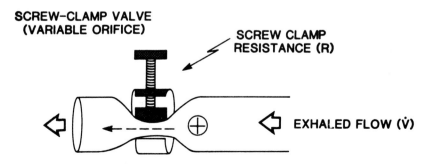

SCREW-CLAMP VALVE (VARIABLE ORIFICE)

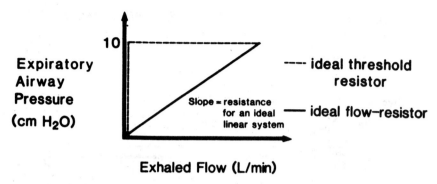

Figure 10-21 An ideal threshold resistor maintains a constant expiratory airway pressure at all flow rates. In contrast with an ideal flow resistor, expiratory airway pressure varies linearly with flow rate.

flow rate,[7] as opposed to a flow resistor, in which deviations in airway pressure occur when gas flow rate through the system is changed (Fig. 10-21).

A third type of expiratory pressure valve is the pneumatic balloon valve described previously (see Fig. 10-12). Balloon valves combine the properties of threshold and flow resistors.[6,8,9]

In actuality, resistance to exhaled flow occurs to a variable degree with all three types of valves.[8-11] When exhaled $\dot{V}$ is high, as occurs with coughing, very high airway pressures may result,[9] possibly predisposing the patient to an increased risk of barotrauma. For example, consider two threshold resistor valves set at a pressure of 10 cm H_2O. If, with valve 1, R is 10 cm H_2O/liter/sec and total flow directed through the valve (system flow plus exhaled flow) is 1 liter/sec (60 liters/min), then expiratory pressure is 20 cm H_2O. In contrast, with valve 2, in which R is 1 cm H_2O/liter/sec and total flow directed through the valve is 1 liter/sec, expiratory pressure is 11 cm H_2O. If valve 1 is used and the patient suddenly coughs, generating a peak exhaled flow of 4 liters/sec, expiratory pressure increases to 50 cm H_2O. Under the same conditions with valve 2, pressure increases to only 14 cm H_2O. As is obvious, resistance, even with threshold resistors, is quite variable. For categorization, high-resistance (e.g., valve 1) and low-resistance (e.g., valve 2) threshold resistors can be designated. Only low-resistance threshold resistors should be used in CPAP systems (eg., Vital Signs, Hamilton, and Emerson)[12] in order to maintain airway pressure essentially constant in the face of variations in expiratory flow rate.

Work of Breathing

The relationship between the rate of gas inflow provided to the breathing circuit and the rate of the patient's inspiratory flow is a factor that determines whether CPAP or sPEEP results. If the rate of gas inflow to a low-resistance breathing circuit is greater than the rate of the patient's spontaneous inspiratory flow, CPAP results (i.e., pressure is always positive). Conversely, when the rate of inflow to the breathing circuit is less than the rate of the patient's inspiratory flow, sPEEP results (i.e., pressure at the peak of inspiration is 0 or subambient; Fig. 10-22). In the latter situation, increased inspiratory work of breathing results (Fig. 10-23).[13] An increase in work required to breathe against the external load of

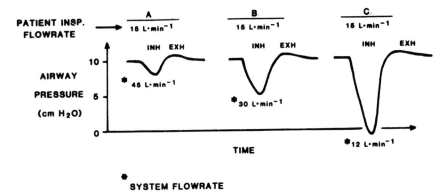

Figure 10-22 Spontaneous breathing with CPAP and sPEEP. In all three examples, the patient's inspiratory flow rate is presumed constant at 15 liters/min and end-expiratory pressure is 10 cm H_2O. *A,* The system flow rate is three times the patient's demand; during spontaneous inspiration, airway pressure decreases to approximately 8 cm H_2O, during expiration pressure returns to 10 cm H_2O. *B,* System flow rate is twice the patient's demand; during inspiration, airway pressure decreases to 5 cm H_2O. *C,* System flow rate is less than the patient's demand; during inspiration airway pressure is less than zero. *A* and *B* represent CPAP while *C* is sPEEP.

Figure 10-23 Work *(W)* required to breathe spontaneously against the external load of the breathing system during CPAP and sPEEP. Airway pressure is 10 cm H_2O, V_T and $\dot{V}$ are equal. During spontaneous inspiration *(I)* with CPAP, P decreases to 8 cm H_2O. With sPEEP, P decreases to -2 cm H_2O. During expiration *(E),* P returns to 10 cm H_2O in both modes. For the same changes in V_T, a greater change in airway pressure occurs during sPEEP, resulting in a larger pressure–volume loop. The areas within these loops represent W. For CPAP, W is 0.25 kg·m/min; for sPEEP, W is 1.56 kg·m/min, a 524% increase.

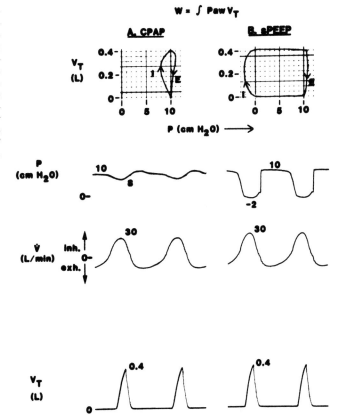

the breathing system (W),* in addition to the patient's intrinsic flow-resistive and elastic work of breathing, is associated with a greater decrement in airway pressure (increased total work of breathing). Because a fundamental goal in treating patients in acute respiratory failure is to reduce respiratory work, careful attention must be paid when delivering CPAP to maintain positive pressure at end-inhalation.[14] A low-resistance breathing system providing high flow on demand (usually greater than 60 liters/min) during spontaneous inhalation usually meets the requirements.[15]

Demand-Flow Valves

Demand-flow valves provide CPAP efficiently. These systems were introduced during World War II as a means of increasing altitude tolerance by delivering oxygen under pressure to face masks worn by pilots. Some 30 years later, Forrest M. Bird and Jack Emerson introduced similar devices as alternatives to the continuous-flow reservoir bag apparatus. Demand-flow valves function as pressurized, high-capacity reservoirs to provide intermittent inspiratory flow at a level sufficient to reduce spontaneous inspiratory work and to maintain high inspiratory positive airway pressure. The rate of gas flow should accelerate and decelerate automatically in response to the patient's requirements for inspiratory flow (Fig. 10-24).

A demand-flow CPAP system offers two theoretical advantages. First, since both the valve and the breathing circuit are pressurized at the same level, inspiratory effort is negligible. Thus, a decrease of 1 cm H_2O or less below the baseline pressure provides instantaneous gas flow at any CPAP level. Second, significant gas loss, inherent in continuous high-flow reservoir bag CPAP systems, does not occur because flow is intermittent and only on demand.

Overall, however, some poorly designed demand-flow valve CPAP systems actually predispose to increased inspiratory work.[16–21] If the flow output is inadequate, greater inspiratory effort results as the patient struggles to meet his peak inspiratory flow requirements (Fig. 10-25). Such demand-flow valves, in combination with high-resistance humidifiers and low-flow air–oxygen blenders, lead to intolerably high resistance to flow and failure of CPAP or in an overly stressed and fatigued patient.

Reports involving healthy volunteers,[16,17] lung models,[18,19] and patients[20] demonstrate significant variability in the operational characteristics of commercially available demand-flow CPAP systems. In some of these reports, a continuous flow (60 liters/min) reservoir bag system with a low-resistance threshold resistor expiratory pressure valve (Emerson) required less inspiratory effort, maintained higher inspiratory airway pressure, and was associated with less work of breathing when compared to several demand-flow systems.[16–18,20] The desirable characteristics of a demand-flow system are listed in Table 10-3.

INTERMITTENT MANDATORY VENTILATION

Originally proposed by Kirby and colleagues as a method to ventilate infants with hyaline membrane disease[22,23] and by Downs and associates for use with adults,[24] IMV allows the patient to breathe spontaneously, with mechanical inflations supplied at regular preset

---

*This terminology has been proposed by Arthur B Otis, Ph.D., to describe the work performed by the patient which is imposed by the apparatus used to provide spontaneous positive-pressure ventilation.

Figure 10-24 Demand flow valve mechanism. At the onset of spontaneous inspiration *(A)*, airway pressure and pressure inside the demand flow valve decrease. The diaphragm immediately moves to the right, opening a ball type outflow valve. Gas flows from a high pressure source to the patient. Increased demand causes increased opening of the outflow valve. During expiration *(B)*, airway pressure returns to its baseline value, pressure inside the demand flow valve increases, and the diaphragm moves to the left, closing the valve and terminating flow.

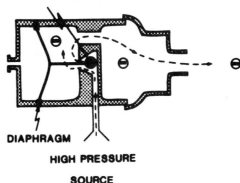

A DEMAND-FLOW VALVE

SPONTANEOUS INHALATION - FLOW

OUTFLOW VALVE

DIAPHRAGM

HIGH PRESSURE

SOURCE

B EXHALATION - NO FLOW

DIAPHRAGM

HIGH PRESSURE

SOURCE

intervals. The mechanical ventilatory rate set by the operator (the IMV breaths) cannot be influenced by the patient. Between sequential mechanical breaths, an unrestricted flow of gas equal to or greater than the patient's peak inspiratory demand must be provided to minimize spontaneous work of breathing.

Several physiological advantages have been proposed for IMV. Spontaneous breathing, with its attendant lower inspiratory intrapleural pressure (Ppl) and decreased rate of mechanical ventilator cycling, lowers mean Ppl below that associated with CMV and continuous positive-pressure ventilation (CPPV). As a result, right ventricular filling and cardiovascular function are better preserved with IMV than with CMV.[25] Moreover, when IMV is combined with CPAP or sPEEP (Fig. 10-26) and contrasted to CPPV, the cardiopulmonary effects differ substantially; IMV allows higher expiratory positive pressure with fewer deleterious effects on venous return and cardiac output.[26] Spontaneous breathing with IMV also promotes more normal matching of ventilation to perfusion ($\dot{V}/\dot{Q}$) than CMV.[27]

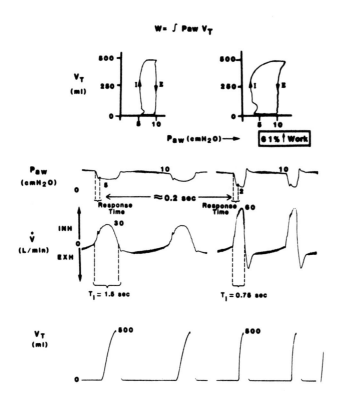

$$W = \int Paw\ V_T$$

Figure 10-25 Response characteristics of an unacceptable demand flow CPAP system. Changes in Paw, $\dot{V}$, and V_T are indicated during spontaneous ventilation with CPAP of 10 cm H_2O. On the left, T_I and peak inspiratory $\dot{V}$ were 1.5 sec and 30 liters/min, respectively. Response time of the valve is approximately 0.2 sec (delay time), after which it opens, and gas flows to the patient at an inspiratory positive pressure of 5 cm H_2O. Work (W) required to breathe against the external load of the CPAP system is represented by the area circumscribed within the pressure–volume loop (top). On the right, the same system again provides 10 cm H_2O CPAP and the same V_T, but T_I and peak inspiratory $\dot{V}$ are 0.75 sec and 60 liters/min, respectively. Valve response time is unchanged, but inspiratory positive pressure decreases to 2 cm H_2O, a 61% increase in W. In the first situation, the demand valve was "off" for 13% of the inspiratory period (0.2/1.5). In the second, it was off for 27% (0.2/0.75), necessitating a lower Paw (triggering pressure).

EQUIPMENT

Sufficient flow through the IMV circuit must be provided to satisfy the patient's peak spontaneous inspiratory flow demand, just as with CPAP circuits. Gas flow rates of two to three times the patient's minute ventilation usually are sufficient. Also, as with CPAP circuitry, the resistance to gas flow through the IMV system must be minimal during spontaneous breathing (*i.e.*, highly resistant humidifiers and one-way valves, narrow-bore

TABLE 10-3   DESIRABLE CHARACTERISTICS OF A DEMAND-FLOW VALVE (DFV) CPAP SYSTEM

Response time	Delay time from the onset of spontaneous inhalation to DFV opening and gas flow to patient (⟨0.2 sec)
Triggering pressure	1–2 cm H_2O below end-expiratory pressure
Flow rate output	≥ 120 liters/min during spontaneous inhalation; must be able to accelerate and decelerate flow on patient demand
CPAP range	0 ≥ 30 cm H_2O (upper limit has not been established)
Expiratory pressure valve	Low-resistance threshold resistor (*e.g.*, Vital Signs, Hamilton, and Emerson)
Air/oxygen blender	High-flow output (≥ 120 liters/min), directly related to flow rate output of DFV
Resistance characteristics of breathing circuit	Low-flow-resistive components in the breathing circuit (*e.g.*, humidifier, one-way valves, properly sized diameter tubing, avoidance of right-angle and narrow-bore endotracheal tube connectors)

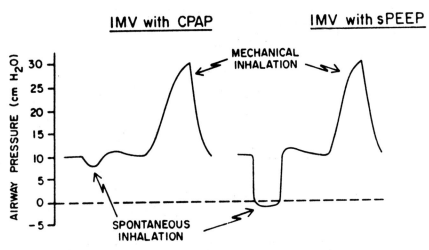

Figure 10-26 Intermittent mandatory ventilation combined with CPAP and sPEEP. Less work of breathing is required with CPAP.

breathing circuit tubing, and right-angled connectors should *not* be used). Systems that cannot provide adequate gas flow on demand increase the patient's work of breathing to intolerably high levels and can result in failure of the technique.

No rebreathing should occur. If the exhalation valve on the expiratory limb of the breathing circuit is only competent (closed) during mechanical inspiration, there is entrainment of ambient air during spontaneous inspiration with rebreathing of exhaled gas. If CPAP and IMV are used simultaneously, gas compression and high circuit-tubing compliance may also cause rebreathing of exhaled gas. Consider a patient receiving 20 cm H_2O CPAP from a system in which circuit compliance results in a gas compression volume of 5 ml/cm H_2O pressure. Under these conditions, approximately 100 ml of exhaled gas can be rebreathed with each breath. This problem may be avoided only if sufficient continuous flow is directed through the IMV system.[14]

Full humidification of inspired gas during spontaneous and mechanical inspiration must be provided. Two problems arise with humidifiers used in IMV systems: the capability to humidify gas sufficiently during high-flow conditions ($\geq$ 60 liters/min), which on occasion is necessary to satisfy spontaneous inspiratory demand; and flow resistance characteristics of the humidifier itself. Poulton and Downs studied several commercially available humidifiers.[28] The Bird heated-wick humidifier delivered acceptable humidity with negligible flow resistance during high-flow conditions. Other humidifiers failed to provide sufficient humidity or imposed excessive resistance to gas flow, either of which precludes their use in an IMV system. High flow resistance is not a problem during CMV because the ventilator provides essentially all the work of breathing. However, during spontaneous inspiration with IMV, the patient must provide this work.[15]

The IMV system should be capable of pressurizing the inspiratory reservoir to the CPAP level. A continuous-flow or demand-flow system (Fig. 10-27) can be used. Most commercially available IMV-CPAP systems today are of the latter design. Here also the demand-flow valves function as pressurized reservoirs and should be capable of providing

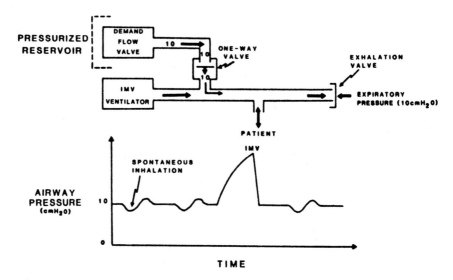

Figure 10-27 IMV–demand flow CPAP system. At the end of spontaneous expiration, the one-way valve closes, and the demand flow valve, breathing circuit, and expiratory pressure valve are pressurized to the same level (10 cm H₂O). The pressure gradient across the one-way valve is zero, since pressure in the demand flow valve and the breathing circuit is the same. Inspiratory effort to open the one-way valve is minimal. Ideally, gas flow is directed through the breathing circuit at a flow rate sufficient to minimize decreases in airway pressure.

high inspiratory flow (up to 120 liters/min) in order to prevent large decreases in airway pressure.

Low-resistance threshold resistor valves are advisable for two reasons. First, high-resistance valves significantly increase expiratory airway pressure (especially during coughing). Second, large decreases in inspiratory airway pressure are likely to occur with continuous gas flow through high-resistance valves. During spontaneous inspiration, some of the continuous flow passing through the valve is diverted to the patient. Since pressure in the circuit is proportional to both resistance and flow, the reduction of flow through the valve results in a substantial reduction of inspiratory pressure and a corresponding increase in the patient's work of breathing.[15]

SYNCHRONIZED INTERMITTENT MANDATORY VENTILATION

This technique also allows spontaneous breathing between mechanically delivered ventilator breaths. At regular intervals, the mandatory breath is synchronized to begin with the patient's next spontaneous inspiratory effort in the same fashion as the pressure-cycled (assisted) termination of exhalation that was described earlier. This technique was introduced because of concern that a mechanical breath might be superimposed on a spontaneous breath ("stacking"), causing increases in peak inspiratory pressure, mean airway pressure, and mean intrapleural pressure. Similar concerns existed if the mechanically delivered volume was added at the peak of spontaneous exhalation.

Subsequently, investigations were conducted to examine the clinical efficacy of synchronized intermittent mandatory ventilation (SIMV). Shapiro and colleagues noted that mean Ppl, assessed with an esophageal balloon, was substantially lower with SIMV than with IMV in normal volunteers.[29] However, Hasten and coworkers compared SIMV with IMV in 25 critically ill patients and found that although peak inflation pressure was greater with IMV than with SIMV, cardiovascular variables (blood pressure, cardiac output, stroke index, central venous pressure, pulmonary artery pressure) did not differ significantly.[30]

In another study, Heenen and colleagues studied anesthetized near-drowned dogs ventilated with IMV or SIMV.[31] Again, no differences between the two modes were noted with respect to cardiac output, stroke volume, Ppl, and intrapulmonary shunt. Peak inflation and mean airway pressures were significantly increased with IMV and some breath stacking occurred, but without demonstrable adverse effects. Based on these data, SIMV does *not* seem to offer any physiological advantages compared with IMV and may be thought of as an expensive solution to a basically nonexistent problem.

PRESSURE SUPPORT VENTILATION

Newer microprocessor-driven mechanical ventilators (*e.g.*, Hamilton Veolar, Puritan-Bennett 7200, Bear-5, and Siemens 900 C) include PS modes that operate in conjunction with their demand-flow valve systems. Work of breathing appears to be decreased by PS, but the technique is based on an entirely different concept than CPAP. In the PS mode, the ventilator is patient-triggered "on," continuing in the inspiratory phase to a preselected positive-pressure limit.[32,33] As long as the patient's inspiratory effort is maintained, the preselected airway pressure stays constant, with a variable flow of gas from the ventilator. Inspiration cycles "off" when the patient's inspiratory flow demand decreases to a preselected percentage of the initial peak mechanical inspiratory flow (Fig. 10-28). The ventilator thus is flow-cycled in the PS mode, following which passive exhalation occurs (Table 10-4).

Figure 10-28 Work of breathing *(W)* with CPAP *(left)* and PS with CPAP *(right)*. At CPAP of 10 cm H_2O, Paw decreases to 5 cm H_2O during spontaneous inhalation *(SI)*; VT is 500 ml, and the patient performs the work of breathing. At PS 5 cm H_2O with CPAP 10 cm H_2O, the ventilator is patient-triggered "On," and an abrupt increase in Paw to 15 cm H_2O follows; VT here is also 500 ml, but the work of breathing is provided by the ventilator *(I)*. At end-inspiration, the ventilator flow cycles "Off" (when the patient's inspiratory flow demand decreases to 25% of the peak mechanical inspiratory flow rate) and passive exhalation occurs.

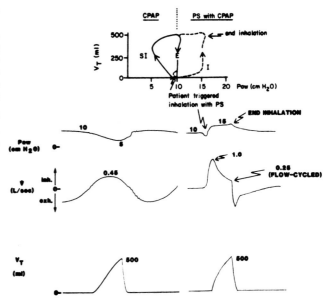

TABLE 10-4 VENTILATORS INCORPORATING PRESSURE SUPPORT

Ventilator	Cycling Mechanism*	Range
Hamilton Veolar	Flow-cycled†	1–50 cm H_2O
Siemens 900 C	Flow-cycled†	1–100 cm H_2O
Bear-5	Flow-cycled†	1–72 cm H_2O
Puritan-Bennett 7200	Variable: exhalation after 300 ms may begin when the inspiratory flow rate is ≤5 liters/min for 100 ms or if airway pressure exceeds the end-expiratory pressure plus the PS level by 1.5 cm H_2O for 100 ms	1–30 cm H_2O

* Refers to the mechanism responsible for the switchover from PS inspiration to expiration.
† Ventilator flow cycles "off" when the inspiratory flow demand decreases to 25% of the initial peak mechanical inspiratory flow rate.

Continuous recording of airway pressure and VT changes during PS yields a pressure–volume loop that moves to the right during inspiration and is indicative of work produced by the ventilator. The patient's spontaneous work of breathing with PS is less compared to breathing with CPAP at the same pressure (see Fig. 10-28). The airway pressure, flow, and lung volume changes during PS are more akin to assisted mechanical ventilation than to spontaneous positive-pressure with CPAP. At constant levels of combined PS and CPAP, peak inspiratory flow rate, flow waveform, inspiratory time, tidal volume, mean airway pressure, and the airway pressure contour depend on the patient's breathing pattern (Fig. 10-29).

Since PS is a form of mechanical ventilation, patients treated with it should not be considered to be breathing spontaneously. Patients receiving PS with CPAP may appear to be assuming the full workload of spontaneous ventilation, and arterial blood gas tensions

Figure 10-29 Variations in patient-triggering pressures *(PT)*, airway pressure contour, mean airway pressure (area under pressure–time curve), peak inspiratory flow, flow wave contour, inspiratory time *(Ti)* and VT despite uniform PS of 5 cm H_2O, and CPAP of 10 cm H_2O.

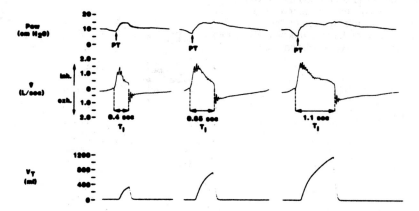

and *p*H values can lead the clinician to conclude erroneously that this is the case. Consider a patient who still has unresolved pulmonary abnormalities (decreased FRC and lung compliance).Treatment with PS of 5 cm H_2O and CPAP of 5 or 10 cm H_2O, with a low inspired oxygen concentration, may result in "normal" blood gas values. However, after tracheal extubation, the patient may become dyspneic and hypercapnic while breathing spontaneously (ambient pressure) in the absence of this support. This point was illustrated in a group of patients treated with PS whose Pa_{CO_2} averaged 40 ± 2 mm Hg. Following extubation, Pa_{CO_2} increased to 47 ± 2 mm Hg.[34]

APPLICATION

Two approaches are described.[35,36] The first employs a low level (*e.g.*, 5 to 10 cm H_2O) of PS as "assisted mechanical ventilation" between IMV breaths, to decrease spontaneous ventilatory work. Poorly designed demand-flow valve systems (low-flow on demand, long response time, low triggering pressure, highly resistant breathing circuit, and a flow-resistor expiratory pressure valve) and endotracheal tube resistance are cited as the rationale for using PS. However, unless the PS level is set precisely to match the pressure drop necessitated by the circuit resistance and demand valve, positive-pressure ventilation results.[32]

The second approach employs PS as a stand-alone mechanical ventilatory mode. Here, the PS level is adjusted to provide the desired tidal and minute volume. Since large variations in tidal and minute volume can occur at a set level of PS (see Fig. 10-30), titration based on volume exchange is sometimes difficult. Capnography is useful in titrating the level of PS

Figure 10-30 During inhalation with HFJV, gas is accelerated through an injector creating subambient pressure at the outlet and causing additional gas to be entrained. Tidal volume is the sum of injector and entrained volumes. Pressure becomes positive further down the endotracheal tube. Passive exhalation occurs through the entrainment of the orifice. No valves are present.

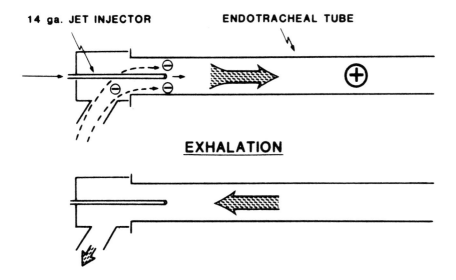

INHALATION

14 ga. JET INJECTOR   **ENDOTRACHEAL TUBE**

EXHALATION

to an appropriate end-tidal P_{CO_2}. When PS serves as a stand-alone technique, there is no safety or back-up mechanism to ventilate the patient in the event of apnea (except with the Hamilton Veolar ventilator).

MANDATORY MINUTE VOLUME

Hewlett and colleagues described a technique called mandatory minute volume (MMV) in which the patient is guaranteed a preselected minute ventilation.[37] If the entire amount is breathed spontaneously, ventilator augmentation does not occur. If not, that portion of the preselected minute ventilation which is not breathed spontaneously is collected by the ventilator and delivered automatically. Ventilators incorporating MMV are the Hamilton Veolar, Bear-5, and Ohmeda CPU 1. The Hamilton Veolar employs PS in its MMV mode. If the patient's expected minute ventilation is less than the preselected value, the ventilator automatically adds PS in 1 to 2 cm H_2O increments until the desired minute ventilation is reached. The Bear-5 and Ohmeda CPU 1 ventilators provide mandatory breaths should the patient fail to achieve the preselected minute ventilation during spontaneous breathing.

HIGH-FREQUENCY JET VENTILATION

The term high-frequency ventilation is a generic one encompassing three primary techniques: high-frequency positive-pressure ventilation (HFPPV), high-frequency jet ventilation (HFJV), and high-frequency oscillation (HFO). Most clinical experience in the United States is with HFJV. Gas is accelerated through an injector cannula and lateral pressure decreases below the ambient level at the nozzle or orifice of the injector. The result, as previously described, is additional gas entrainment, which contributes significantly to the inspiratory flow of V_T (see Figs. 10-2, 10-3, 10-30).[38,39]

Inspiratory flow and pressure waveforms with HFJV presumably are rectilinear and linear, respectively; however, as lung-thorax compliance decreases and/or airway resistance increases, peak flow delivery and V_T are decreased and airway pressure is increased (at the same jet drive pressure and inspiratory time) (Fig. 10-31).[40] Tidal volume also decreases as the level of PEEP/CPAP is increased,[41] probably because jet entrainment is inhibited by increased airway/alveolar back pressure.[42,43]

Three controls are common to all high-frequency jet ventilators: drive pressure, frequency, and percent inspiratory time (%T_I). The drive pressure directly affects V_T and PIP (*i.e.*, the increased drive increases V_T and PIP). The %T_I control regulates the duration of inspiration. At a frequency of 100 breaths/min, the entire ventilatory cycle is 0.6 second; if a 20% T_I is selected, inspiratory time is 0.12 second and expiratory time is 0.48 second. Thus, the inspiratory-to-expiratory time ratio (I:E) is approximately 1:4 or 0.25. Such values commonly are employed in adult and pediatric patients. Overall characteristics of HFJV are summarized in Table 10-5.

A special endotracheal tube with a jet injector lumen embedded in its side wall frequently is used for HFJV (Fig. 10-32) in lieu of the "traditional" 14-gauge jet injector. At the same ventilator settings, the latter demonstrates significantly greater PIP, peak-entrained flow, and exhaled V_T than the injector lumen endotracheal tube.[44]

Another technique employs a sliding Venturi device (Bird).[45] This system is similar to that for HFJV; however, the pulsatile jet flow is delivered into a Venturi tube that provides

Figure 10-31 HFJV evaluation under conditions of: normal compliance *(C)* and normal resistance *(R)*; decreased C and normal R; and normal C and increased R. With a tenfold *increase* in R, a 27% decrease in V_T resulted compared to the control. Rate 100 breaths/min, 20% inspiratory time, jet drive pressure 25 psig. *Paw,* airway pressure measured inside the endotracheal tube (10–15 cm distal to the jet nozzle); P_{ENTR}, changes in pressure at the entrainment port of the jet injector; $\dot{V}$, entrained and total exhaled flows; and V_T exhaled tidal volume.

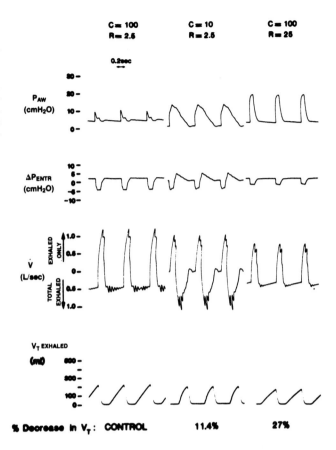

gas entrainment (Fig. 10-33). Comparisons of the sliding Venturi device, the 14-gauge injector, and the injector lumen endotracheal tube methods at identical ventilator settings in subjects with acute respiratory failure reveal that V_T is greatest with the sliding Venturi, less with the 14-gauge injector, and least with the injector lumen endotracheal tube. Arterial P_{CO_2}

TABLE 10-5   CHARACTERISTICS OF HIGH-FREQUENCY JET VENTILATION

Frequency	100–150 breaths/min
Injector type	(1) 14-gauge steel cannula (internal diameter = 1.7 mm; length = 10 cm)
	(2) Lumen embedded in side wall of a special endotracheal tube (see Fig. 10–17)
	Time
Cycling mechanism	20%–30% respiratory cycle
% Inspiratory time	5–50 psig (directly affects airway pressure, tidal volume, and minute volume)
Drive pressure	
	Injector flow plus entrained flow (100–300 ml)
Tidal volume	Square
Inspiratory flow pattern	Passive
Exhalation	

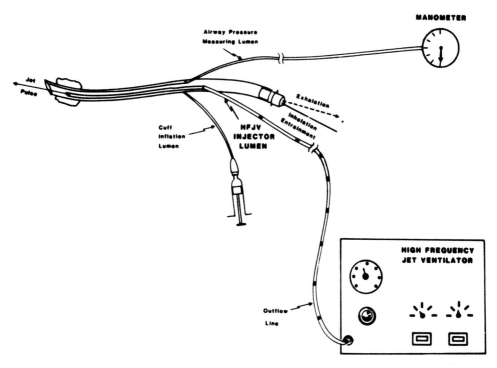

Figure 10-32 HFJV applied with a special endotracheal tube (Hi-Lo Jet Orotracheal Tube, NCC–Malinkrodt) containing three lumens in its sidewall: one to inflate the cuff, one to inject pulses of gas, and one to measure airway pressure. The lumen used for HFJV is attached to a solenoid valve-actuated high frequency jet ventilator. The large central lumen serves as a conduit for entrained gas during inhalation and for exhalation.

shows the reverse, that is, CO_2 pressure is lowest with the sliding Venturi and greatest with the injector lumen endotracheal tube.[46]

Indications and complications of HFJV are listed in Table 10-6. Inadequate humidification is one of the more common problems reported. Anhydrous gas delivered at high rates of flow causes secretions to "cake," particularly in the endotracheal tube; in some instances, total occlusion has occurred, requiring immediate extubation and reintubation. Deleterious effects on the respiratory mucosa and the airways result from breathing dry gas. To minimize this problem, water is infused into the jet stream and nebulized directly into the airway. Humidity is easily controlled by regulating the drip rate of the water infusion pump; however, care must be taken to avoid fluid overload. An infusion rate of approximately 20 to 30 ml/hr appears satisfactory for most patients.

Another potential complication arises with the injector lumen endotracheal tube. If the tip of the endotracheal tube is at or near the carina, and the orifice of the injector lumen is "aimed" toward a mainstem bronchus, the bulk of the insufflated flow is directed to one lung, predisposing to maldistribution of ventilation. This problem can be minimized by positioning the endotracheal tube an appropriate distance (approximately 6 cm) from the carina.[47]

Figure 10-33 Sliding Venturi mechanism for high-frequency ventilation (Bird). During inspiration, gas flow pressurizes a diaphragm, which slides the Venturi mechanism to the right and occludes the exhalation port. Acceleration of gas flow through the Venturi decreases lateral pressure and causes gas entrainment. During expiration, cessation of the drive flow depressurizes the diaphragm and a spring causes the Venturi mechanism to move leftward, allowing exhalation.

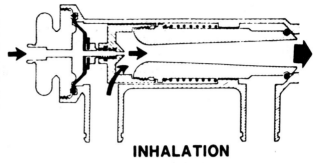

INHALATION

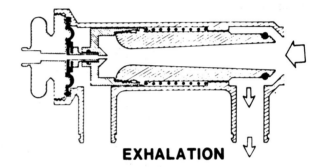

EXHALATION

MONITORING

Quantitative and qualitative assessment of ventilatory function is of paramount importance in critically ill patients. Respiratory monitoring can be partitioned into pulmonary mechanics (volume–pressure–flow relationships) and gas exchange. Despite recent advancements and sophisticated technology, visual observation by experienced practitioners remains the primary and essential form of respiratory surveillance. The human interface is necessary to optimize the usefulness of and appropriate response to monitored data. Assessment of the breathing pattern and respiratory rate remains the "gold standard."

TABLE 10-6   INDICATIONS FOR AND COMPLICATIONS OF HIGH-FREQUENCY JET VENTILATION

Established Indications
Bronchopleural fistula
Bronchoscopy
Laryngoscopy

Possible Indications
Excessive PIP—may predispose to pulmonary barotrauma, decreased cardiac output, and increased intracranial pressure; lower airway pressures with HFJV might minimize these problems.

Hyaline membrane disease—Low PIP with HFJV may decrease the incidence of bronchopulmonary dysplasia.
Emergency percutaneous transtracheal jet ventilation—for upper airway obstruction, crushed larynx, and similar conditions.

Complications
Inadequate humidification
Damage to tracheal mucosa—shear forces from the high-velocity jet pulses may damage these tissues.

Periodic objective biochemical studies provide a secondary level of monitoring. Foremost among these are analyses of arterial blood gas tensions and *p*H. In their absence, one can only speculate regarding the status of oxygenation, ventilation, and acid–base regulation. Chest radiography also is frequently employed. However, this clearly has limitations, including the fact that changes often lag behind clinical alterations by as much as 24 hours.

A third level of respiratory monitoring is provided by spirometry and respiratory gas analysis (capnography and mass spectrometry), which can be obtained periodically or continuously.

MECHANICS

Tidal Volume

Tidal volume delivery from a mechanical ventilator may be inadequate as a result of improper ventilator adjustments, mechanical failure, and circuit leaks or disconnection. Measurements of this value should be taken from the expiratory limb at the proximal airway to detect the gas actually coming from the patient's lungs. Small, portable meters (*e.g.*, Wright respirometer) are commonly used for VT assessment. Gas flow into the instrument spins a flat, two-bladed rotor (vane). The flow-generated rotation is converted by a gear drive to a volume measurement that is displayed on the face of the instrument. Because moisture impairs its performance, the instrument is most appropriate for intermittent monitoring.

Continuous VT monitoring is facilitated with an electronic pneumotachometer, consisting of a tube with a pressure port on each side of a hydraulic resistance (Siemens) or variable orifice hinged membrane (Hamilton) (Fig. 10-34). During ventilation, the variable orifice size increases or decreases on either side of the membrane corresponding to the direction of gas flow. The pressure change across the membrane is proportional to $\dot{V}$. A microprocessor converts this differential pressure into a flow signal and integrates it against time to calculate VT.

Another pneumotachometer incorporates ultrasonic vortex detection technology (Bear-1,2,5). Vortices (waves) are generated by gas tumbling over a strut placed in the airstream (Fig. 10-35). A piezoelectric transducer transmits an ultrasonic sound wave across the flow stream. The vibrating airstream intermittently alters the frequency of the ultrasonic beam, and this variation is converted into electronic signals directly proportional to flow. A microprocessor integrates the signal against time to derive VT.

Volume measurements must exclude gas compressed in the breathing circuitry at end-inspiration. Although previously discussed, this fact deserves reiteration. The product of PIP

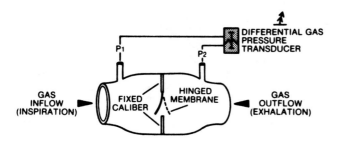

Figure 10-34 Variable orifice pneumotachometer. A transducer measures the differential pressure which is proportional to the gas flow across the orifice (see text).

Figure 10-35 Tidal volume measurement by ultrasonic detection of flow-generated vortices (see text).

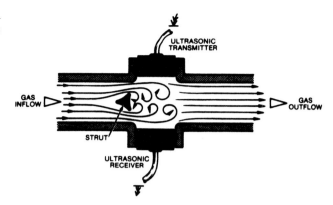

(cm H_2O) × 5 (ml/cm H_2O) provides an estimate of the compression volume of most circuits. In patients requiring high PIP, considerable volume "loss" occurs.

Alarms for low minute volume (MV) or V_T are available on most ventilators. Some also include surveillance for high MV. The low V_T threshold (alarm limit) usually is adjusted to monitor the predominant breathing pattern (e.g., for adults, 100 ml less than the mechanical V_T, or 50 to 75 ml less than the spontaneous V_T). When the preselected threshold is not maintained, an audible alarm and a visual indicator are activated, serving as presumptive evidence that a condition of hypoventilation warrants immediate attention.

Airway Pressure

Airway pressure should be monitored continuously in the ventilated patient. Most ventilators have a mechanism whereby the PIP threshold (limit) can be adjusted. If this limit is exceeded, inspiration is automatically terminated and gas is vented from the circuit. Recently available ventilators incorporate a pressure transducer to measure and display breathing circuit pressure.

Once the desired V_T is verified, PIP should be noted. Some ventilators not only permit adjustment of the PIP limit but also incorporate a low inspiratory pressure alarm and an alarm signaling loss of PEEP/CPAP. The PIP and low inspiratory pressure alarm ranges should be set 5 to 10 cm H_2O above and below the initial PIP. An abrupt decrease of 5 to 10 cm H_2O may be indicative of a circuit leak. An acute rise of pressure can signify a number of problems, including partial or complete airway obstruction, bronchospasm, tension pneumothorax, patient–ventilator phasing problems, or improper valving of gas when optional or test apparatus is incorporated into the breathing circuit.

The threshold of the PEEP/CPAP alarm should be set 3 to 5 cm H_2O below the selected end-expiratory pressure to provide leak detection during low-rate IMV/SIMV or spontaneous CPAP modes. It can also indicate failure to provide adequate flow during spontaneous ventilation, which is detailed later.

RESPIRATORY GAS MONITORING

Capnography is used increasingly to monitor carbon dioxide concentration. Mass spectrometry is also used to monitor inspired and expired oxygen and carbon dioxide (as well as nitrogen and nitrous oxide and volatile anesthetics agents). It is now used primarily in the operating room but will, no doubt, be seen more often in the ICU.

REFERENCES

1. Instruction Manual, Bear-2 Ventilator. Riverside, CA, Bear Medical Systems, 1981
2. Operator's Manual, Veolar Ventilator. Reno NV, Hamilton Medical Corporation, 1985
3. Instruction Manual, Bear-5 Ventilator. Riverside, CA, Bear Medical Systems, 1985
4. Service Manual, 7200 Series Microprocessor Ventilator. Los Angeles, CA, Puritan-Bennett Corporation, 1985
5. Kacmarek RM. Dimas S, Reynolds J, et al: Technical aspects of positive end-expiratory pressure (PEEP): 1. Physics of PEEP devices. *Resp Care* 1982; 27:1478
6. Kirby RR: Positive airway pressure: System design and clinical application. In Shoemaker WC (ed): *Critical Care: State of the Art*, vol 5, p G1. Shoemaker WC Fullerton, CA, Society of Critical Care Medicine, 1985
7. Mushin WW, Rendell-Baker L, Thompson PW: *Automatic Ventilation of the Lungs*, 3rd ed. pp 105, 127. Oxford, Blackwell Scientific Publications, 1969
8. Marini JJ, Culver BH, Kirk W: Flow resistance of exhalation valves and positive end-expiratory pressure devices used in mechanical ventilation. *Am Rev Respir Dis* 1985; 131:850
9. Banner MJ, Lampotang S, Boysen PG, et al: Flow resistance of expiratory positive pressure valve systems. *Chest* 1986; 90:212
10. Hall JR, Rendleman DC, Downs JB: PEEP devices: Flow dependent increases in airway pressure (abstr). *Crit Care Med* 1978; 6:100
11. Nunn JF: *Applied Respiratory Physiology*, 2nd ed, p 100. London, Butterworths, 1977
12. Banner MJ, Lampotang S, Boysen PG, et al: Resistance characteristics of expiratory pressure valves. *Anesthesiology* 1986; 65:A80
13. Douglas M, Downs JB: Special correspondence. *Anesth Analg* 1978; 57:347
14. Downs JB: Mechanical ventilatory therapy. *Curr Rev Respir Ther* 1981; 3:82
15. Downs JB: Ventilatory patterns and modes of ventilation in acute respiratory failure. *Respir Care* 1983; 28:586
16. Gibney RTN, Wilson RS: Pontoppidan H: Comparison of work of breathing on high gas flow and demand valve continuous positive airway pressure systems. *Chest* 1982; 82:692
17. Cox D, Niblett DJ: Studies on continuous positive airway pressure breathing systems. *Br J Anaesth* 1984; 56:905
18. Op't Holt TB, Hall MW, Bass JB, et al: Comparison of changes in airway pressure (CPAP) between demand valve and continuous flow devices. *Respir Care* 1982; 27:1200
19. Gjerde GE, Katz JA, Kramer RW: Inspiratory work and airway pressure with continuous positive airway pressure delivery systems (abstr). *Crit Care Med* 1984; 12:272
20. Henry WC, West GA, Wilson RS: A comparison of the oxygen cost of breathing between a continuous flow CPAP system and a demand-flow CPAP system. *Respir Care* 1983; 28:1273
21. Kirby RR: Continuous positive airway pressure; To breathe or not to breathe. *Anesthesiology* 1985; 63:578
22. Kirby RR, Robison E, Schulz J: Continuous flow ventilation as an alternative to assisted or controlled ventilation in infants. *Anesth Analg* 1972; 51:871
23. Kirby RR, Robison E, Schulz J: A new pediatric volume ventilator. *Anesth Analg* 1971; 50:533
24. Downs JB, Klein EF, Desautels D: Intermittent mandatory ventilation. A new approach to weaning patients from mechanical ventilators. *Chest* 1973; 64:331
25. Kirby RR, Perry JC, Calderwood HW: Cardiorespiratory effects of high positive end-expiratory pressure. *Anesthesiology* 1975; 43:533
26. Kirby RR, Downs JB, Civetta JM: High level positive end-expiratory pressure (PEEP) in acute respiratory insufficiency. *Chest* 1975; 67:156
27. Banner MJ, Gallagher TJ: Respiratory failure in the adult, ventilatory support. In Kirby RR, Smith RA, Desautels DA (eds): *Mechanical Ventilation*, p 209. New York, Churchill Livingstone, 1985
28. Poulton TJ, Downs JB: Humidification of rapidly flowing gas. *Crit Care Med* 1981; 9:59
29. Shapiro BA, Harrison RA, Walton JR: Intermittent demand ventilation (IDV), a new technique for supporting ventilation in critically ill patients. *Respir Care* 1976; 21:521
30. Hasten RW, Downs JB, Heenen TJ: A comparison of synchronized and nonsynchronized intermittent mandatory ventilation. *Respir Care* 1980; 25:554
31. Heenan TJ, Downs JB, Douglas ME: Intermittent mandatory ventilation—Is synchronization important? *Chest* 1980; 77:598
32. Down JB: New modes of ventilatory assistance. *Chest* 1986; 90:626
33. Banner MJ, Kirby RR: Pressure support ventilation. *Crit Care Med* 1986; 14:665
34. Prakash O, Meiji S: Cardiopulmonary response to inspiratory pressure support during spontaneous ventilation vs. conventional ventilation. *Chest* 1985; 83:403
35. MacIntyre N: Pressure support ventilation. *Respir Care* 1986; 31:189
36. MacIntyre N: Respiratory function during pressure support ventilation. *Chest* 1986; 89:677
37. Hewlett AM, Platt AS, Terry VG: Mandatory minute volume. A new concept in weaning from mechanical ventilators. *Anaesthesia* 1977; 32:163

38. Froese AB: High frequency ventilation, A critical assessment. In Shoemaker WC (ed): *Critical Care, State of the Art*, vol 5, p V(A):1. Fullerton, CA, Society of Critical Care Medicine, 1984

39. Banner MJ: Technical aspects of high frequency ventilation. *Curr Rev Respir Ther* 1985; 7:91

40. Carlon GC, Miodownik S, Ray C: High frequency jet ventilation. In Carlon GC, Howland WS (eds): *High Frequency Ventilation in Intensive Care and During Surgery*, p 77. New York, Marcel Dekker, 1985

41. Banner MJ, Gallagher RC, Desautels DA, et al: A manifold to measure exhaled tidal volume during high frequency jet ventilation. *Crit Care Med* 1985; 14:730

42. Schlacter MD, Perry ME: Effect of continuous positive airway pressure on lung mechanics during high frequency jet ventilation. *Crit Care Med* 1984; 12:755

43. Hamilton LH, Londino JM, Linehan JH: Pediatric endotracheal tube designed for high frequency ventilation. *Crit Care Med* 1984; 12:988

44. Banner MJ, Boysen PG: Comparison of two flow injector devices to deliver high frequency jet ventilation. *Crit Care Med* 1986; 14:374

45. Mikhail MS, Banner MJ: Hemodynamic effects of positive end-expiratory pressure during high frequency ventilation. *Crit Care Med* 1985; 13:733

46. Gallagher RC, Banner MJ, Modell JM: Comparison of delivery systems for high frequency jet ventilation. *Crit Care Med* 1985; 13:313

47. Kessler H: High frequency jet ventilation. In Carlon GC, Howland WS (eds): *High Frequency Ventilation in Intensive Care and During Surgery*, p 175. New York, Marcel Dekker, 1985

CHAPTER ELEVEN

MONITORING OF NEUROLOGIC FUNCTION

Robert R. Kirby

INTRODUCTION

Unlike hemodynamic or respiratory function monitoring in the intensive care unit (ICU), no objective method for continuously monitoring the brain's electrical activity is widely accepted. The neurologic examination, Glasgow Coma Score (GCS), and standard electro-encephalogram (EEG) assess the patient's neurologic status intermittently and have major limitations. Newer techniques including processed EEGs, somatosensory evoked responses (SERs), and auditory brain stem evoked responses (ABRs), popularized in the operating theater, have not yet been integrated on a regular basis in the ICU.

Prevention of secondary damage due to ischemia and hypoxia is essential. Critical threshold levels for blood pressure/flow which maintain cerebral function in a normal individual may not be appropriate for the progressively failing brain in a patient with cerebral vasospasm following a subarachnoid hemorrhage.

Maintenance of normal cerebral perfusion pressure (CPP), which is mean arterial blood pressure (MAP) minus mean intracranial pressure (ICP), over a wide range of blood pressure (autoregulation)[1] is lost in a variety of pathologic states. Autoregulation may be disrupted in the damaged areas and in areas remote from the injury site. Moderate hypotension of little consequence in normal patients can lead to cerebral ischemia, while sudden hypertension predisposes to an abnormal increase in cerebral blood flow (CBF) and cerebral edema.

Twenty percent of the cardiac output is directed to the brain which comprises only 2% of the adult body weight. When CBF falls below 23 ml/100 g/min, a neurologic deficit results in awake monkeys.[2] If it decreases below 18 to 21 ml/100 g/min in anesthetized animals, EEG recordings are altered, while below 15 ml/100 g/min, SERs are reduced. Nevertheless, an evoked response can still be obtained when CBF is reduced by 80%.[3] Synaptic failure may be reflected by subtle changes such as a decrease in the amplitude of the cortical SER or loss of fast EEG activity. As CBF decreases below 10 ml/100 g/min, effluxes of cellular potassium and edema formation are common. At even lower CBF levels, these abnormalities increase.[2-4] If prompt action is not taken, infarction and cellular death occur, depending on the degree and duration of ischemia.[2] Total ischemia at normal body temperature of more than 15 minutes' duration is usually associated with brain cell death.

However, at least experimentally, cellular survival may be possible after as much as 2 hours of incomplete focal ischemia. Thus, absence of the EEG or cortical SERs indicates that severe ischemia is present but does not mean necessarily that cellular death has occurred. Prompt reversal of ischemia and the associated electrophysiologic abnormalities usually can be achieved by improvement of CPP. Nevertheless, an estimate of CBF based on the CPP, which generally is adequate for the normal brain, is of little help in a damaged brain with loss of autoregulation.

MONITORS OF NEURAL FUNCTION

Irreversible brain damage may be prevented by aggressive intervention. Successful intra-operative neurologic monitoring suggests a natural extension of such techniques to the ICU for the early detection of cerebral failure due to hypotension, hypoxia, increased ICP, or mass lesions.[5]

Direct monitoring techniques test the function of central nervous system (CNS) structures and pathways and include the neurologic examination, ABRs, SERs, and standard or processed EEG recordings. The computed tomographic (CT) scan, conversely, provides anatomic information (although functional changes often can be inferred from observed structural alterations). Blood pressure, pulse, serum electrolytes and glucose, arterial blood gas values and pHa indirectly reflect the metabolic environment of the brain. Clinicians who use electrophysiologic monitoring must keep these factors, other physiologic variables, and the patient's medications in mind. A flat EEG obtained from a patient in barbiturate coma or one who is profoundly hypothermic is not indicative of brain death, but absent evoked responses strongly support such a diagnosis.

NEUROLOGIC EXAMINATION

The neurologic examination is always available for precise and frequent monitoring. However, patients' responses to verbal commands are compromised by muscle relaxants, tran-quilizers, barbiturates, narcotics, and other medications, making its use unsatisfactory in many clinical circumstances. Numerous drugs given routinely in most ICUs impair cognitive function.

In trauma patients alcoholic intoxication is a frequent predisposing factor further complicating neurologic examination. Nevertheless, a decreased level of consciousness should not be attributed to alcohol alone unless other drugs and intracranial pathology have been ruled out. A CT scan should be performed as soon as possible if the effects of alcohol obscure the neurologic examination.

"Classical" physical findings may not be present to ascertain the presence or absence of increased ICP. Cushing's triad, the association of increased ICP with systemic hypertension and bradycardia, is present less than 25% of the time even when ICP is greater than 30 mm Hg.[6] If a value greater than 15 mm Hg is accepted as abnormal, the detection rate of under 25% is clearly unsatisfactory and has resulted in increased utilization of direct ICP monitoring.

GLASGOW COMA SCORE (SCALE)

The Glasgow Coma Score[7,8] (Table 11-1) is a clinical grading system commonly used for determining severity of brain injury. Coma is defined as an inability to obey commands,

TABLE 11-1   MODIFIED GLASGOW COMA SCORE[8]

Sign	Evaluation	Score
Eye opening	Spontaneous	4
	To speech	3
	To pain	2
	None	1
Best verbal response	Oriented	5
	Confused	4
	Inappropriate	3
	Incomprehensible	2
	None	1
Best motor response	Obeys commands	6
	Localizes pain	5
	Withdrawal to pain	4
	Flexion to pain	3
	Extension to pain	2
	None	1

speak, or open the eyes. The accepted value for severe brain injury is a GCS of 8 or less. Patients with a score of 7 or less require immediate tracheal intubation and possibly hyperventilation. A GCS of 3 is assigned to ventilator-dependent patients with no response to verbal or painful stimulation. Because the GCS reflects the patient's ability to process and act on information presented, it is a useful tool for assessing depth of coma and predicting outcome.[9]

Because of the widespread use of tracheal intubation, pharmacologically induced neuromuscular paralysis, and mechanical ventilator-induced hyperventilation, the GCS can only be accurately ascertained before and after but not during such therapy. In any event, it is artifactually low since patients' verbal responses cannot be determined while they are intubated. A score of 3 assigned to a mechanically ventilated, paralyzed patient may reflect drug effect rather than neurologic status. Patients with a GCS of 3 often have a poor outcome and are frequently treated expectantly.[9]

STANDARD ELECTROENCEPHALOGRAM

The EEG reflects spontaneous and on-going electrical activity recorded on the surface of the scalp. Changes in the EEG are closely linked to critical thresholds in CBF but also result from altered Pa_{O_2}, temperature, and external stimulation (Table 11-2).[10] However, standard EEG recording is not routinely performed in the ICU due to insufficient technical personnel, the difficulty of on-line EEG interpretation, numerous electrically induced artifacts, and drug-induced suppression of cortical activity. Standard recordings use 20 electrodes and 16 separate traces, and at the common EEG paper speed of 30 mm/sec, 4 hours of recording yields 432 m of paper. They are less commonly used for verification of brain death today because of the problems of obtaining artifact-free recordings in the ICU. Nuclear perfusion scans and cerebral angiography, to assess the absence of CBF, and ABRs are preferred in many institutions.

TABLE 11-2 EEG ALTERATIONS

Depression	Activation
Hypoxia	Hyperoxia
($Sa_{O_2} < 65\%$; $Pa_{O_2} < 40$ mm Hg)	
Hypocapnia	Hypercapnia
Anesthetics	Anesthetics
	(*i.e.*, enflurane)
Postseizure	Stimulation
Hypotension	Seizure
Hypoglycemia	
Hypothermia	

PROCESSED ELECTROENCEPHALOGRAMS

To simplify EEG recording and to make it more useful for clinical application in the operating room and ICU, some monitors process the raw data automatically. These monitors analyze the frequency content of the brain's electrical activity with a limited number of channels (2–8), displaying the results and producing a hard copy. Typically, they use a process called Fourier analysis which is based on the concept that all periodic waveforms can be constructed from an infinite number of sinusoidal waves of differing frequencies (Fig. 11-1).

Since these waves do not all start on the same part of the sine wave cycle, they are out of phase. Each must be expressed in terms of phase, amplitude, and frequency. The amplitude and phase of a sinusoidal waveform can be described as the sum of a sine and cosine wave of identical frequencies (Fig. 11-2). A mathematical process termed discrete

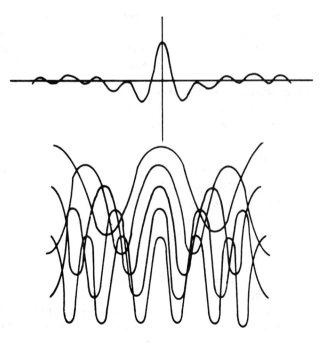

Figure 11-1 Construction of a periodic waveform (*top*) from the summation of numerous sine waves of varying frequencies (*bottom*). (Health Devices 1986; 15:71. Used with permission of ECRI, Inc.)

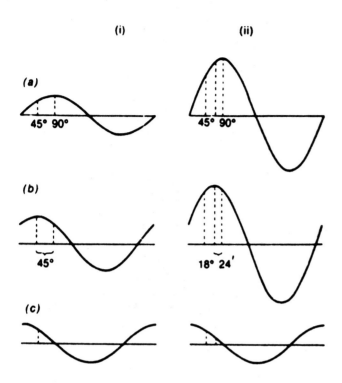

Figure 11-2 Sine and cosine waves. The addition of the sine and cosine signals yields a sinusoid. The sum of the first signals (*i*) produces a 45° shift, while the second set (*ii*) with a larger amplitude sine component produces a shift of 18°24'. (Health Devices 1986; 15:71. Used with permission of ECRI, Inc)

Fourier analysis (DFA) calculates the amplitude of the sine and cosine waves of all frequencies present in the original waveform. However, the mathematical calculations are so great that an algorithm called fast Fourier transform (FFT) is used. It combines predictably identical terms and can be calculated in real time simultaneously with data collection. Such computer-processed FFT analysis forms the basis of two popular processed EEG monitors.

Compressed Spectral Array

A three-dimensional representation of power and frequency plotted against time (frequency domain plot) is known as the compressed spectral array (CSA)[11] and is seen in Figure 11-3. Several minutes of EEG activity can be recorded on a single sheet, and changes are apparent even to physicians not trained in standard EEG interpretation.

A CSA can be used for bedside screening. Limited cortical activity is recorded which does not allow precise localization of cerebral pathology, but such monitoring is valuable to detect seizure activity, cortical ischemia, and burst suppression during barbiturate coma. Processed EEG monitoring should accompany SER recordings to document global cortical activity. However, beware of artifacts which also can be "processed" leading to erroneous interpretation.

Density Modulated Spectral Array

A computer-processed EEG can also be represented in a dot matrix format. Horizontal size and density of the dots are functions of particular frequencies of the EEG, the density modulated spectral array (DSA),[12] seen in Figure 11-4. Data which may be "lost" behind large amplitude peaks of the CSA can often be detected by DSA analysis.

Figure 11-3 Compressed spectral array plotting of power and frequency against time. This frequency domain display allows easy recognition of frequency concentration shifts over long periods. However, the large amplitude of some traces can obscure activity in others. (Health Devices 1986; 15:71. Used with permission of ECRI, Inc)

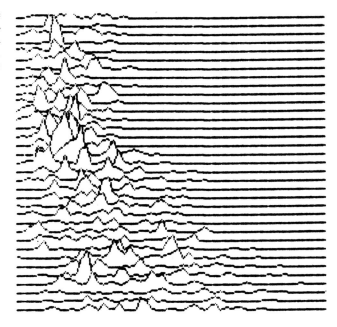

COMPUTED TOMOGRAPHY

An increase of ICP or decrease of intracranial compliance is suggested when a CT scan reveals a mass lesion with a 0.5-cm or greater midline shift or encroachment on the major cerebrospinal fluid (CSF) cisterns.[13] Absence of the basal cisterns on a CT scan is associated with high mortality, particularly when the GCS is 3 or 4. Initial CT visualization of the basal cisterns does not guarantee a good outcome, since later ischemia and hypoxia can rapidly change the prognosis. Mass lesions demonstrated in the posterior, frontal, and temporal lobes frequently are associated with brain stem compression.

INTRACRANIAL PRESSURE

The only direct assessment of ICP is obtained by measurement. Accurate monitoring of ICP depends on the type of monitor placed and the criteria used for determining abnormal values.[14] The Richmond subarachnoid bolt is popular since it does not require brain tissue penetration or knowledge of ventricular positions. However, it requires constant attention to maintain an unobstructed pathway to the subarachnoid space. Ventriculostomy catheters may be impossible to place when cerebral edema causes shifting or collapse of the lateral ventricle system. Subdural or epidural catheters placed through a burrhole can also be used, as can implanted ICP transducers. The latter are beset by numerous technical difficulties related to calibration and stability, however, and are not widely used.[14]

Normal ICP is less than 15 mm Hg. Prolonged uncontrollable ICP above 29 mm Hg is associated with a poor outcome. Patients may exhibit increases in ICP due to pain, suctioning, laryngoscopy, tracheal intubation, and venous obstruction related to head positioning rather than because of intracranial pathology.

In patients with an intracranial mass effect and a shift of the ventricular system, small fluctuations in ICP can produce considerable deterioration in neurologic function. Intracra-

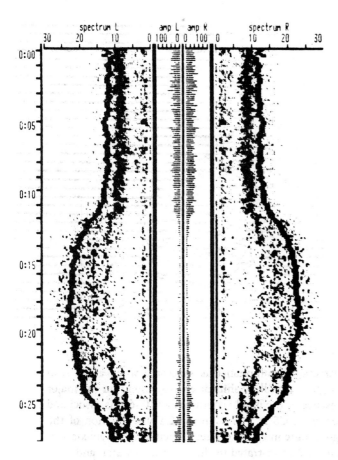

Figure 11-4 Density modulated spectral array in mirror-image format. (Health Devices 1986; 15:71. Used with permission of ECRI. Inc)

nial pressure reaches the phase of rapid rise prior to clinical signs of pupillary dilatation.[15] Thus a normal ICP does not exclude a mass lesion. Monitoring of patients during the acute phase of injury when the ICP is normal is more important than later monitoring when it is uncontrollable. A high ICP suggests decreased CPP and the possibility of regional or global ischemia. As cerebral edema increases, the microvascular network around the neurons collapses and ischemia results. Intracranial compliance determinations are felt by some investigators to have greater prognostic value than the mean ICP.[16]

EVOKED RESPONSES

Unlike EEG recordings which reflect on-going cerebral activity, evoked responses are associated with specific external stimuli. Somatosensory evoked responses commonly use median, peroneal, and posterior tibial nerve stimulation and, ideally, recordings from the peripheral nerve, dorsal spinal cord, and sensory cortex (Fig. 11-5). Auditory brain stem evoked responses use cochlear nerve stimulation and recording of brain stem transmission.

Both modalities can be recorded at the bedside, and allow immediate, quantitative interpretation of the data. The former are affected minimally by the level of consciousness or sedation, neuromuscular paralysis, intoxicants, anesthetics, and anticonvulsant drugs.

Figure 11-5 Recording of SERs. At least two channels are used, each consisting of a pair of electrodes. One electrode is placed along the anatomic pathway; the other serves as a reference. Following median or posterior tibial stimulation, recordings of interest include Erb's point, CII (cervical cord) and cortical areas: C3', Cz, C4'. C3' is contralateral to the stimulation site, 3 cm posterior to C3 (not shown); C4' is ipsilateral to the stimulation site, 3 cm posterior to C4 (not shown). Cz is recorded at the cortex. (Gravenstein JS, Paulus DA: *Clinical Monitoring Practice*, 2nd ed, p 27. Philadelphia, JB Lippincott, 1987)

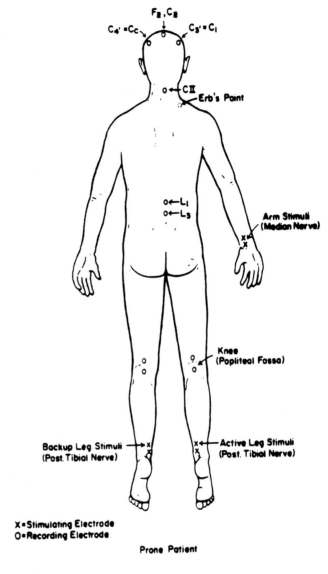

Auditory responses can be used to detect posterior fossa ischemic events. However, since they reflect subcortical function, they can be normal despite severe cortical abnormalities.

Electromagnetic interference and 60-Hz line noise resulting from fluorescent lights, thermal blankets, mechanical ventilators, monitoring devices, other electrical equipment, and shared power lines are common in the ICU and often make data interpretation difficult at best.

Somatosensory Evoked Responses

In comatose patients, SERs are usually recorded following median nerve stimulation. Erb's point, to monitor intact peripheral conduction, is recorded on one channel, while the arrival of the afferent volley at the contralateral sensory cortex is recorded on the second channel (Fig. 11-5). The SER (Fig. 11-6) has a brain stem component 13 to 16 msec after stimulation of the median nerve which is useful when the ABR is absent because of otologic pathology. The first cortical event is a waveform recorded over the contralateral sensory cortex approximately 20 msec after stimulation. Some questions still exist as to the exact generator sites of the SER. However, experimental data linking loss of the cortical SER to critical CBF values make it an excellent means to detect cerebral ischemia.

Lack of a cortical response to a peripheral stimulus can occur after injury to the peripheral nerve (*i.e.*, brachial plexus avulsion), from white matter ischemia that affects axonal conduction of the afferent volley to the cortical cell bodies, with lesions at the thalamic level (intraventricular hemorrhage), or by a direct effect on the cortical cellular activity (subdural hematoma).

Somatosensory evoked responses can be used to monitor spinal cord function during surgical procedures or following trauma. Motor deficits (anterior cord) can be present even though SER recordings (posterior cord) are normal. Also, a lower spinal cord injury will not be detected by SER testing from the median nerve.

Abnormal SERs (and ABRs) in comatose patients with normal visual evoked responses (VERs) suggest cortical function is better than that of the brain stem. Conversely, abnormal SERs and VERs in the presence of maintained ABRs indicate that cortical dysfunction is responsible for the comatose state.

Auditory Brain Stem Evoked Responses

Short latency ABRs (Fig. 11-7), recorded in the first 10 msec following auditory stimulation, reflect brain stem transmission. Central transmission is divided into a rostral component (waves III–V), representing pons to midbrain conduction (superior olive, lateral lemniscus, and inferior colliculis, respectively), and a caudal component (waves I–II), representing conduction from the auditory nerve to the pons (auditory nerve and cochlear nucleus, respectively).[17] Waves VI and VII reflect thalamic transmission and thalamocortical radiations to the primary auditory cortex. Although the exact generator sites of the ABR, like SERs, are not proven, this division of brain stem central transmission is useful to localize

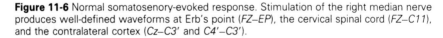

Figure 11-6 Normal somatosenory-evoked response. Stimulation of the right median nerve produces well-defined waveforms at Erb's point (*FZ–EP*), the cervical spinal cord (*FZ–C11*), and the contralateral cortex (*Cz–C3'* and *C4'–C3'*).

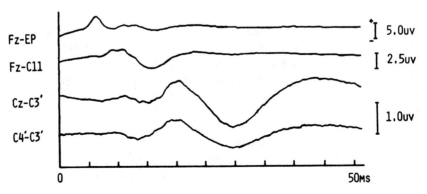

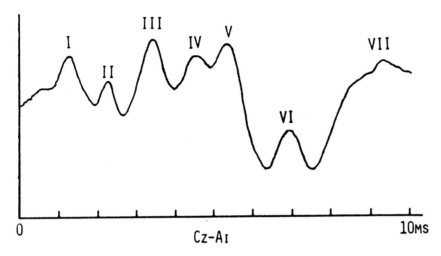

Figure 11-7 Normal short latency auditory brain stem evoked response (first 10 msec following auditory stimulation). The displayed waves, I to VII, represent recordings at various sites from the eighth nerve through the auditory pathway to the cortex.

pathologic lesions. Auditory brain stem responses are highly resistant to sedatives, anticonvulsants, and barbiturates (Table 11-3).

Middle latency responses generated 10 to 60 msec after stimulation have a limited role in acute management but should not be overlooked. In the absence of barbiturates, decreased amplitude of the response may suggest cortical ischemia, especially when it is associated with a similar decrease in the cortical SER amplitude. Middle latency responses also appear to have prognostic value in predicting cognitive outcome. They are profoundly influenced by barbiturates (see Table 11-3).

Multimodality Evoked Responses

The multimodality evoked potential battery[18,19] may be more accurate than the neurologic examination, CT scan, or other physiologic parameters, and compares favorably with the

TABLE 11-3 COMPARISON OF ELECTROPHYSIOLOGIC MONITORING OF CNS FUNCTION

	VER	SER	ABR	EEG	CSA
Drug sensitivity	+	−	−	−	+
Monitor pathways	+	+	+	−	−
Quantitation	+	+	+	−	+
Diagnose seizures	−	−	−	+	+
Altered by temperature	+	+	+	+	+

GCS, ICP, and CT scan as a prognostic indicator. It uses ABR and early SER recordings together with central conduction time (CCT). The latter modality represents the time delay between evoked potentials in brain stem or cervical spinal cord structures and the first recordable cortical waveforms. Changes are associated with cortical dysfunction, synaptic delay in the thalamus or cortex, or slowed axonal conduction. Narayan was able to predict outcome 1 year following severe head injury with 81% accuracy with this battery.[19] Such data may be misleading, since the initial electrophysiologic measurements usually are made several days after injury,[18] thereby increasing the overall prognostic accuracy. During the critical 24 to 48 hours after injury, prognosis remains extremely difficult to ascertain.

CLINICAL APPLICATIONS

BRAIN STEM ISCHEMIA

Abnormal ABRs are associated with brain stem ischemia, CT scan evidence of compressed cisterns around the brain stem, transtentorial herniation of the brain stem, and brain death.[20,21] Brain stem ischemia from hypotension or midbrain compression can be reflected by ABR testing before ICP increases and brain stem CBF falls. An increased ABR, with CCT not localized to either the caudal or rostral components, may be the only evidence of neuronal dysfunction.

Patients with brain stem ischemia due to early transtentorial herniation present with unilateral or bilaterally dilated pupils, high ICP, and MAP that may be normal, low, or high. Confirmation of midbrain compression depends on an abnormality of waves III to V, which appears early but reverts to normal if medical/surgical management is effective. If treatment is not effective, a rostral-caudal deterioration of the ABRs occurs until only wave I, from the extracranial portion of the acoustic nerve, can be recorded (Fig. 11-8). Patients with evidence of transtentorial herniation but with normal ABRs should be aggressively treated.

BRAIN DEATH

Auditory evoked responses are particularly useful to predict an unfavorable outcome in head trauma patients as well as in other patients being assessed for brain death.[20,21] However, unless a peripheral SER is also recorded, no conclusion can be drawn concerning brain stem function if wave I is absent. Otologic pathology occurring with bilateral basilar skull fracture may account for absence of a response despite intact brain stem function. The only ABR assessment associated unequivocally with brain death is the presence of bilateral peripheral components (wave I), but no brain stem response (see Fig. 11-8).

If the ABRs demonstrate brain stem function, a nuclear cerebral perfusion scan will document CBF. In the late stages of cerebral failure, blood flow may be present only in the saggital sinus, but this finding does not establish brain death. Only a demonstrated absence of blood flow satisfies the criteria. Absence of wave I on initial assessment is reported in 13% to 77% of brain-injured patients. A well-formed ABR is strong evidence for brain stem function, even in the absence of brain stem reflexes.

In the SER pathway (see Fig. 11-5), a recordable Erb's point following median nerve stimulation reflects intact peripheral nerve conduction. A more central SER recorded over the cervical area (CII) demonstrates intact cervical conduction (spinal cord dorsal columns). Finally, a normal cortical SER indicates that conduction through the brain stem to the cortex is present. A recordable Erb's point in a patient without demonstrable cervical pathology and with no brain stem and cortical SERs supports a diagnosis of absent brain stem and

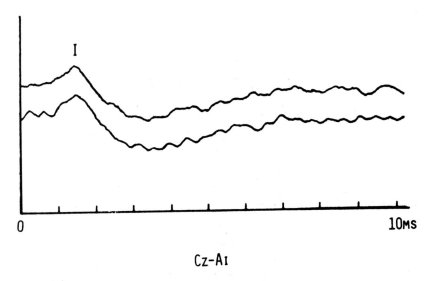

Cz-Aɪ

Figure 11-8 Abnormal ABR in a patient with a clinical diagnosis of brain death. Only wave I (eighth nerve) is recorded following maximal auditory stimulation. The remaining brain stem components (waves II–VII) are absent. Compare with Figure 11-7.

cortical function (Fig. 11-9). Lack of EEG activity, except in the setting of pharmacologic sedation or hypothermia, further substantiates the diagnosis of brain death.

BARBITURATE COMA

During barbiturate coma, neurologic status cannot be determined by either clinical examination or the EEG. Middle latency ABRs, representing auditory cortex activity, are abolished by barbiturate therapy and are also of no use. Short latency ABRs are very resistant to the effects of barbiturates and sedation (see Table 11-3), leaving this monitoring as the primary means to follow brain stem function. Cortical SER activity is unaffected by barbiturate therapy except at very high serum levels. The effects of cortical ischemia can be monitored with SERs even when the CSA demonstrates only burst suppression.

Compressed spectral array monitoring is extremely effective in titrating barbiturate therapy in patients with uncontrollable ICP in whom barbiturate coma is the only remaining therapy. If barbiturates are to be used, their effect on cortical activity must be monitored continuously whenever possible. Some patients require considerably higher serum levels of barbiturates than others before cortical burst suppression is achieved. Once this point is reached, further increase is unwarranted because of adverse cardiovascular side-effects.

OTHER ORGAN SYSTEMS

The emphasis in this chapter is on neurologic monitoring, *per se*. However, other organ system functions can be important and may play a major role in the patient's ultimate outcome. This fact is easily recognized in cases of multisystem trauma or failure (shock, sepsis, and so forth), but is just as true in many episodes of primary CNS dysfunction.

An excellent example involves subarachnoid hemorrhage from a ruptured cerebral

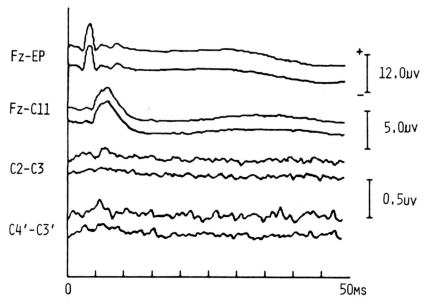

Figure 11-9 Abnormal SER in a patient with a clinical diagnosis of cortical death. Only Erb's point and cervical cord potentials are noted following median nerve stimulation. Cortical responses are absent. Compare with Figure 11-6.

aneurysm. In an attempt to prevent secondary cerebral vasospasm and a worsening of the ischemic insult, many neurosurgeons favor vigorous fluid administration with colloids and crystalloids to augment cardiac output and presumably CBF, particularly to the involved areas. Although the efficacy of this treatment is not fully documented, its use appears to be increasing. Patients with otherwise normal cardiopulmonary function tolerate this regimen reasonably well. Those with marginal function may not. I have seen several episodes of pulmonary edema resulting from overly zealous fluid therapy which necessitated vigorous diuretic therapy and positive-pressure ventilatory support. Rather than awaiting the rather insensitive endpoint of fluffy pulmonary infiltrates appearing on a chest radiograph, one might consider the selective use of pulmonary artery catheterization to evaluate cardiovascular and pulmonary integrity more precisely.

The importance of this and other monitoring is self-evident to anybody involved in critical care medicine. Nunn has addressed the exacerbation of cerebral hypoxia and some implications for care in a theoretical but very provocative chapter in his classic textbook.[22] Anybody embarking on the care of critically ill patients with neurologic impairment is advised to read it. The ultimate goal is support of all systems without associated impairment of brain activity.

SUMMARY

Accuracy, speed, and immediate interpretation of ABR/SER/CSA waveforms are crucial. The usefulness of these recordings must be considered in the context of the underlying neuropathologic (CT scan) and neurophysiologic (MAP, ICP, Pa_{O_2}) factors. Other variables such as drug administration, otologic pathology, and peripheral nerve injuries must be considered, and a basic appreciation of the concepts of brain pathophysiology and rationale for the use of ABR/SER/CSA monitoring in acute management is critical. A team approach and cooperation between the service recording the electrical data, the clinician responsible for the patient's management, and the ICU personnel are essential if such data are to contribute significantly to immediate decision-making.

The full cost–benefit ratio of such monitoring is yet to be proven and is questioned by some experts. Controlled clinical studies are needed before the clinical utility of these techniques can be evaluated or routinely recommended. Equipment with trending capabilities for continuous on-line monitoring and inclusion of automated alarm parameters may help to answer these questions.

CONCLUSION

Frequent clinical and peripheral physiologic assessment of the ICU patient with intracranial pathology remains the mainstay of neuromonitoring in the ICU. The role of electrophysiologic monitors of brain status is currently being refined and assessed. It appears that evoked potentials (ABR, SER) and the processed EEG (CSA, DSA) will play important roles in the near future, assuming that benefit from such monitoring can be established.

Figures 11-6 through 11-9 were kindly supplied by William A. Friedman, M.D., Assistant Professor of Neurosurgery, University of Florida College of Medicine. Dr. Friedman also reviewed the chapter and made numerous suggestions to improve its content. His help is gratefully acknowledged.

REFERENCES

1. Lassen NA: Cerebral blood flow and oxygen consumption in man. *Physiol Rev* 1959; 39:183
2. Javes TH, Morowitz RB, Krowell RM, et al: Thresholds of cerebral ischemia in awake monkeys. *J Neurosurg* 1981; 54:773
3. Astrup J, Symon L, Branston NM, et al: Cortical evoked potential and extracellular potassium and hydrogen at critical levels of brain ischemia. *Stroke* 1977; 8:51
4. Siesjo BK: Cerebral circulation and metabolism. *J Neurosurg* 1984; 60:883
5. Pashayan AG: Monitoring the neurosurgical patient. In Gravenstein N (ed): *Problems in Anesthesia: Monitoring*, pp 104–120. Philadelphia, JB Lippincott, 1987
6. Marshall LF, Smith RW, Shapiro HM: The influence of diurnal rhythms in patients with intracranial hypertension: Implications for management. *Neurosurg* 1978; 2:100
7. Teasdale G, Jennett B: Assessment of coma and impaired consciousness. A practical scale. *Lancet* 1974; 2:81
8. Jennett B: Assessment of the severity of head injury. *J Neurol Neurosurg Psychiatry* 1976; 39:647
9. Jennett B, Teasdale G, Galbraith S, et al: Severe head injuries in three countries. *J Neurol Neurosurg Psychiatry* 1977; 49:291
10. Sundt TM Jr, Sharbrough FW, Piepgras DG, et al: Correlation of cerebral blood flow and electroencephalographic changes during carotid endarterectomy. With results of surgery and hemodynamics of cerebral ischemia. *Mayo Clin Proc* 1981; 56:533
11. Bickford RG, Billinger TW, Flemming NI, et al: The compressed spectral array—A pictorial EEG. *Proc San Diego Biomed Symp* 1975; 11:365
12. Flemming RA, Smith NT: An inexpensive device for analyzing and monitoring the electroencephalogram. *Anesthesiology* 1979; 50:456
13. Tabaddor K, Danziger A, Whisoff HS: Estimation of intracranial pressure by CT scan in closed head trauma. *Surg Neurol* 1982; 18:212
14. Shapiro HM: Neurosurgical anesthesia and intracranial hypertension. In Miller RD (ed): *Anesthesia*, p 1563. Philadelphia, JB Lippincott, 1986

15. Sullivan HG, Becker DP: Intracranial pressure monitoring and interpretation. In *Anesthesia and Neurosurgery*, p 58. St. Louis, CV Mosby, 1980
16. Lorenzo AV, Bresnan MJ, Barlow CF: Cerebrospinal fluid absorption deficit in normal pressure hydrocephalus. *Arch Neurol* 1974; 30:387
17. Tsubokawa T, Ramsay RE: Evoked responses: Use in a neurological intensive care unit. In Green B, Marshall LF, Gallagher TJ (eds): *Intensive Care for Neurological Trauma and Disease*, pp 201–215. Orlando, Academic Press, 1982
18. Greenberg RP, Newlan PG, Hyatt MS, et al: Prognostic implications of early multimodality evoked potentials in severely head-injured patients. *J Neurosurg* 1981; 55:227
19. Narayan RK, Greenberg RP, Miller JD, et al: Improved confidence of outcome prediction in severe head injury. A comparative analysis of the clinical examination, multimodality evoked potentials, CT scanning and intracranial pressure. *J Neurosurg* 1981; 54:751
20. Starr A: Auditory brainstem responses and brain death. *Brain* 1976; 99:543
21. Goldie WB, Chiappa KH, Young RR, et al: Brainstem auditory and short latency somatosensory evoked responses in brain death. *Neurology* 1981; 31:248
22. Nunn JF: *Applied Respiratory Physiology*, pp 471–477. London, Butterworths, 1977

PART TWO

PROCEDURES

CHAPTER TWELVE

VASCULAR CANNULATION

William E. Kaye
Howard G. Dubin

Cannulation must always be considered an invasive procedure, which entails significant risks, both immediate and long term, to the patient. The indication for catheter, the choice of catheter, and the optimal route of insertion must be assessed carefully. The operator should be skilled in the technique and familiar with the indications and complications of each route. In practice, since both skills and detailed knowledge must be developed, the learner must have studied relevant anatomy, understand technique, observed others, assisted with insertion, and then be considered ready to perform procedures under supervision. The philosophy of "See one, do one, teach one" was never really clever, and in today's world it is totally inappropriate. In general, venous cannulation is indicated for fluid and drug administration, to obtain blood specimens for laboratory determinations, for physiologic monitoring, and for access to the central circulation whereas arterial cannulation is used for hemodynamic monitoring and to allow frequent arterial blood sampling. Pulmonary artery catheterization is used for hemodynamic monitoring, mixed venous blood sampling, and determination of cardiac output.

Many brands of catheters are now on the market, but essentially they can be placed into three groups: [1] those that consist of hollow needles (including those attached to a syringe); [2] plastic catheters inserted over a hollow needle; and [3] indwelling catheters inserted either through a hollow needle or over a guidewire that has been placed previously. The length of the catheter chosen depends on the site of insertion and is discussed later. The gauge and the length of the catheter determines its flow characteristics. The flow rate through a 14-gauge catheter of 5-cm length averages 125 ml/min, whereas the flow rate through a 16-gauge 20-cm long catheter may be one-half as much,[1] since resistance to flow is inversely proportional to the fourth power of the conduit radius (Table 12-1).

The catheters themselves are made from various polymers. Early catheters were often made of polyethylene, polyvinylchloride, or nylon. These polymers may, however, be thrombogenic. The stiffness of the catheter may affect the risk of thrombus formation in that stiffer catheters are associated with increased thrombus formation.[2-5] Fluorocarbons were introduced as Teflon TFE (tetrafluoroethylene) and Teflon FEP (a copolymer of hexofluoropropylene and tetrafluoroethylene) in an attempt to produce a less thrombogenic polymer. Silicone elastomer is nonthrombogenic and extremely pliable; however, this very pliability makes insertion difficult without use of an insertion stylet. Silicone catheters appear to have

TABLE 12-1   AVERAGE FLOW RATES FOR VENOUS CATHETERS

	AVERAGE FLOW RATES (in ml/min) FOR TAP WATER	
	Pressure (200 mm Hg 95% ci[*])	*Gravity (95% ci)*
Central Venous Catheter		
USCI 9 French Introducer Internal Diam. 0.117". Length 5 1/2"	566($\pm$16)	247($\pm$2)
USCI & French Introducer Internal Diam. 0.104". Length 5 1/2"	540(n/c)[†]	566($\pm$5)
Deseret Angiocath Gauge 14. Length 5 1/4"	341($\pm$6)	157($\pm$6)
Deseret Angiocath Gauge 16. Length 5 1/4"	195($\pm$4)	91($\pm$2)
Deseret Angiocath Gauge 16. Length 12"	142($\pm$4)	54($\pm$3)
Peripheral Venous Catheter		
IV Extension Tubing Internal Diam. 12" Length 12"	500($\pm$21)	222($\pm$4)
Argyle Medicut Gauge 14. Length 2"	484($\pm$8)	194($\pm$5)
Deseret Angiocath Gauge 14. Length 2"	405($\pm$2)	173($\pm$4)
Viera Quick - Cath Gauge 14. Length 2 1/4"	—	167($\pm$1)
Argyle Medicut Gauge 16. Length 2"	353($\pm$4)	151($\pm$3)
Deseret Angiocath Gauge 16. Length 2"	231($\pm$1)	108($\pm$1)
Viera Quick - Cath Gauge 16. Length 2"	—	108($\pm$1)

(Reproduced with permission from Hoelzer MF: Recent advances in intravenous therapy. *Emerg Clin North Am* 1986; 4:487)
[*] Confidence interval.
[†] No measurement.

a decreased incidence of thrombus formation as compared to polyethylene catheters.[6,7] Full heparinization may be necessary, however, to reduce completely the incidence of clot formation.[8]

In this chapter general principles are described and applied in descriptions of the various procedures used as examples. Chapters 13 and 14 contain more detailed information as to sites and complications.

VENOUS CANNULATION

The percutaneous routes of catheter insertion can be divided into two categories: peripheral and central. Peripheral venipuncture can be performed percutaneously by means of an arm or leg vein or the external jugular vein. Central venipuncture can be performed percutaneously by means of the femoral vein, internal jugular vein, or subclavian vein.

VENOUS ACCESS—PERIPHERAL

Any visible or palpable vein can be used for peripheral venous cannulation. However, certain sites are preferable. The following points should be considered while chosing a peripheral access site.[9] In general, the long veins of the forearm and dorsum of the hand are the most accessible and most easily stabilized IV sites. The use of the nondominant forearm not only increases patient comfort but also reduces the risk of accidental cannula removal. Avoid veins near joints to reduce the need for splinting and provide greater patient comfort. The antecubital fossa should also be avoided so that the veins may be preserved for venipuncture or potential shunts. Leg veins should not be used because of the risk of subsequent deep vein thrombosis and to protect potential veins for coronary artery bypass surgery.

Many techniques are available to help in locating and subsequently distending veins. The tourniquet functions to obstruct venous return while arterial filling continues. Hence, the pressure applied by the tourniquet must be less than arterial pressure (an often forgotten point in the hypotensive patient). Other techniques to help locate veins include holding the arm in a dependent position, hand exercise, vasodilation with nitroglycerin,[10] venous distension devices,[11] and sequential cannulation.[12] The most important issue, however, is a thorough understanding of the anatomy.

Anatomy: Upper Extremities

On the dorsum of the hand, a series of veins arise from the digital veins that run parallel to the long axis of the hand, interconnected by a series of arches that form the dorsal plexus. At the radial side of the dorsal plexus, a thick vein, the superficial radial vein, runs laterally up to the antecubital fossa and joins the median cephalic vein to form the cephalic vein. Other superficial veins on the ulnar aspect of the forearm run to the elbow and join the median basilic vein to form the basilic vein. The median vein of the forearm bifurcates into a Y in the antecubital fossa, laterally becoming the median cephalic and medially becoming the median basilic. The basilic vein passes up the inner side of the arm, becoming deep at the lower third of the arm. As it continues cephalad, it joins the brachial vein to become the axillary vein (Fig. 12-1).[13]

Anatomy: Lower Extremities

The long saphenous vein begins on the inner side of the foot, receiving branches from the dorsal venous arch of the foot. It travels upward in front of the medial malleolus of the tibia to the groove between the upper medial end of the tibia and the calf muscle, and passes backward behind the internal condyle of the femur. It then runs somewhat outward and upward on the inner side of the front of the thigh to 1.5 in (3.8 cm) below the inguinal ligament, where it pierces the saphenous opening to end in the femoral vein (Fig. 12-2).[13]

Anatomy: External Jugular Vein

The external jugular vein is formed below the ear and behind the angle of the mandible where a branch of the posterior facial vein joins the posterior auricular vein. The external jugular vein then passes downward and obliquely backward across the surface of the sternocleidomastoid muscle and pierces the deep fascia of the neck just above the middle of the clavicle, ending in the subclavian vein lateral to the anterior scalene muscle. Valves and

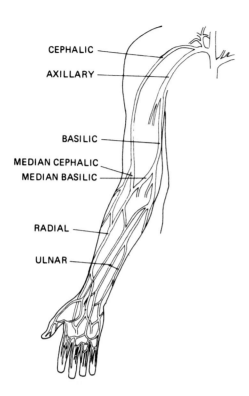

CEPHALIC

AXILLARY

BASILIC

MEDIAN CEPHALIC

MEDIAN BASILIC

RADIAL

ULNAR

Figure 12-1 Anatomy of the veins of the upper extremity. (Reproduced with permission from Kaye[13] by permission of the American Heart Association, Inc.)

other veins enter the external jugular vein at the entrance to the subclavian vein. There are also valves in the external jugular vein about 4 cm above the clavicle (Fig. 12-3).[13]

Technique. As mentioned, there are three general techniques for venous access.[13] The common steps for all these techniques are outlined below.

Technique for Peripheral IV Cannulation

1 Apply a tourniquet (or other venous distending devices) proximal to the anticipated IV site.
2 Locate the vein and cleanse the overlying skin with either an alcohol or povidone-iodine solution.
3 Anesthetize the skin if a large-bore cannula is to be inserted in an awake patient.
4 Hold the vein in place by applying pressure on the vein distal to the point of entry (Fig. 12-4).
5 Puncture the skin with the bevel of the needle upward at a position about 0.5 to 1.0 cm from the vein; enter the vein either from the side or from above (Fig. 12-5).
6 Note blood return and proceed as discussed later.

If a catheter-over-needle device is used (Fig. 12-6), make the venipuncture with the catheter and needle inserted together. Withdraw the needle so that the point is covered by the catheter (about 0.5 cm) and advance the catheter an additional 0.5 cm. Aspirate or observe for continued dripping of blood to confirm intravenous location. Then remove the

Figure 12-2 Anatomy of the long saphenous vein of the leg. (Reproduced with permission from Kaye[13] by permission of the American Heart Association, Inc.)

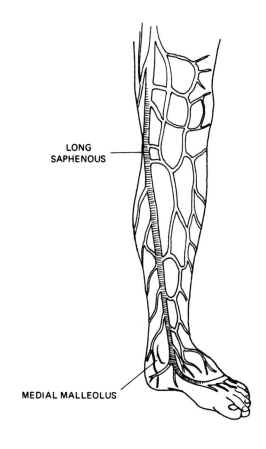

Figure 12-3 Anatomy of the external jugular, internal jugular, and subclavian veins. (Reproduced with permission from Kaye[13] by permission of the American Heart Association, Inc.)

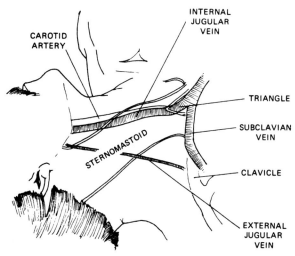

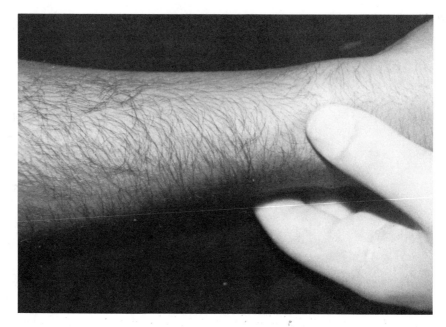

Figure 12-4 After a tourniquet has been applied and the vein has become distended, grasp the vein with the thumb and apply traction distally to hold it in place.

Figure 12-5 After the skin has been punctured, advance the catheter-over-needle device. When the vein wall is encountered, thrust the needle tip forward slightly to achieve venous puncture.

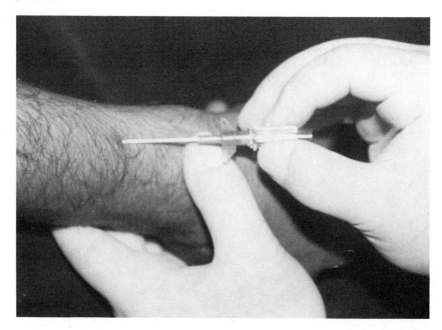

Figure 12-6 Insertion of a catheter over a needle. (Reproduced with permission from Kaye[13] by permission of the American Heart Association, Inc.)

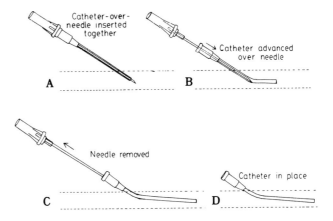

needle and advance the catheter as in Fig. 12-7. Connect the end of the IV tubing directly to the end of the catheter. The length of the catheter is limited by the length of the needle required, but the puncture in the vein is exactly the size of the external catheter, which reduces the possibility of blood leaking around the venipuncture site.

If a catheter-inside-the-needle approach is used (Fig. 12-8), insert the needle into the vessel, advance the catheter through the needle into the vessel, then pull the needle itself

Figure 12-7 While maintaining a grip on the needle, advance the catheter with your fingers. Alternatively, if you have assistance, someone else can maintain traction on the vein and you can use the hand, previously used to grasp, now to advance the catheter.

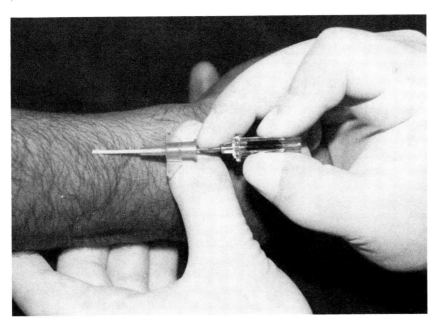

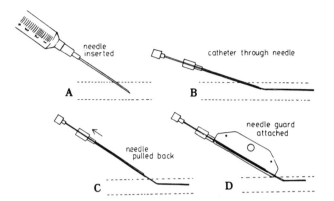

needle
inserted

catheter through needle

A

B

needle guard
attached

needle
pulled back

C

D

Figure 12-8 Insertion of a catheter through a needle. (Reproduced with permission from Kaye[13] by permission of the American Heart Association, Inc.)

back to a position outside the vessel and place a needle guard over the needle. Attach the IV tubing to the catheter. Do not retract the catheter forcibly through the needle. The sharp bevel of the needle *will* clear the catheter, producing a catheter-fragment embolus. These emboli have had to be removed from arms, the heart, and pulmonary circulation. This technique is rarely used today because of this problem among others. Commercially available kits using a small needle and guidewire are safer and easier, and end up with a large catheter size for small needle puncture. This technique is described next.

A third alternative is to insert the catheter over a guidewire (modified Seldinger technique) (Fig. 12-9). Though this technique can be used for peripheral veins, it is most commonly used for central vein cannulation. The guidewire must be several centimeters longer than the catheter to be placed, and the diameter of the wire must be small enough to allow it to pass through both the needle and the catheter. At all times during the insertion of a catheter over a guidewire the end of the guidewire must extend beyond the end of the catheter that remains outside the patient; this prevents the wire from sliding all the way into the catheter and being lost within the circulation. The tip of the guidewire must be flexible; a J-tip facilitates passage of the wire through the tortuous vessels. After the venipuncture is made with the needle, remove the syringe and insert the flexible-tipped or J-tipped guidewire through the needle into the vessel. The wire should pass easily without

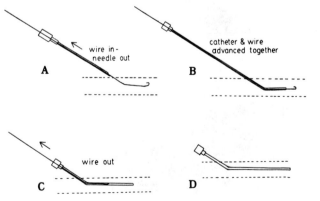

wire in-
needle out

A

catheter & wire
advanced together

B

wire out

C

D

Figure 12-9 Insertion of a catheter over a guide wire (Seldinger technique). (Reproduced with permission from Kaye[13] by permission of the American Heart Association, Inc.)

resistance. If resistance is met, remove the wire and confirm the intraluminal status of the needle placement by aspiration. Once the guidewire is placed through the needle into the vein, remove the needle and insert the catheter over the guidewire, being sure to control the proximal end of the guidewire. When the catheter is in place, remove the guidewire and connect the infusion tubing to the catheter. The use of a guidewire eliminates the hazard of a catheter-fragment embolus; it allows the wire to be withdrawn if it does not pass into the vein easily and permits repositioning of the needle within the vein without having to remove the needle altogether.

A guidewire may be used to introduce a dilator and sheath for insertion of an intra-cardiac catheter. Once the guidewire is in the vein, remove the needle. Make a small incision in the skin at the insertion site and pass the dilator and sheath over the wire into the vein. Remove the dilator and guidewire, leaving the sheath in place. The size of the sheath is determined by the size of the catheter to be introduced.

Complications. The three principle complications of peripheral cannulation are thrombosis, infection, and fluid extravasation into the tissues. Although thrombosis has been common, the use of the newer catheters may decrease this risk. The thrombosis may be secondary not only to the catheter construction, but also to chemical irritation, that is, hypertonic solutions. Infection of the skin site, septic thrombophlebitis, and bacteremia may also occur. Getzen and Pollack[14] report an incidence of infection of 3.3% in peripheral cannulations. The Centers for Disease Control in Atlanta[15] recommend that catheters be replaced every 48 to 72 hours.

VENOUS ACCESS—CENTRAL

Femoral Vein

Femoral vein cannulation is an underutilized approach for access to the central circulation. This may be related to early reports of excessive complications of infection and thrombo-sis.[16,17] However, with the increasing use of femoral catheters in dialysis centers, there is a renewed interest in the approach. It should rarely be used in patients with abdominal sepsis or those who have a heightened risk of venous thrombosis, before femoral vein cannulation.

Anatomy. The femoral vein lies in the femoral sheath, medial to the femoral artery imme-diately below the inguinal ligament. If a line is drawn between the anterior superior iliac spine and the symphysis pubis, the femoral artery runs directly across the midpoint; medial to that point is the femoral vein. If the femoral artery pulse is palpable, the artery can be located with a finger, and the femoral vein will lie immediately medial to the pulsation (Figs. 12-10 and 12-11). The femoral vein is formed from both the deep and the superficial (saphenous) veins of the legs; it extends above the inguinal ligament as the external iliac and becomes the common iliac after being joined by the internal iliac. Both common iliacs join to become the inferior vena cava.

Technique. The steps for initiating IV therapy of the femoral vein follow.

    1 If the puncture is being performed electively, shave the hair around the area. Cleanse the overlying skin vigorously with povidone–iodine solution. Drape as for any sur-

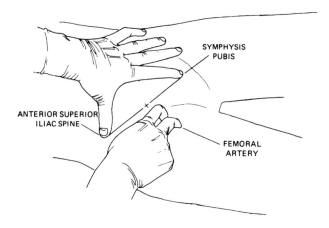

Figure 12-10 The femoral artery runs directly across the midpoint of a line drawn between the superior iliac spine and the symphysis pubis. (Reproduced with permission from Kaye[13] by permission of the American Heart Association, Inc.)

gical procedure. Wear sterile gloves. Ideally, a face mask and a hair cover should be worn as well.

2 Locate the femoral artery either by its pulsation or by finding the midpoint of a line drawn between the anterior superior iliac spine and the symphysis pubis (see Fig. 12-10).

3 Infiltrate the skin with lidocaine if the patient is awake.

4 Make the puncture with the needle attached to a 5- or 10-ml syringe two finger breadths below the inguinal ligament, medial to the artery, directing the needle

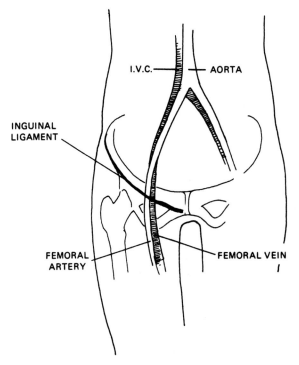

Figure 12-11 Anatomy of the femoral vein. The femoral vein lies medial to the femoral artery below the inguinal ligament. (Reproduced with permission from Kaye[13] by permission of the American Heart Association, Inc.)

cephalad at a 45° angle with the skin (some prefer to enter at a 90° angle) until the needle will go no further (see Fig. 12-11).

5 Maintain suction on the syringe and pull the needle back slowly until blood appears in the syringe, indicating that the lumen of the vein has been entered.

6 Lower the needle more parallel to the frontal plane and proceed as previously described, depending on the type of needle-catheter device used.

7 Cover the puncture site with a povidone–iodine ointment and a sterile dressing. Tape the dressing in place.

Complications. As reviewed by Dailey,[18] the success rate of insertion is high and the complication rate low when large-bore catheters are placed for short periods of time. The major risks include thrombosis, hemorrhage, and infection.

Recent studies report a remarkably low incidence of thrombophlebitis in patients cannulated femorally. Getzen and Pollack[14] reported no instance of thrombosis in their study of 759 patients. Erban[19] showed no clinical thrombosis in his series of 2368 heparinized patients. In the same study, 4 patients who had received femoral catheters were noted to have thrombosis at autopsy compared to 10 episodes of thrombosis in 2494 subclavian lines (not a significant difference).

Hemorrhage is not a very significant problem in femoral cannulation, although it can occur. Getzen and Pollack[14] reported an incidence of "major hematoma" of 1.6% for peripherals and of 1.3% for femoral lines. Infection of the site may occur. There remains a general misconception that femoral lines are more prone to local infection and bacteremia than other sites. However, two studies tend to refute this. Gertner and co-workers[20] studied the risk of infection in subclavian, internal jugular, basilic, external jugular, and femoral lines left in place for a mean of 5.15 days. Twenty-five percent of the subclavian lines were culture positive as compared to 19% of femoral lines. Although 19% is an unacceptably high percentage the incidence was not greater than the other routes of cannulation. Getzen and Pollack[14] reported an incidence of infection at the venipuncture site of 1.4% in femoral lines, 1.1% in subclavian lines, and 3.3% in peripheral lines. As discussed for peripheral lines, all femoral lines should be discontinued at 48 to 72 hours. In our institution we allow these lines to be changed by a guidewire technique (see discussion on central lines). Other complications include arteriovenous fistulas,[21] bowel perforation,[22] and laceration of the inferior epigastric artery.[23]

Internal Jugular and Subclavian Veins

Anatomy *Internal Jugular Vein.* The internal jugular vein (see Figs. 12-3 and 12-12) emerges from the base of the skull, enters the carotid sheath posterior to the internal carotid artery, and runs posteriorly and laterally to the internal and common carotid artery. At its end, the internal jugular vein is lateral and slightly anterior to the common carotid artery. The internal jugular vein runs medial to the sternocleidomastoid muscle in its upper part, posterior to it in the triangle between the two inferior heads of the sternocleidomastoid in its middle part, and behind the anterior portion of the clavicular head of the muscle in its lower part. Here it ends just above the medial end of the clavicle being joined by the subclavian vein.[13]

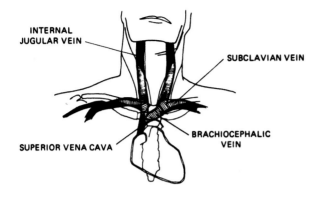

INTERNAL
JUGULAR VEIN

SUBCLAVIAN VEIN

SUPERIOR VENA CAVA

BRACHIOCEPHALIC
VEIN

Figure 12-12 Anatomy of the internal jugular and subclavian veins. (Reproduced with permission from Kaye[13] by permission of the American Heart Association, Inc.)

Anatomy *Subclavian Vein.* The subclavian vein (see Figs. 12-3, 12-12, and 12-13) which in adults is about 3 to 4 cm long and 1 to 2 cm in diameter, begins as a continuation of the axillary vein at the lateral border of the first rib, crosses over the first rib, and passes in front of the anterior scalene muscle. The anterior scalene muscle is about 10 to 15 mm thick and separates the subclavian vein from the subclavian artery, which runs behind the anterior scalene muscle. The vein continues behind the medial third of the clavicle where it is immobilized by small attachments to the rib and clavicle. At the medial border of the anterior scalene muscle and behind the sternocostoclavicular joint, the subclavian unites with the internal jugular to form the innominate, or brachiocephalic, vein. The large thoracic duct on the left and the smaller lymphatic duct on the right enter the superior margin of the subclavian vein near the internal jugular junction. On the right, the brachiocephalic vein descends behind the right lateral edge of the manubrium, where it is joined by the left brachiocephalic vein, which crosses over behind the manubrium. On the right side, near the sternal–manubrial joint, the two veins join to form the superior vena cava. Medial to the anterior scalene muscle, the phrenic nerve, the internal mammary artery, and the apical pleura are in contact with the posteroinferior side of the subclavian vein and the jugulosubclavian junction.[13]

Technique *General Principles.* The steps for initiating IV therapy of the internal jugular and subclavian veins follow.[13] (Figures illustrate internal jugular cannulation.)

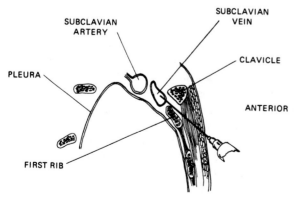

SUBCLAVIAN
ARTERY

SUBCLAVIAN
VEIN

PLEURA

CLAVICLE

ANTERIOR

FIRST RIB

Figure 12-13 Sagittal view through the medial third of the clavicle. (Reproduced with permission from Kaye[13] by permission of the American Heart Association, Inc.)

1 A needle at least 6 cm long with a catheter at least 15 to 20 cm long is usually selected. If the Seldinger technique is used, a thin-wall 18-gauge needle will accept a standard guidewire. A 15-cm catheter is generally used for an internal jugular approach from the right side, whereas a 20-cm catheter is used for any other approach.

2 Identify landmarks. For both the internal jugular approach[24] and subclavian[25] approach, ultrasound guided techniques have been advocated.

3 Determine the depth of catheter placement. The tip of the catheter should be above the right atrium (Fig. 12-14).

4 Place the patient in a supine, head-down position (Trendelenburg) of at least 15° to distend the veins and reduce the chance of air embolism. Extend the patient's head and turn it away from the side of venipuncture (Fig. 12-15).

5 Cleanse the area around the site of puncture with a povidone–iodine solution and drape as for any surgical procedure. Wear sterile gloves. Ideally, a face mask and a hair cover should be worn as well.

6 If the patient is awake, infiltrate the skin with 1% lidocaine without epinephrine.

7 Mount the needle on a 5- or 10-ml syringe containing 0.5 to 1.0 ml saline solution or lidocaine. After the skin has been punctured with the bevel of the needle upward, flush the needle to remove an occasional skin plug.

8 As the needle is slowly advanced, maintain negative pressure on the syringe. As soon as the lumen of the vein is entered, blood will appear in the syringe (Fig. 12-16). Advance the needle a few millimeters further to obtain a free flow of blood. Rapid backward movement of the plunger and the appearance of bright red blood indicate that an artery has been entered, and the needle should be removed and pressure held on the venipuncture site for 5 to 10 minutes. Remember, color of arterial blood will depend upon oxygenation; in the ICV arterial blood often is *not* bright red.

9 Occasionally, the vein will not be entered despite the fact that the needle has been inserted to the appropriate depth. Maintain negative pressure on the syringe and slowly withdraw the needle; blood may suddenly appear in the syringe, indicating that the needle is now in the lumen of the vein. If no blood appears, completely

Figure 12-14 Surface markers on the chest wall to determine the depth of catheter placement: *(a)* sternoclavicular joint–subclavian vein; *(b)* midmanubrial area–brachiocephalic vein; *(c)* manubrial-sternal junction–superior vena cava; and *(d)* 5 cm below the manubrial-sternal junction–right atrium. (Reproduced with permission from Kaye[13] by permission of the American Heart Association, Inc.)

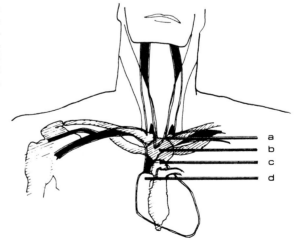

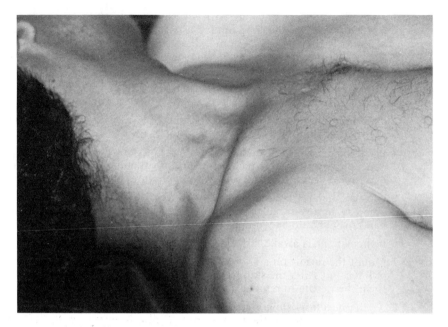

Figure 12-15 The patient has been placed in an appropriate position for internal jugular puncture. For purposes of illustration, the patient has tensed his neck making the sterno-cleidomastoid muscle visible.

Figure 12-16 Using appropriate landmarks (see text), the skin insertion site has been chosen and infiltrated with xylocaine. Introduce the needle (or catheter-needle device) to be used for passage of the guidewire. Advance the tip in the direction of the internal jugular vein, maintaining suction on the syringe. When the needle point punctures the internal jugular vein, blood will enter the syringe.

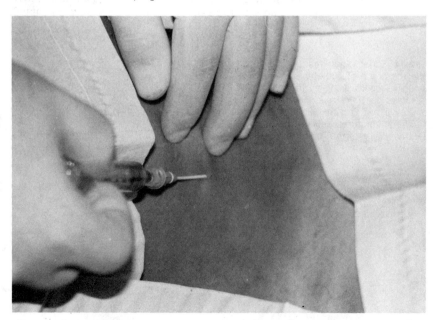

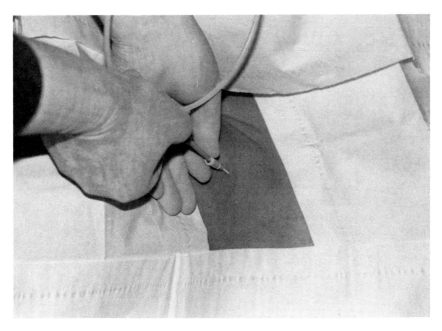

Figure 12-17 Grasping the guidewire in one hand, disconnect the syringe and quickly introduce the guidewire. This may be done through the needle itself or through the plastic catheter, if a needle-catheter device is used.

remove the needle and reinsert it, directing it at a slightly different angle depending on the site of venipuncture.

10 Remove the syringe from the needle, with the finger occluding the needle to prevent air embolism. (A 5-cm water pressure difference across a 14-gauge needle will allow the introduction of about 100 ml of air per second.) If the patient is breathing spontaneously, remove the syringe during exhalation. If the patient is being artificially ventilated with a bag-valve unit or with a mechanical ventilator, remove the syringe during the inspiratory (positive pressure) cycle. Quickly insert the guidewire through the needle to the predetermined point and remove the needle.

11 Insert the guidewire through the needle into the vein. If the guidewire does not pass freely into the vein, remove the guidewire, attach the syringe, and, while maintaining negative pressure on the syringe, reposition the needle until it is in the vein; remove the syringe and insert the guidewire once again. If the guidewire passes freely into the vein, remove the needle (Fig. 12-18) and then pass the catheter over the guidewire into the vein (Fig. 12-19).

12 The catheter should be sutured to the skin, making certain that the catheter is not compressed by the suture (Fig. 12-20).

13 Apply povidone-iodine ointment to the puncture site and tape the catheter in place.

14 The catheter through needle may also be used but has passed from common usage because of risks and the kits now available.

Technique. *Internal Jugular.* The right side of the neck is preferred for venipuncture for three reasons:

1 The dome of the right lung and pleura is lower than the left.

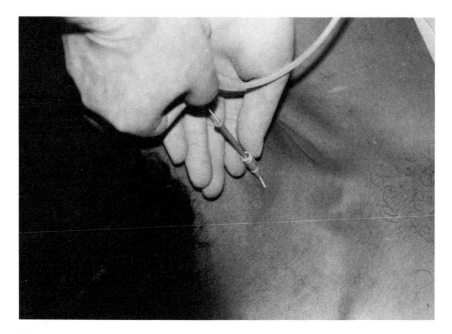

Figure 12-18 Advance the guidewire until about 10–12 cm. are estimated to be below the level of the skin. This should insure that the tip of the guidewire is within the lumen of the internal jugular vein and not run the risk of perforation of the superior vena cava, right atrium, or right ventricle. Holding the guidewire in place, withdraw the needle. When the tip of the needle exits the skin, grasp the guidewire at the skin insertion point and completely remove the needle from the guidewire.

2 There is more or less a straight line to the atrium.

3 The large thoracic duct is not endangered.

I prefer the central approach for internal jugular vein cannulation (Fig. 12-21). The steps for internal jugular cannulation follow.

1 Locate by observation and palpation the triangle formed by the two heads (sternal and clavicular) of the sternocleidomastoid muscle and the clavicle. It may be helpful to have the awake patient lift his head slightly off the bed to make the triangle more visible. In some patients with large or obese necks, it may be difficult to identify the triangle. Palpate the suprasternal notch and slowly move laterally, locating first the sternal head of the sternocleidomastoid muscle, the clavicle, the triangle itself, and, finally, the clavicular head of the sternocleidomastoid muscle.

2 Occasionally the carotid arterial pulse will be palpable within the triangle. Place two fingers along the artery and retract it medially. This maneuver identifies both the location of the artery (so that inadvertent puncture is avoided) and the position of the internal jugular vein, which is lateral to the artery.

3 Insert the needle at a site 0.5 to 1 cm above the apex of the triangle formed by the two heads of the sternocleidomastoid muscle and the clavicle.

4 Direct the needle caudally and laterally, parallel to the medial border of the clavicular head of the sternocleidomastoid muscle toward the ipsilateral nipple at a 45° to 60° angle with the frontal plane.

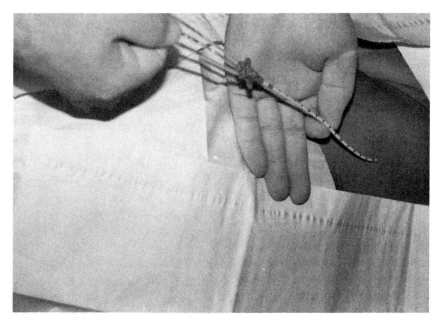

Figure 12-19 Using a scalpel blade, enlarge the needle puncture site so that it will accommodate the catheter. Place the end of the catheter over the tip of the guidewire and advance it through the skin insertion site. Grasp the guidewire distal to the catheter hub and advance the catheter. From the right internal jugular position approximately 15 cm. of catheter should be introduced.

5 If the vein is not entered after the needle has been inserted a few centimeters, slowly withdraw the needle, maintaining negative pressure on the syringe. If the vein is still not entered, withdraw the needle completely; reinsert it, directing it 5° to 10° laterally. If still unable to enter the vein, direct the needle more in line with the sagittal plane. However, do not direct the needle medially (across the sagittal plane) because the carotid artery will be punctured.

Subclavian Vein. I prefer the infraclavicular subclavian puncture for cannulation of the subclavian vein.[13] The subclavian approach should not be used in [1] uncooperative patients, [2] patients with bleeding diathesis, [3] patients with pulmonary bullae, [4] patients with abnormal anatomy, and [5] patients with previous clavicular fractures.

Technique. *Infraclavicular Subclavian Approach.* Steps in the infraclavicular subclavian approach (Fig. 12-22) follow.

1 The patient must be in a supine, head-down position of at least 15°. Some people prefer to place a rolled-up towel vertically between the scapulae and along the vertebral column.

2 Prepare the skin with antiseptic sutures (Fig. 12-23).

3 Introduce the needle 1 cm below the junction of the middle and medial thirds of the clavicle.

4 Hold the syringe and needle parallel to the frontal plane.

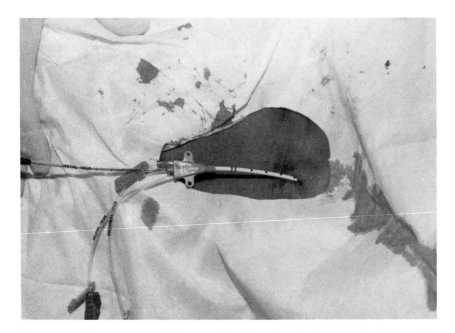

Figure 12-20 The catheter should be sutured in place using the flange attached. Depending upon the type of catheter, the flange may be attached to the catheter away from the insertion site. In these instances, the catheter should be sutured in place at the skin insertion site as well.

5 Direct the needle medially and slightly cephalad, behind the clavicle toward the posterior–superior aspect of the sternal end of the clavicle.

6 Establish a good point of reference by firmly pressing the fingertip into the suprasternal notch to locate the deep side of the superior aspect of the clavicle, and direct the course of the needle slightly behind the fingertip.

7 Once the lumen of the vein has been entered, rotate the bevel of the needle caudally and clockwise 90°, thus facilitating the downward turn that the catheter must negotiate into the brachiocephalic vein.

8 Suture in place (Fig. 12-24).

Complications. Percutaneous placement of central lines by means of the internal jugular or subclavian approach are commonly performed procedures. Both approaches, however, have an overall complication rate ranging from 0.4% to 22%.[26–29] The complications can be divided into two categories: that of mechanical complication usually occurring during placement, and that of long-term complication related to the duration of the catheter remaining in place.

In general, mechanical complications can be divided into vascular injury (hematoma, carotid artery laceration, subclavian artery perforation, internal mammary artery laceration, brachiocephalic false aneurysm, arteriovenous fistula), pleural injury (pneumothorax, hemothorax, hemomediastinum), venous cannulation injury (air embolism, retained catheter fragment); lymphatic injury (thoracic duct injury); neurologic injury (phrenic nerve, brachial

Figure 12-21 Central internal jugular approach. (Reproduced with permission from Kaye[13] by permission of the American Heart Association, Inc.)

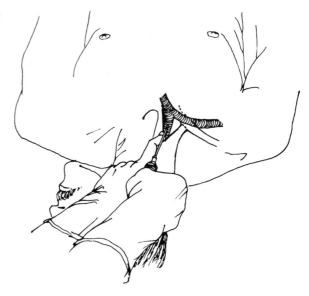

plexus, recurrent laryngeal nerve injury, Horner syndrome); trachea (endotracheal cuff deflation); and thyroid injury (penetration of a thyroid cyst).[30] The mechanical complication rate ranges from 1% to 10%.[28–32]

Success rates for venous cannulation vary with the experience of the operator and the site chosen. In a study by Sznajder and colleagues,[28] the internal jugular approach had a

Figure 12-22 Infraclavicular subclavian approach. (Reproduced with permission from Kaye[13] by permission of the American Heart Association, Inc.)

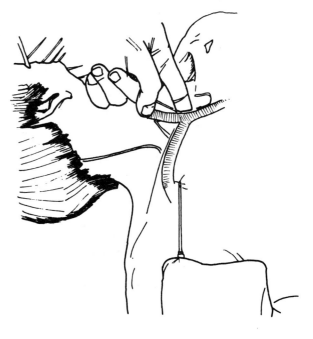

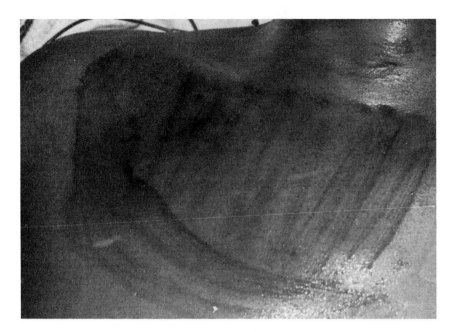

Figure 12-23 The patient has been positioned for infraclavicular subclavian venous puncture and the skin prepared for insertion.

failure rate of 7% by experienced operators and a failure rate of 22% with inexperienced operators. The subclavian approach yielded a failure rate of 7.5% with experienced operators and 15% with inexperienced operators. The complication rates for internal jugular approach (arterial puncture, pneumothorax, hematoma, hemothorax, arrhythmia) were 4.7% for experienced operators and 22% for inexperienced operators. For the subclavian approach the complication rate was 6% for experienced operators and 9.4% for the inexperienced operators. Other studies, however, report success rates for the internal jugular approach of 97% to 100%, with 83% on first attempt. Burr and Ainefeld[33] reviewed the experience of 17 authors and 10,013 subjects who had internal jugular cannulation and found a lower complication rate than with the subclavian approach. They again found that the risk decreased with experience. These figures should be interpreted to mean that learners must know as much as possible about anatomy and technique beforehand. They should observe and assist before performing, and when performing for the first *times,* they should be assisted by experienced personnel. While everyone must acquire experience, the patient must not be subjected to unnecessary risks during the process.

Catheters can be malpositioned on initial placement, with the incidence varying by approach, ranging from 30% malposition by external jugular approach, 5.7% by internal jugular approach, and 5.5% by infraclavicular subclavian approach.[34,35] Although malposition is often easily noted and corrected upon reviewing the post-procedure chest radiograph, the aberrant catheter may yield a host of problems, as reviewed by Dunbar and associates.[36]

Long-term complications related to the duration of time the catheter is in place can be divided into those involving [1] thrombosis and [2] infection. Thrombosis of the central vessels is an often overlooked complication of central venous access. Grant[37] found an

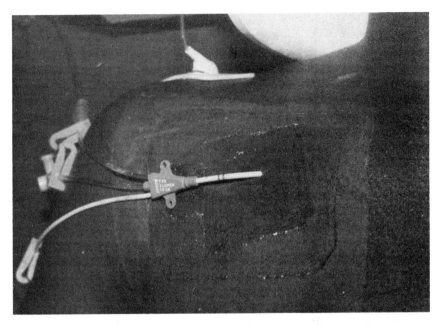

Figure 12-24 Final positioning of the catheter on the chest wall after it has been inserted into the subclavian vein. The catheter should be sutured at the insertion site. If a flange is present (often fixed to the catheter at 20 cm), it may be necessary to suture the catheter at the puncture site and the flange separately in order to avoid introducing too great a length of catheter into the subclavian vein.

incidence of 2.9% of clinical suspicion of thrombosis of the subclavian vessel in his series, whereas in studies using phlebography or radionuclide venography the incidence was as high as 35%.

The other major complication of central venous catheters is the increased risk of catheter-related infections which increases dramatically with the length of time the line is in place and with the number of breaks in sterile technique.[38] Lines placed by percutaneous approach may have an incidence of bacteremia nine times less than those placed by direct cutdown.[38] The current availability of multilumen central venous access lines raises concerns over their risk of catheter-related sepsis.[39–41] It appears that single lumen lines designated for TPN can remain in place for long periods of time if strict adherence to insertion protocol is maintained, as well as maintenance by trained intravenous or nutrition teams and strict prohibition of line violation for any reason. A 1.7% incidence of catheter sepsis in TPN lines maintained an average of 18.8 days has been demonstrated. Recent studies have shown marked differences in assessment of risk of infection of single lumen versus triple lumen central venous lines. Kelly and co-workers[40] found a 3.1% risk of catheter-associated bacteremia in triple lumen catheters, whereas Miller and colleagues[39] found a 33% risk of catheter-induced sepsis in triple lumen catheters compared to only 10% of single lumen catheters in their institution.

The risk of infection appears to increase dramatically after the line has been in place for 3 days. The incidence of positive catheter cultures and associated bacteremia increases markedly after 2 to 3 days.[42] Studies by Bozzetti and colleagues[43] and Pettigrew and co-workers[44] suggest that catheter exchanges by means of guidewire technique has an acceptably low risk of sepsis, if the site is not infected. However, exchange should be performed primarily to obtain a specimen of the catheter originally in place for semi-quantitative culture. In this manner, the site and route of cannulation is maintained, in most cases the removed segment is sterile when obtained, and the patient has not been subjected to an unnecessary second cannulation. See Chapter 2, "Clean and Aseptic technique at the Bedside" for details.

ARTERIAL CANNULATION

Arterial cannulation (see also Chapter 13 "Hemodynamic Monitoring: Arterial Catheters") is indicated for both hemodynamic monitoring and to avoid the discomfort and injury from multiple arterial blood sampling. An indwelling arterial cannula also allows the monitoring of moment-to-moment variations in blood pressure in hemodynamically unstable patients, as well as more accurate monitoring in those patients with unreliable indirect blood pressure monitoring. The patient in shock with elevated systemic vascular resistance may register a significant discrepancy between pressure obtained by auscultatory and palpatory methods and pressure obtained intra-arterially.

An artery suitable for placement of an indwelling catheter for continuous monitoring of intra-arterial pressures should have the following characteristics: [1] the vessel should be large enough to measure pressure accurately without the catheter occluding the artery or producing thrombosis; [2] the artery should have adequate collateral circulation; [3] there should be easy access to the site for nursing care; and [4] it should not be an area prone to contamination. The most common sites used are the radial artery followed by the femoral artery, dorsalis pedis, and the axillary artery. Occasionally the brachial artery is used.

The radial artery is the most commonly used site for cannulation and is probably safe and free from significant potential complications if careful attention is directed to demonstrating adequate ulnar collateral flow before cannulation.[45,46] However, if the patient develops shock or a low output state after cannulation, the flow through the collateral circulation may be inadequate. Thus, one should ascertain that collateral flow is adequate when first performing arterial cannulation, but this should not be regarded as a guarantee if hemodynamic instability develops later. Even though thrombosis of the radial artery at the catheter site is common, ischemic injury of the hand is rare if there is adequate ulnar collateral flow, although a recent report suggests that the risk is small even if collateral flow is poor.[47] The dorsal pedal arteries are without significant cannulation hazards if collateral flow is demonstrated to the remainder of the foot through the posterior tibial artery. The axillary artery is a large artery with excellent collateral flow, suggesting that thrombosis would not lead to any serious sequelae. However, embolism of air or thrombus that forms around the catheter tip may produce ischemic injury to the brain or the hand. The femoral artery is a large artery that is frequently used for monitoring pressures but should be avoided in the presence of abdominal sepsis or occlusive arterial disease of the lower extremity. The femoral pulse still may be palpable when the radial pulses are lost in patients with marked hypotension. Since thrombosis that might follow brachial artery cannulation may lead to ischemic injury of the lower arm and hand, the brachial artery is not used routinely in my institution.

DETAILS OF CANNULATION (RADIAL ARTERY)

Anatomy

The radial artery, a branch of the brachial artery, extends down the anterior radial aspect of the forearm where, after sending a branch to the palm, it disappears deep to the abductor pollicis longus tendon just beyond the distal end of the radius. From there, it continues across the floor of the anatomic snuffbox into the dorsum of the hand. At the wrist, the radial artery is palpable in a longitudinal groove formed by the tendon of the flexor carpi radialis medially and the distal radius laterally. The ulnar artery, the other major branch of the brachial artery, extends down the ulnar aspect of the forearm to the wrist, where it is sheltered by the tendon of the flexor carpi ulnaris. At the wrist, the ulnar artery is palpable just lateral to this tendon. The superficial palmar arch is formed from a continuation of the ulnar artery into the hand; both the deep palmar arch and the dorsal arch are a continuation of the radial artery.[46]

Technique for Radial Artery Cannulation

Steps for radial artery cannulation follow.[46]

1 The patient's hand should be supported and dorsiflexed at the wrist approximately 60° with both the hand and the lower forearm secured to a board. A roll of gauze behind the wrist will maintain dorsiflexion (Fig. 12-25).

2 Locate the radial artery just proximal to the head of the radius.

3 Cleanse the area with povidone–iodine solution.

Figure 12-25 The patient's hand has been supported and fixed to a small arm board prior to insertion of the radial artery catheter.

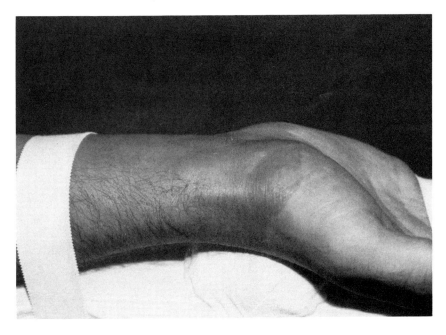

4 Wear sterile gloves and drape the area with sterile towels.

5 Infiltrate the skin over and to the sides of the radial artery with 1% lidocaine without epinephrine if the patient is awake.

6 Use a 20-gauge 2-inch catheter. Insert the catheter-over-needle device at about a 30° angle to the surface of the skin (Fig. 12-26). Advance the catheter and needle stylet into the artery until blood appears in the hub of the needle (Fig. 12-27).

7 While holding the needle in the fixed position, advance the catheter over the needle into the artery. (Fig. 12-28).

8 Remove the needle and attach the hub of the catheter to the connecting tubing.

9 Tie the catheter securely in place with 3-0 or 4-0 monofilament sutures.

10 Remove packing, if used, from under the back of the wrist and fix the wrist in a neutral position to the board (Fig. 12-29). This is essential because one or two full flexions of the wrist joint can completely destroy an arterial line, and securing the hand in a dorsiflexed position may lead to neuromuscular injury to the hand.

11 Apply povidone–iodine ointment to the skin at the site of insertion and cover with a sterile dressing.

Complications of Arterial Catheterization

Certain risk factors may increase the complication rate of arterial lines. Factors that may predispose to increased risk include decreased hemodynamic stability, that is, hypotension, low cardiac output, and use of vasopressors; intrinsic vascular disease (atherosclerosis, severe

Figure 12-26 Palpate the right radial pulse with the fingers of your left hand. Choose a site approximately 0.5 to 1 cm. distal to the palpation point for insertion of the needle-catheter device.

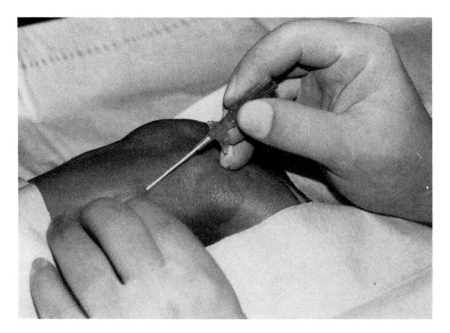

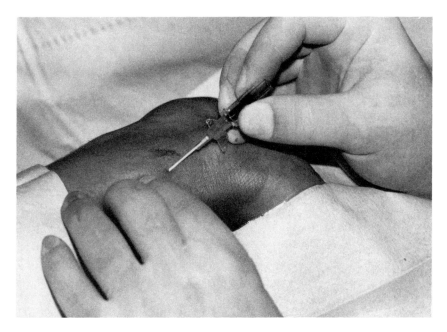

Figure 12-27 After puncturing the skin, advance the needle directly towards the palpated pulse. Sometimes the pulsations can be sensed through the needle; often the change from subcutaneous fat to muscular arterial wall can be sensed. Advance the needle until blood appears in the needle hub.

hypertension, Raynaud's, autoimmune disorders); and contamination (sepsis, break-in technique, prolonged intravascular stay).

The most common complication is thrombosis. The risk of thrombosis increases with length of time the line is in place. Radial lines left in place longer than 48 hours have an increased risk of thrombosis over those left in place for shorter times.[48,49] The size of the cannula also plays a role in the risk of thrombosis. The larger the size of the cannula relative to the diameter of the vessel, the greater is the risk of thrombosis.[50,51] The risk of thrombosis also increases with tapered catheters and differs depending on the catheter material (Teflon being less thrombogenic than polyethylene).[49–52]

Intermittent flushing also increases the risk of thrombosis, and a continuous heparin flush with a pressurized heparinized system is recommended. Jones and colleagues[53] and Bedford[49] have shown that 5% to 8% of thrombosis formation can be expected with intra-arterial monitoring. However, most patients with asymptomatic occlusion recanalize. The incidence of surgical intervention for symptomatic occlusion is only about 1%.[54]

The other major complication with arterial lines is infection. The factors include length of time the line is in place and technique of insertion. There is an increased risk of infection in lines that remain in place longer than 72 hours.[42] Percutaneously inserted catheters have a decreased incidence of infection as compared to those placed by surgical cutdown.[38] Intra-arterial lines may be responsible for as much as 10% to 30% of nosocomial bacteremias[55] and may also serve as sites for secondary infection. In Band and Maki's study,[56]

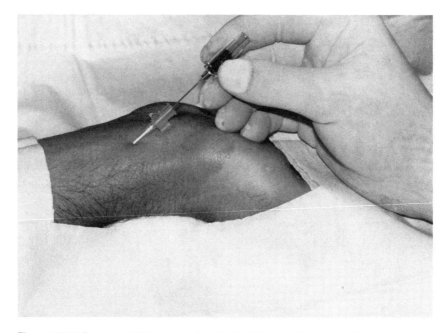

Figure 12-28 Once blood fills the needle hub, hold the needle in place. Push the catheter into the arterial lumen over the stationary needle.

of 37 catheters exposed to bacteremia 5 were tip-culture positive for the same organism. In our institution, all arterial lines are removed after 72 hours and sent for culture. New sites are chosen after careful assessment of vascular patency.

Other complications noted with arterial lines are embolism, skin necrosis, and possible exsanguination from a disconnected line.

PULMONARY ARTERY CATHETERIZATION

INDICATIONS FOR PULMONARY ARTERY CATHETERIZATION

There are several general indications for pulmonary artery catheterization (see also Chapter 14, "Hemodynamic Monitoring: Pulmonary Artery Catheters") in critically ill patients,[57] including [1] measurement of right atrial (RA), pulmonary arterial (PA), and pulmonary artery occlusion (PAOP) pressures; [2] assessment of cardiac function by measuring cardiac output; and [3] sampling of pulmonary arterial (mixed venous) blood. With data derived from these measurements, one can evaluate both right and left ventricular function, which includes defining hemodynamic subsets, determining the response to therapeutic interventions with serial measurements, and separating cardiogenic from noncardiogenic pulmonary edema.

DESCRIPTION OF THE PULMONARY ARTERY CATHETER

The catheter is constructed of polyvinylchloride, and the standard length for adults is 110 cm. It is available in both a 7 French and 7.5 French size. The catheter is marked with black rings at 10-cm intervals measured from the tip. It can contain three or four lumens and a

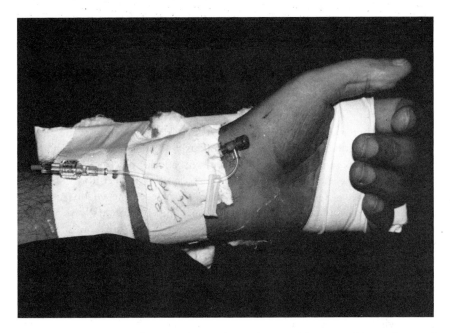

Figure 12-29 After the catheter has been advanced to a satisfactory position and sutured in place, apply povidone-iodine ointment and cover with an occlusive dressing. Remove the material used to dorsiflex the hand and tape the hand to the armboard in a more natural and comfortable position. This photograph shows the hand two days after the dressing was placed to illustrate natural position and method of taping in use.

wire. In the standard 7 French triple lumen catheter the distal lumen ends at the tip of the catheter and is used for measurement of pulmonary artery and pulmonary artery occlusion pressures and for sampling of pulmonary artery mixed venous blood. A proximal lumen ends about 30 cm from the tip of the catheter and is used for injecting the thermal bolus into the right atrium for thermodilution cardiac output, measurement of right atrial pressure, fluid and drug administration, and blood sampling. In the 7.5 French catheter a third lumen terminates at either the 20- (right ventricle) or 30-cm mark (extra right atrial port) and can be used for fluid and drug administration and for sampling of right atrial blood. A pacing wire can also be inserted through the right ventricular port to allow right ventricular pacing. A fourth lumen ends in a balloon near the catheter tip. The balloon, when inflated with 1.5 cm of air, protrudes over the catheter tip and decreases the risk of endomyocardial stimulation and induction of arrhythmias during the passage of the catheter tip through the right heart. The inflated balloon guides the catheter from the intrathoracic veins through the right heart to the pulmonary artery, where its progress is stopped as the balloon impacts the pulmonary vessel. The balloon then occludes the pressure from the pulmonary artery. The catheter tip can then, if properly zeroed and calibrated, give a measurement of PAOP that is an approximation of left atrial pressure. The wire terminates in a thermistor bead 3.5 to 4.0 cm proximal to the tip and provides electrical connections between the thermistor and the cardiac output computer. The thermistor allows continuous measurement of pulmonary artery blood temperature (body core temperature) and measurement of cardiac output by thermodilution (see Chapter 5, "Cardiac Output Measurement Technology). In my institution a sterile sleeve adapter is also attached to the pulmonary artery catheter, and when the line is placed one end is fastened to the introducer and the other end is stretched to encompass the pulmonary artery catheter and then tightened into place. This allows for minor repositioning of the catheter in a sterile fashion.

SITE OF INSERTION

The pulmonary artery catheter originally was inserted through a cutdown into the antecubital fossa. Now it is more frequently inserted percutaneously by an introducer through the internal jugular vein, subclavian vein, or femoral vein. As a rule, percutaneous catheter insertion can be performed in a shorter period of time than can a venous cutdown and may decrease the risk of infectious complications. However, the use of the venous cutdown avoids the hazards of pneumothorax and hemorrhage, especially in patients with existing bleeding diathesis, that exist with internal jugular or subclavian insertions, although arm immobilization is necessary. It may be more difficult to insert the catheter through the femoral vein; the catheter has to travel a long distance before reaching the right heart and may be deflected by the various veins entering the inferior vena cava.

PULMONARY ARTERY CATHETER INSERTION

If the patient is receiving mechanical ventilation before catheter insertion, the ventilatory settings and alarms should be checked, the connecting tubing emptied of water, and the trachea suctioned. Lidocaine, atropine, and a defibrillator must be available at the bedside, and the patient should be monitored continuously with an EKG. The equipment should be readied and calibrated according to hospital protocol.

Meticulous sterile technique is mandatory. The area of insertion should be prepared as for any surgical procedure, with as large an area of the bed draped as possible. The operator and assistants should wear hair covers, masks, and sterile gowns and gloves for the insertion. If the catheter is to be placed through a central access route, a percutaneous introducer is placed (using the techniques described for the subclavian approach or the internal jugular approach). I also attach a three-way stopcock to the introducer line so that, if necessary, this line can be used for IV access.

The balloon is tested by inflating it to the recommended volume. Generally the balloon should be inflated with air. Filtered carbon dioxide should be used if there is any possibility of a right-to-left shunt where a systemic air embolus might occur. Liquids should never be used for balloon inflation. To be certain that there are no leaks in the balloon, it can be inflated under water. Three-way stopcocks should be attached to the CVP (proximal) and pulmonary artery (distal) lumens (and to the additional third lumen if present) and pressure monitoring lines attached to the stopcocks. The stopcock in the third lumen can be closed after flushing. All lumens should be flushed with sterile saline solution containing 2 to 4 units of heparin per milliliter so that fluid remains in the catheter and the lumens are free of air bubbles.

To avoid damage to the catheter or the balloon when inserting it through a cutdown, use a vessel dilator or disposable vein guide. Forceps should not be used on the balloon. To avoid damaging the balloon during percutaneous insertions through a catheter introducer, use an 8 French catheter sheath for the 7 French pulmonary artery catheter (8.5 sheath for a 7.5 catheter). During insertion, the balloon should be fully inflated when the catheter is in the central circulation. This will aid its passage as implied by the name "flow-directed, balloon tipped" catheter. It should remain inflated while it is in the right ventricle; this will minimize ventricular irritability. The recommended volume for balloon inflation should not be exceeded because balloon rupture may result. The balloon should always be deflated before withdrawing the catheter to avoid damage to intracardiac structures.

TECHNIQUE OF INSERTION

Steps in the technique of pulmonary artery catheter insertion follow.[57]

1 Identify a site for emergency access of drugs in the event that they need to be used during the line insertion.

2 Identify space in the room for the emergency defibrillator to be placed in the event that it needs to be used during the line insertion.

3 Confirm that there is no preexisting left bundle branch block. Transient right bundle branch block may occur as the catheter tip passes through the right ventricle. This condition may be especially hazardous in a patient who has preexisting left bundle branch block because it causes complete heart block.[58,59] In such patients it is prudent to insert a temporary transvenous pacing catheter before attempting insertion of a pulmonary artery catheter or to use a pulmonary artery catheter with pacing capabilities.

4 Check the ventilator alarms and circuits and make any adjustments needed before beginning the line insertion (if applicable).

5 Set up the transducers; calibrate and level them.

6 Shave the insertion site (if applicable).

7 Using sterile technique (including hair cover, mask, and gloves), vigorously prep the insertion site.

8 Change to new sterile gloves.

9 Drape the insertion site.

10 Assemble the pulmonary artery catheter, flush all lumens with a heparinized solution, check the balloon, and apply a sterile sleeve adapter, if desired.

11 Anesthetize the insertion site with lidocaine 1% without epinephrine.

12 Cannulate the vessel of choice.

13 Insert a flexible J-tipped guidewire through the needle and remove the needle. (Be careful that ventricular ectopy is not induced, since the guidewire may touch the right ventricle).

14 Make a small skin incision over the guidewire to facilitate insertion of the introducer/dilator.

15 Thread the introducer/dilator assembly over the guidewire. Remove the guidewire and dilator together, leaving the introducer in place. Aspirate back on the introducer lumen from the sidearm to document intravascular position and to eliminate any air, and then inject a heparinized solution to maintain line patency.

16 Insert the pulmonary artery catheter through the introducer while monitoring the pressure waveform from the distal lumen. Since the pulmonary artery catheter has a preformed tip, it is important to insert the catheter with the curve pointing in such a way as to pass easily through the right atrium, the right ventricle, and into the pulmonary artery. Generally, if the catheter is inserted from the internal jugular or the subclavian vein, it should be in the right atrium after about 15 to 20 cm, and often 40 cm if inserted from the left antecubital fossa. Once the catheter is in the central vein, inflate the balloon to its full volume. There should be a slight resistance to inflation of the balloon. If no resistance is felt, the balloon may have ruptured, and it should be removed and retested. If a great deal of resistance is met, the balloon is probably malpositioned and should be repositioned.

17 With continuous waveform monitoring, advance the catheter carefully through the right atrium into the right ventricle, the pulmonary artery, and to the pulmonary artery occlusion position (Fig. 12-30). When the catheter is in the vena cava, the waveform is usually relatively damped. If the patient is asked to cough, there should be an abrupt increase in the pressure, indicating that the catheter tip is within the veins of the thorax. When the catheter enters the right atrium, the amplitude of the waveform should be unchanged, but venous waves should still be recognized. As the catheter passes the tricuspid valve and enters the right ventricle, there is an abrupt increase in systolic pressure, which falls rapidly toward zero and then plateaus before the next abrupt rise with systole. The diastolic waveform in the right ventricle has the appearance of a square root sign. When the catheter enters the pulmonary artery, the systolic pressure remains the same (in the absence of obstruction at the pulmonic valve), but the waveform is that of an arterial pressure with a dicrotic notch and a gradual fall during diastole before the next abrupt upstroke. The diastolic pressure is higher in the pulmonary artery than in the right ventricle. When the catheter reaches the occlusion position, the waveform should again become damped with the appearance of a and v waves; mean occlusion pressure should be equal to or less than pulmonary artery diastolic pressure. Once this position is reached, the balloon should be deflated, at which time the waveform should abruptly change from occlusion to that of the pulmonary artery.

In the average-sized adult, if the catheter is inserted from the internal jugular or the subclavian vein, the pulmonary artery should be entered after about 50 cm of the catheter has been inserted; if from the arm or the femoral vein, the pulmonary artery should be entered after about 70 cm of catheter has been inserted. Insertion of the catheter beyond this length without reaching the pulmonary artery suggests that the catheter is coiling up either in the right atrium or the right ventricle. If the pulmonary artery is not entered, deflate the balloon and withdraw the catheter to the right atrium. In conditions of low-output state, tricuspid regurgitation, or pulmonary hypertension, it may be difficult or impossible to pass the catheter into the pulmonary artery. On occasion, having the patient take deep breaths will facilitate the passage of the catheter; if unsuccessful, fluoroscopy will have to be used. As the catheter remains in the vascular compartment, it softens. At times it may be necessary to flush the catheter with cold solution to stiffen it and make passage easier. In addition, if several attempts at passage are unsuccessful, it may be necessary to remove and replace the catheter. The patient's position should also be changed. On occasion, right lateral, upright, or left lateral decubitus has been

Figure 12-30 Pressure waveforms recorded as the pulmonary artery catheter is advanced through the right atrium *(RA)*, right ventricle *(RV)*, into the pulmonary artery *(PA)*, and to wedge *(PCW)* position. (Reproduced with permission from Kaye[57] by permission of the American Heart Association, Inc.)

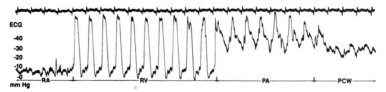

successful when other manipulations have failed. Also, in low output states, inotropic agents or calcium chloride may increase cardiac output and permit passage of the catheter.

The following are criteria to confirm the occlusion position:[57] [1] the ability to flush the catheter before inflating the balloon, which excludes the possibility of catheter obstruction; [2] the disappearance of the typical pulmonary artery pressure tracing when the balloon is inflated and its reappearance promptly after deflation; [3] the presence of an occlusion pressure lower than or equal to pulmonary artery diastolic pressure; and [4] oxygen tension or saturation of blood drawn from the occlusion position greater than or equal to that of pulmonary artery blood (specimen obtained with balloon deflated). In patients with arterial hypoxema, the aspirated PAO oxygen tension may even be higher than systemic arterial blood.

18 Once the occlusion position has been reached, alternately inflate and deflate the balloon and position the catheter so that occlusion waveform can be obtained with full inflation of the balloon.

19 Once the catheter is in place in the pulmonary artery, secure the catheter with suture. As soon as the catheter is secured, obtain a chest radiograph to document the location of the catheter tip. This procedure will exclude the presence of pneumothorax or other complications if the insertion was by way of the internal jugular or subclavian technique. If the catheter was inserted from the arm, immobilize the arm. Remember, however, that pneumothorax may not appear for some hours if only a small air leak is present. Therefore even if a patient's clinical condition deteriorates later, it may be prudent to repeat the chest radiograph, even if an earlier film did not show a pneumothorax.

20 The pulmonary artery waveform must be continuously monitored so that inadvertent wedging can be recognized immediately and the catheter withdrawn. Failure to withdraw the catheter from a wedge position may lead to pulmonary infarction.

21 If the catheter has been in place for some time and the tip has slipped back toward the pulmonic valve so that occlusion pressures can no longer be obtained, do not advance the catheter unless it is covered by a catheter sleeve. Bacteria may be introduced from either that part of the catheter outside the patient or from the skin insertion site itself. Special catheter sheaths have been developed that allow the catheter to be repositioned aseptically.

COMPLICATIONS

The list of potential complications associated with pulmonary artery catheterization can be divided into six categories.

1 Those associated with insertion

2 Pulmonary infarction or pulmonary artery perforation

3 Thrombosis and thromboembolism

4 Arrhythmias

5 Valvular damage

6 Infection

Pulmonary artery catheter insertions have the same risks associated with internal jugular line or subclavian line insertions. These risks include pneumothorax, hematoma, and laceration of the vein or carotid artery with subsequent hemorrhage. Although balloon rupture is rarc, it may yield a systemic air embolus in the presence of a right-to-left intracardiac shunt. Further, the ruptured balloon cannot provide protection to the vascular wall or myocardium if catheter repositioning is necessary. Knotting of the catheter most often occurs when there is looping of the catheter in the right ventricle. The knot may also form around an intracardiac structure such as a papillary muscle.[60–63] Generally the knotted catheter can be removed without much difficulty, but occasionally a surgical approach is neccesary[64] (Fig. 12-31).

Pulmonary infarction may occur if it migrates distally and an undetected wedge pattern persists.[65] The extent of the pulmonary infarction depends on the degree of blood flow obstructed and the amount of time the catheter is left in wedge position. In addition to pulmonary infarction, pulmonary artery rupture should be considered in any patient with hemoptysis. The reported incidence of pulmonary artery rupture is 0.2%.[66] The risk of pulmonary artery perforation is increased with distal placement of the catheter, vigorous balloon inflation, or flushing. The risk is also increased in patients with pulmonary hypertension, with mitral valve disease, and those receiving anticoagulant therapy.[67–71]

As the pulmonary artery catheter sits in the vascular space, thrombus formation around the catheter and at sites of endocardial contact may occur.[65,72–74] This may potentiate thromboembolic events. The risk of thrombus formation is increased by the same events mentioned previously that increase the risk of thrombus formation for central venous and arterial cannula. The ruptured balloon may also increase the risk of thrombus formation. The risk of thromboembolic events is decreased with the use of heparin bonded catheters, although it is unclear for how long.[75]

Atrial and ventricular arrhythmias are common during pulmonary artery catheter

Figure 12-31 A two-lumen pulmonary artery catheter did not traverse the pulmonary valve. Attempts to advance the catheter resulted in this knot. Because of its size, surgical exposure of the internal jugular vein and venotomy was necessary in order to extricate the knotted catheter for removal.

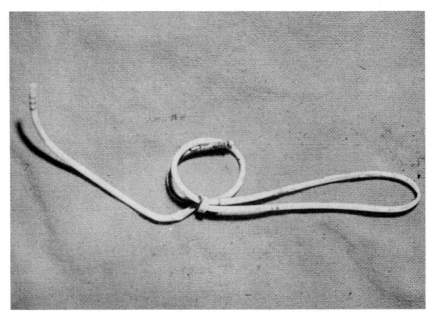

insertions. The incidence of ventricular ectopy in a recent study was 45%;[76] however, the risk of sustained ventricular ectopy seems small. The incidence may be reduced by assuring that the balloon adequately encloses the tip of the catheter and that the time of exposure of the tip of the catheter to the right ventricle is small.[77] As mentioned previously, there is an increased incidence of transient right bundle branch block during pulmonary artery catheter insertion, and in the patient with a preexisting left bundle branch block a pacing catheter (or a catheter that allows a pacer to be placed quickly through one of the pulmonary artery catheter lumens) should be placed before inserting the pulmonary artery catheter. Autopsy evidence confirms that mechanical damage to the tricuspid and pulmonic valves may occur as the result of prolonged catheterization, though no known clinical correlates have been defined in most patients.[61,76,78]

As with other central lines, pulmonary artery catheters are at risk for infection, both at the insertion site and systemically. These risks are increased with repeated breaks of the closed system for blood drawing (mixed venous sample), thermodilution cardiac output measurements, and catheter repositioning. The length of time the line is in place is also an important factor, with an increased risk of a culture-positive catheter segment after 72 hours.[42,79] Rates range from 3% to as high as 35%.[76,79–82] Systemic evidence of infection was found to be 8% in one study.[79]

REFERENCES

1. Graber D, Dailey RH: Catheter flow rates updated. *J Am Coll Emerg Physicians* 1977; 6:518
2. Indar R: The dangers of indwelling polyethylene cannulae in deep veins. *Lancet* 1959; 1:284
3. Hoshal VL, Ause RG, Hoskin PA: Fibrin sleeve formation on indwelling subclavian central venous catheters. *Arch Surg* 1971; 102:353
4. Jones MV, Craig DB: Venous reaction to plastic intravenous cannulae; influence of cannulae composition. *Can Anesth Soc J* 1972; 19:491
5. Spanos HG, Hecker JF: Thrombus formation on indwelling venous cannulae. *Anaesth Intensive Care* 1976; 4:217
6. Welch GW, McKeel DW, Silverstein P, et al: The role of catheter composition in the development of thrombophlebitis. *Surg Gynecol Obstet* 1974; 138:421
7. Ross AH, Griffith CD, Anderson JR, et al: Thromboembolic complications with silicone elastomer subclavian catheters. *J Parenteral Enteral Nutr* 1982; 6:61
8. Ruggiero RP, Aisenstein TJ: Central catheter fibrin sleeve–heparin effect. *J Parenteral Enteral Nutr* 1983; 7:270
9. Clutton–Brock TH: How to set up a drip and keep it going. *Br J Hosp Med* 1984; 132:162
10. Moore PL: Nitroglycerin improves venous cannulation. *Anesthesiology* 1986; 64:533
11. Hedges JR, Weinshenker E, Dirksing R: Evaluation of venous distension device: Potential aid for venous cannulation. *Ann Emerg Med* 1986; 15:540
12. Jarvis AP: Aids for easy venous cannulation. *Anesthesiology* 1986; 65:448
13. Kaye W: Intravenous techniques. In *Textbook of Advanced Cardiac Life Support*, pp 151–161. Dallas, Texas, American Heart Association, 1981
14. Getzen LC, Pollack EW: Short term femoral vein catheterization. *Am J Surg* 1979; 138:875
15. Guidelines for the prevention and control of nosocomial infection. In *Center for Disease Control Working Group Guidelines for Prevention of Intravascular Infections.* Washington, DC, US Department of Health and Human Services, Public Health Service, 1981
16. Bansmer MD, Keith BA, Tesluk MD: Complications following use of indwelling catheters of inferior vena cava. *JAMA* 1958; 167:1606
17. Moncrief JA: Femoral catheters. *Am Surg* 1958; 147:166
18. Dailey RH: Femoral vein cannulation: A review. *J Emerg Med* 1985; 2:367
19. Erban J: Long term experience with the technique of subclavian and femoral vein cannulation in hemodialysis. *Artif Organs* 1979; 2:241
20. Gertner J, Herman B, Pescio M, et al: Risk of infection in prolonged central venous catheterization. *Surg Gynecol Obstet* 1979; 149:567
21. Committee on Cardiac Catheterization and Angiocardiography: American Heart Association Report. *Circulation* 1953; 7:769

22. Nidus BD, Matalon R, Katz LA, et al: Hemodialysis using femoral vessel cannulation. *Nephron* 1974; 13:416
23. Sung JP, Bikangaga AW, Abbott JA: Massive hemorrhage to scrotum from laceration of inferior epigastric artery following percutaneous femoral vein catheterization: Case report. *Milit Med* 1981; 146:362
24. Yonei A, Nonoue T, Sari A: Real time ultrasonic guidance for percutaneous puncture of the internal jugular vein. *Anesthesiology* 1986; 64:830
25. Peters JL, Belsham P, Garrett CPO, et al: Doppler utrasound, an aid to percutaneous infraclavicular subclavian vein catheterization. *Am J Surg* 1982; 143:391
26. Bernard RW, Stahl W: Subclavian vein catheterizations. A prospective study. I. Non-infectious complications. *Ann Surg* 1971; 173:184
27. Bernard RW, Stahl W, Chase RM: Subclavian vein catheterizations: A prospective study. II. Infectious complications. *Ann Surg* 1971; 173:191
28. Sznajder JI, Zveibil FR, Bitterman H, et al: Central vein catheterization failure and complication rate by three percutaneous approaches. *Arch Intern Med* 1986; 146:259
29. Moosman DA: The anatomy of infraclavicular subclavian vein catheterization and its complications. *Surg Gynecol Obstet* 1973; 136:71
30. Hassett JM, Babikian G, Flint LM: Complications of subclavian lines. *Curr Concepts Trauma Care.* 1985;17
31. Borja AR, Masri Z, Shruck L, et al: Unusual and lethal complications of infraclavicular subclavian vein catheterization. *Int Surg* 1972; 57:42
32. Herbst CA Jr: Indications, management, and complications of percutaneous subclavian catheters. *Arch Surg* 1978; 113:1421
33. Burr C, Ainefeld EW: *The Caval Catheter*, pp 39–65. Berlin, Springer-Verlag, 1978
34. Peters JL, Gossett CPO: Complications of central venous catheterization. In Peters JL (ed): *A Manual of Central Venous Catheterization and Parenteral Nutrition*, Chap 12. Littleton, Massachusetts, John Wright & Sons, 1983
35. Malatinsky J, Kadlic T, Majek M, et al: Misplacement and loop formation of central venous catheters. *Acta Anaesthesiol Scand* 1976; 20:237
36. Dunbar RD, Mitchell R, Lavine M: Aberrant locations of central venous catheters. *Lancet* 1981; 1:711
37. Grant JG. *Handbook of Total Parenteral Nutrition*, Philadelphia, WB Saunders, 1980
38. Maki DG: Infections associated with intravascular lines. In Remington J, Shwartz M (eds): *Current Clinical Topics in Infectious Disease*, vol 3, p 309. Philadelphia, WB Saunders, 1982
39. Miller JJ, Bahman V, Mathru M: Comparison of the sterility of long term central venous catheterization using single lumen, triple lumen and pulmonary artery catheters. *Crit Care Med* 1984; 12:634
40. Kelly CS, Ligas JR, Smith CA, et al: Sepsis due to triple lumen central venous catheters. *Surg Gynecol Obstet* 1986; 163:14
41. Pemberton LB, Lyman BL, Lander V, et al: Sepsis from triple vs single lumen catheters during total parenteral nutrition in surgical or critically–ill patients. *Arch Surg* 1986; 121:591
42. Kaye W, Wheaton M, Potter–Bynoe G: Radial and pulmonary artery catheter-related sepsis. *Crit Care Med* 1983; 11:249
43. Bozzetti F, Terno G, Bonfanti G, et al: Prevention and treatment of central venous catheter sepsis by exchange via a guide wire. *Ann Surg* 1983; 198:48
44. Pettigrew RA, Lang SD, Haydock DA, et al: Catheter related sepsis in patients on intravenous nutrition: A prospective study of quantitative catheter cultures and guidewire changes for suspected sepsis. *Br J Surg* 1985; 72:52
45. Weiss M, Gattiker RI: Complications during and following radial artery cannulation: A prospective study. *Int Care Med* 1986; 12:424
46. Kaye W: Intravenous techniques. In *Textbook of Advanced Cardiac Life Support*, pp 165–178. Dallas, Texas, American Heart Association, 1981
47. Wilkins RG: Radial artery cannulation and ischaemic damage: A review. *Anaesthesia* 1985; 40:896
48. Mandel MA, Dauchot PJ: Radial artery catheterization in 1000 patients: Precautions and complications. *J Hand Surg* 1977; 2:482
49. Bedford RF: Radial arterial function following percutaneous cannulation with 18 and 20 gauge catheters. *Anesthesiology* 1977, 47:37
50. Davis FM: Radial artery cannulation. Influence of catheter size and material on arterial occlusion. *Anaesth Intens Care* 1978; 6:49
51. Downs JB, Rackstein AD, Klein EF Jr, et al: Hazards of radial-artery catheterization. *Anesthesiology* 1973; 38:283
52. Downs JB, Chapman RL Jr, Hawkins IF Jr: Prolonged radial-artery catheterization. An evaluation of heparinized catheters and continuous irrigation. *Arch Surg* 1974; 108:671
53. Jones RM, Hill AB, Nahrwold MC, et al: The effect of method of radial artery cannulation on post cannulation blood flow and thrombus formation. *Anesthesiology* 1981; 55:76
54. Bartlett RH, Munster AM: An improved technique for prolonged arterial cannulation. *N Engl J Med* 1968; 279:92
55. Maki DG: Nosocomial bacteremia, an epidemiologic overview. *Am J Med* 1981; 70:719

56. Band JD, Maki DG: Infections caused by arterial catheters used for hemodynamic monitoring. *Am J Med* 1979; 67:735

57. Kaye W: Intravenous techniques: In *Textbook of Advanced Cardiac Life Support*, pp 179–193. Dallas, Texas, American Heart Association, 1981

58. Thompson IR, Dalton BC, Lappas DG, et al: Right bundle branch block and complete heart block caused by the Swan-Ganz catheter. *Anesthesiology* 1979; 51:359

59. Abernathy WS: Complete heart block caused by the Swan-Ganz catheter. *Chest* 1974; 65:349

60. Lipp H, O'Donoghue K, Resnekov L: Intracardiac knotting of a flow directed balloon catheter. *N Engl J Med* 1971; 284:220

61. Smith WR, Glauser FL, Jemison R: Ruptured chordae of the tricuspid valve. The consequences of flow directed Swan-Ganz catheterization. *Chest* 1976; 70:790

62. Schwartz KV, Garcia FG: Entanglement of Swan-Ganz catheter around an intracardiac structure (letter). *JAMA* 1977; 237:1198

63. Daum S, Schapira M: Intracardiac knot formation in a Swan-Ganz catheter. *Anesth Analg* 1973; 52:862

64. Mond HG, Clark DW, Nesbitt SJ, et al: A technique for unknotting an intracardiac flow directed balloon catheter. *Chest* 1975; 67:731

65. Foote GA, Schabel SI, Hogdes M: Pulmonary complications of the flow directed balloon tipped catheter. *N Engl J Med* 1974; 290:927

66. McDaniel DD, Stone JG, Faltas AN, et al: Catheter-induced pulmonary artery hemorrhage. *J Thorac Cardiovasc Surg* 1981; 82:1

67. Barash PG, Nardi D, Hammond G, et al: Catheter induced pulmonary artery perforations mechanisms, management and modifications. *J Thorac Cardiovasc Surg* 1981; 82:5

68. Pape LA, Haffajee CI, Markis JE, et al: Fatal pulmonary hemorrhage after use of the flow-directed balloon tipped catheter. *Am Intern Med* 1979; 90:344

69. Page DW, Teres D, Hartshorn JW: Fatal hemorrhage from Swan-Ganz catheter. *N Engl J Med* 1979; 291:260

70. Chun GMH, Ellestad MH: Perforation of the pulmonary artery by a Swan-Ganz catheter. *N Engl J Med* 1971; 284:1041

71. Lapin ES, Murray JA: Hemoptysis with flow directed cardiac catheterization. *JAMA* 1972; 220:1246

72. Yorra FH, Oblath R, Jaffe H, et al: Massive thrombosis associated with use of a Swan-Ganz catheter. *Chest* 1974; 65:682

73. Pace NL, Horton W: Indwelling pulmonary artery catheters—their relationship to aseptic thrombotic endocardial vegetations. *JAMA* 1975; 233:893

74. Greene JF, Cummings KC: Aseptic thrombotic endocardial vegetations—a complication of indwelling pulmonary artery catheters. *JAMA* 1973; 225:1525

75. Hoar PF, Wilson RM, Mangano DT, et al: Herparin bonding reduces thrombogenicity of pulmonary artery catheters. *N Engl J Med* 1981; 305:993

76. Elliott CG, Zimmerman GA, Clemmer TP: Complications of pulmonary artery catheterization in the care of critically ill patients—a prospective study. *Chest* 1979; 76:647

77. Geha DG, Davis NJ, Lappas DG: Persistent atrial arrhythmias associated with placement of a Swan-Ganz catheter. *Anesthesiology* 1973; 39:651

78. O'Toole JD, Wurtzbacher JJ, Wearner NE, et al: Pulmonary valve injury and insufficiency during pulmonary artery catheterization. *N Engl J Med* 1979; 301:1167

79. Applefield JJ, Caruthers TE, Reno DJ, et al: Assessment of the sterility of long-term cardiac catheterization using the thermodilution Swan-Ganz catheter. *Chest* 1978; 74:377

80. Puri VK, Carlson RW, Bander JJ, et al: Complications of vascular catheterization in the critically ill: A prospective study. *Crit Care Med* 1980; 8:495

81. Sise MJ, Hollingsworth P, Brimm JE: Complications of the flow directed pulmonary catheter: A prospective analysis in 219 patients. *Crit Care Med* 1981; 9:315

82. Hoelzer MF: Recent advances in intravenous therapy. *Emerg Clin North Am* 1986; 4:487

CHAPTER THIRTEEN

HEMODYNAMIC MONITORING: ARTERIAL CATHETERS

Cheryl A. Clark
Eloise M. Harman

Arterial catheters are often used in the intensive care unit (ICU) for hemodynamic monitoring and blood gas determinations. Blood pressure in shock patients should be obtained with an arterial catheter, since sphygmomanometric measurements in such patients with a high systemic vascular resistance significantly underestimate systolic pressure. In shock patients with a normal or low systemic vascular resistance and in normal patients, the cuff blood pressure and arterial catheter blood pressure correlate well.[1] Occasionally, patients with severe atherosclerosis have increased blood pressures when it is measured with a sphygmomanometer, but direct intra-arterial measurement reveals a normal value. This phenomenon is referred to as "pseudohypertension" and is thought to be caused by severely sclerotic arterial walls that cannot be compressed by the blood pressure cuff. Accurate intra-arterial blood pressure measurement can avoid inappropriate treatment for hypertension.[2]

IMMEDIATE CONCERNS

PRESSURE WAVEFORMS

Ventricular systole causes a rapid rise in arterial pressure, which is followed by a brief, sustained high level of pressure referred to as the anacrotic shoulder. At the end of systole, pressure falls in both the aorta and left ventricle, resulting in a sharp downward deflection known as the incisura. When left ventricular pressure falls below aortic pressure, the aortic valve closes, resulting in a small increase in arterial pressure followed by a gradual fall in pressure until the next systole.

Because smaller arteries are less compliant than the aorta and different components of the arterial waveform are transmitted at different rates, the waveform undergoes a change in shape as it is transmitted peripherally. The waveform develops a steeper upstroke; the systolic peak is higher; the diastolic pressure is lower; and the dicrotic notch becomes less pronounced. As the pressure wave encounters the noncompliant peripheral arteries, it is unable to travel forward and is reflected backward. When this reflected wave strikes an oncoming one, the two summate and produce the dicrotic wave, represented by a small increase in pressure following the dicrotic notch.

In a normal patient, the more peripherally an arterial catheter is placed, the higher the systolic and the lower the diastolic pressures will be.[3] Because of their small size and peripheral location, the radial or dorsalis pedis arteries are not ideal sites for hemodynamic monitoring. The dicrotic wave is markedly elevated in patients with a low cardiac output and increased peripheral resistance.

INSERTION SITES

Radial Artery

The radial artery is most commonly used, despite the aforementioned limitation for pressure monitoring primarily because of the ease of cannulation, convenience, and widespread experience. Other sites include the dorsalis pedis, femoral, brachial, and axillary arteries. Radial insertion usually is safe because the artery is superficial and has many collateral anastomoses with the ulnar artery. Before radial artery cannulation, however, this collateral circulation should be evaluated with a modified Allen's test. The radial and ulnar pulses are occluded simultaneously, and the patient's fist is repeatedly clenched and unclenched until the palm becomes pale (Fig. 13.1). The ulnar artery is released and the time until palmar blushing noted (Fig. 13.2). If more than 5 to 7 seconds elapse before the blush, ulnar collateral circulation may be inadequate, and another insertion site should be selected.[4] Proper positioning of the patient's hand is important; if the hand is hyperextended at the wrist and fingers, fascial tension obliterates the microcirculation and gives the erroneous impression of inadequate ulnar collateral circulation.[5]

Figure 13-1 Apply pressure over the radial and ulnar arteries and have the patient make a tight fist and release it repeatedly until the fingers are blanched. This may be done passively if necessary.

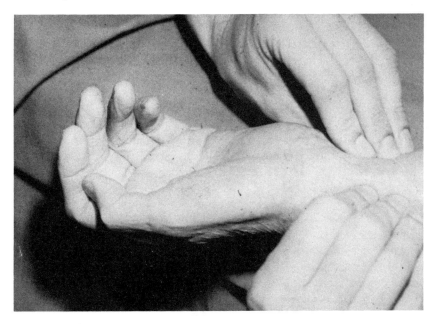

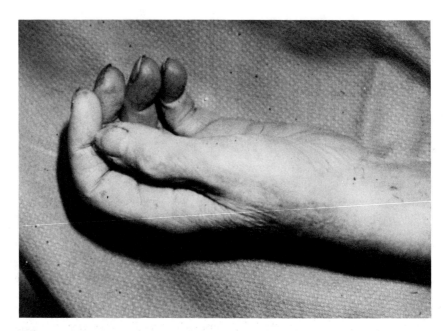

Figure 13-2 Release the pressure over the ulnar artery and watch for the return of color to the fingers, particularly the index finger and thumb. Flushing should occur within 5 to 7 seconds. Satisfactory flushing in a patient without hemodynamic abnormalities does *not* ensure that there would be sufficient collateral circulation if a low output state or shock were to develop.

Some investigators suggest that the traditional visual modified Allen's test is not a sensitive indicator of collateral circulation. Clarke found that only 86% of patients with a *normal* visual Allen's test (palmar blush within 7 seconds after releasing the ulnar artery) have Doppler ultrasonic evidence of adequate ulnar collateral flow to the thumb. Further, 6% of patients with a *borderline* visual Allen's test (palmar blush within 8 to 14 seconds after release of the ulnar artery) have Doppler evidence of adequate ulnar collateral circulation.[6]

The superficial palmar arch is the main source of blood for the fingers and in most patients is supplied predominantly by the ulnar artery (with collateral circulation from the radial artery). In about 12% of hands, the superficial arch arises predominantly from the radial artery; most of these patients have inadequate or no ulnar collateral flow. Radial artery catheterization is hazardous in these patients. Available evidence suggests that at least one digit had *no* blood flow in 19% of cases after radial artery compression, whereas a visual Allen's test detected abnormal flow in only 2%.[7] These data may help to explain why arterial catheterization can result in digital ischemia despite a previously normal visual Allen's test.[8] However, in practice, ischemia is most commonly associated with shock and/or low output states. During rise episodes, collateral flow previously demonstrated to be adequate may diminish to a level that does not support tissue viability. Because many arterial lines are placed before these episodes, even the most careful intubation cannot prevent future difficulties. Thus, while no artery should be cannulated if collateral flow is inadequate, adequate flow when a patient is hemodynamically stable does not eliminate the possibility of ischemia should a low flow state develop.

Placement of a Doppler flow probe over the radial artery, followed by occlusion of both the radial and ulnar arteries and then release of the ulnar artery, is suggested to evaluate adequacy of the collateral circulation. Others recommend Doppler evaluation of the interdigital clefts or the superficial palmar arch. Since the radial artery sends its tributaries to the superficial palmar arch before it enters the anatomic snuffbox, it is suggested that cannulation of the radial artery in this location may carry a lower risk of digital ischemia.[9] Preliminary experience with this technique is encouraging.

Dorsalis Pedis Artery

Before cannulation of the dorsalis pedis artery, collateral flow through the posterior tibial artery should be evaluated. The dorsalis pedis and posterior tibial arteries are occluded, and the great toe is repeatedly compressed until it blanches. If adequate collateral circulation exists, it will become erythematous within 5 seconds after releasing the posterior tibial artery.[10] No published studies compare Doppler and visual examinations of the dorsalis pedis artery. Dorsalis pedis blood pressure often underestimates the true blood pressure in patients with severe peripheral vascular disease, and, as mentioned previously, blood pressure measured in the dorsalis pedis artery differs from that measured in more central arteries. If peripheral vascular disease is present, another site should be selected if possible. Recall also that this artery is congenitally absent in 12% of patients. The steps for cannulation are illustrated in Figures 13-3 through 13-7.

Femoral Artery

The femoral artery often is selected for cannulation because it frequently is palpable in shock patients when no other pulses can be found. The artery should be punctured *below* the inguinal ligament since punctures above this level are associated with significant retroperitoneal hemorrhage. Recent evidence suggests no increase in the risk of complications when the femoral site is chosen. However, the types of complications differ from radial catheterization. The latter are associated with pseudoaneurysm formation (1%) and sepsis (1.5%), whereas femoral catheterization predisposes to infected hematoma (0.9%) and bleeding from the puncture site requiring transfusions (1.8%). Although the femoral artery is a large-caliber vessel, catheters larger than 20 gauge should not be used because of increased incidence of local hematomas and distal emboli. This site should not be used in cases of peripheral vascular disease and in the presence of open, infected abdominal wounds.

Brachial Artery

The brachial artery is a continuation of the axillary artery and gives rise to the radial and ulnar arteries in the antecubital fossa. Because of the high complication rate associated with use of the brachial artery for cardiac catheterization, many physicians are reluctant to use it for arterial cannulation. The most frequently reported complication is embolic occlusion (usually temporary) of the radial or ulnar artery, which occurs in 5% to 41% of cases.[11] Before brachial artery cannulation, flow through the radial and ulnar arteries should be evaluated with a Doppler-assisted Allen's test. If flow in either is compromised, brachial artery cannulation should not be performed. This artery probably should be avoided if another can be used. It should not be used in anticoagulated patients because bleeding into the fascial planes around the antecubital fossa can cause a median nerve compression neuropathy with a resultant Volkmann's contracture.[12] There are no series documenting long-term use of the brachial artery and, if used, duration should be limited to 1 or 2 days at most.

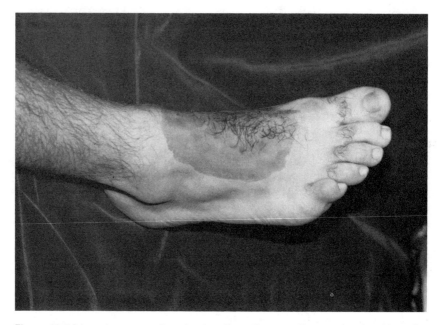

Figure 13-3A In order to cannulate the dorsalis pedis artery, first prepare the skin surface with povidone-iodine solution.

Figure 13-3B Cover the area with sterile drapes.

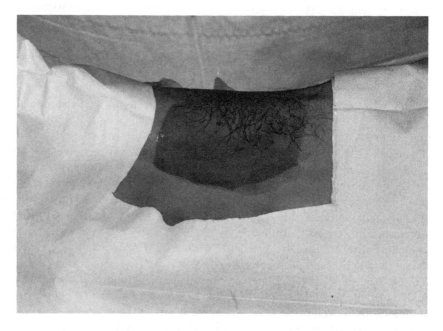

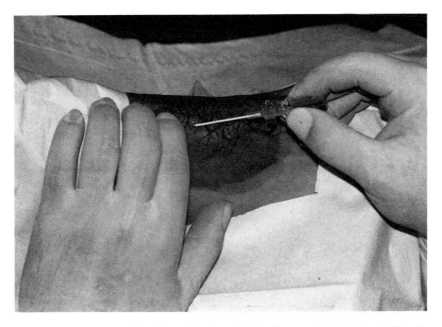

Figure 13-4 Palpate the dorsalis pedis pulse with the fingers of the left hand. Take the catheter-needle assembly and puncture the skin approximately 0.5 to 1 cm distal to the palpated pulse.

Figure 13-5 Advance the needle tip toward the maiximum pulsation. Continue advancing slowly until blood appears in the needle.

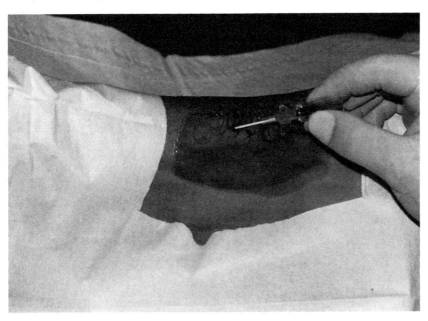

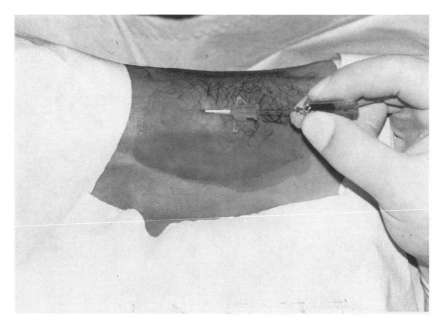

Figure 13-6 Keep the hub of the needle as stationary as possible and advance the catheter into the artery. Withdraw the needle and attach to the pressure monitoring system.

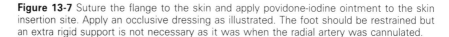

Figure 13-7 Suture the flange to the skin and apply povidone-iodine ointment to the skin insertion site. Apply an occlusive dressing as illustrated. The foot should be restrained but an extra rigid support is not necessary as it was when the radial artery was cannulated.

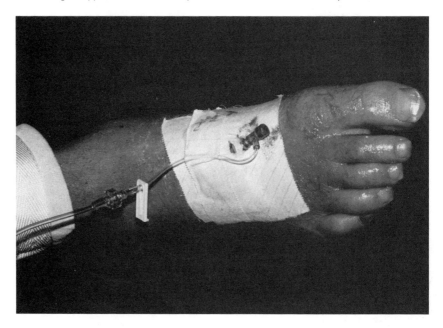

Axillary Artery

The axillary artery is a continuation of the subclavian artery. Because it has a rich anastomotic network surrounding it, thrombosis usually does not cause ischemia to the distal arm. However, thromboembolism from the catheter tip to the radial or ulnar artery has resulted in transient loss of pulse or local parasthesias.

Since the right axillary artery is a continuation of the right subclavian artery, which in turn arises from the brachiocephalic trunk, air or particulate matter can embolize to the brain through the carotid artery during flushing of the axillary arterial catheter. The left axillary artery has a less direct communication with the brain; thus this site may be safer. In either event, flushing should be done gently with minimal volumes to avoid embolization. This site is slightly more difficult to cannulate than others, but, because it is a large central artery, it usually is palpable even in the presence of intensive peripheral vasoconstriction. Long-term patency rates are excellent and complications infrequent. It is also easy to mobilize patients and the technique has much to recommend it for use in long-term ICU patients. Cannulation of the axillary artery is illustrated in Figures 13-8 through 13-11.

COMPLICATIONS

THROMBOSIS

Arterial catheterization is a technically simple procedure, and the incidence of complications appears to be operator-independent, unlike pulmonary artery catheterizations.[13] Multiple punctures, prolonged catheterization, a low cardiac output, hypertension, atherosclerosis, anticoagulant therapy, and severe aortic insufficiency seem to increase the risk of compli-

Figure 13-8 The patient has been positioned for axillary artery cannulation. It may be necessary to shave the area, especially to ensure firm tape fixation after cannulation.

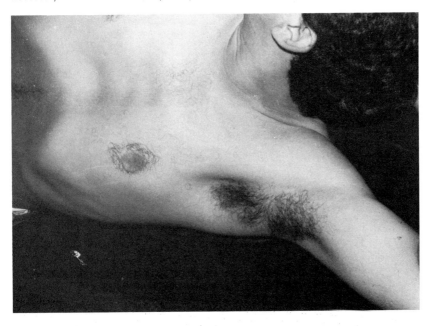

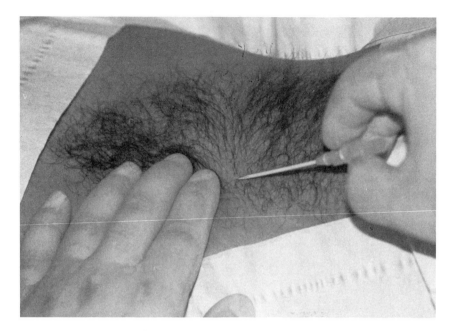

Figure 13-9 Palpate the axillary pulse with the fingers of your left hand. Select an insertion point approximately 1.5 cm distal to the palpated pulse.

Figure 13-10 Advance the tip of the needle directly toward the maixmal pulsation felt by the fingers of the opposite hand. Because the artery is not as superficial and not as well fixed by surrounding structures, it is often more difficult to locate with the needle point. Once the arterial puncture has been made, blood will appear in the hub of the needle. Insert a guidewire.

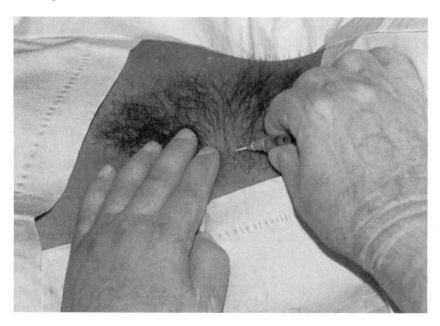

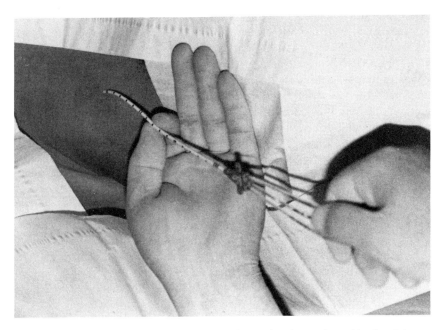

Figure 13-11 In this illustration, a catheter has been placed over the guidewire. Advance the catheter over the guidewire. Suture the catheter in place and apply povidone-iodine ointment.

cations. Patients younger than 10 years of age also apparently have an increased risk of complications (possibly because of the small arterial size), but, in the absence of other risk factors, elderly patients do not.

Arterial thrombosis is more common with catheters larger than 20 gauge, tapered catheters, polypropylene (as opposed to Teflon) catheters, intermittent (rather than continuous) flush systems, and catheterization lasting more than 4 days.[14] Radiopaque catheters do not increase the incidence of thrombosis. Patients with small wrists tend to have small arteries and are at increased risk for radial artery thrombosis.[15] Although arterial thrombosis can induce ischemia of the distal limb, it is completely asymptomatic in 96% of patients.

Radial artery Doppler studies reveal thrombosis in 25% of patients who have 18-gauge arterial catheters in place for less than 20 hours; the thrombosis rate is 50% for catheters in place 20 to 40 hours.[16] Twenty-gauge radial artery catheters in place for 3 days or fewer have an 11% thrombosis rate; those in place from 4 to 10 days have a 29% thrombosis rate.[4] Because of collateral circulation from the ulnar artery, most of these patients continue to have a palpable radial pulse. Thrombus is present at the time of catheter removal in 43% of patients destined to develop radial artery thrombosis and will develop within the next 24 hours in another 30%. Of the remaining patients who sustain thrombosis, most do so within a week of catheter removal.[16] Although recanalization of the thrombosed artery usually occurs, it generally takes from 2 to 3 weeks but can require up to 75 days.[4] One study showed that pretreatment with aspirin decreases the incidence of radial artery thrombosis in patients undergoing elective surgery. However, the average duration of catheterization in that study was only 26 hours; whether this protection extends to longer catheterization times is unknown.[17] The small dorsalis pedis artery also has a high incidence of thrombosis of 6.7% for 20-gauge catheters in place less than 24 hours.[3,10] Heparinization of the flush system decreases the incidence of arterial thrombosis.

Although arterial catheters usually are inserted percutaneously, a surgical cutdown procedure occasionally may be necessary. A much higher incidence of arterial thrombosis occurs within the first 24 hours when a cutdown is performed (48% versus 23% with the percutaneous method), but the incidence of arterial thrombosis at 1 week is the same for both methods. Transfixing and direct threading are two methods commonly used for percutaneous arterial cannulation. When the transfixing method is used, the posterior wall of the artery is deliberately punctured, after which the catheter is withdrawn slightly to ensure its intraluminal placement. When the direct threading method is used, the artery is punctured and the catheter advanced without perforating the posterior wall. No difference in the incidence of arterial thrombosis is reported with either method.

As an arterial catheter is removed, a syringe should be attached to it and suction applied while an assistant presses both proximally and distally to the insertion site. This technique decreases the incidence of arterial thrombotic occlusion following catheter removal when an 18-gauge catheter is used. This same technique can be applied to smaller gauge catheters. Because the incidence of clot formation is lower and it is more difficult to aspirate clot through the smaller catheters, it is unclear whether the incidence of arterial occlusion will be decreased when a 20-gauge or smaller catheter is used.

Emboli can occur as a result of small clots forming around the catheter tip or from air in the flush system. These emboli can migrate distally and remain asymptomatic, or they may cause signs of ischemia. Emboli can also move retrograde into the central nervous system circulation, producing neurologic deficit. Only 6 to 7 ml of flush solution is needed to cause a retrograde embolus from the radial artery to the subclavian–vertebral artery junction.[18] Damping of the arterial waveform may result from thrombosis at the catheter tip, air in the transducer dome, excessive tubing between the catheter and the transducer, or loss of pressure on the bag of flush solution. If thrombosis is suspected, the catheter should be aspirated with a syringe; forceful large-volume flushing should not be performed.

Ischemic necrosis of the skin overlying the catheter occurs in up to 3% of cannulations and in 10% of all instances of thrombosed radial arteries (Fig. 13-12). Thrombosis around the catheter leads to occlusion of the small cutaneous arteries that supply the skin.[4] Smaller catheters are associated with a decreased incidence of this complication. A high likelihood of skin necrosis may be present if a localized area of intense blanching occurs in the skin overlying the catheter when it is flushed. Slight adjustment of the catheter tip usually results in a less localized, more transient pallor, possibly reducing this problem.

INFECTION

Infections continue to be a common complication of arterial catheterization. Important factors include inflammation at the insertion site, catheters left *in situ* for more than 4 days, and catheters placed by surgical cutdown.[19] A ninefold increase in the incidence of bacteremia occurs when a cutdown is performed. Lack of inflammation at the catheter insertion site does not exclude the arterial catheter as the cause of sepsis. Forty percent of arterial catheter-induced septicemias and 72% of patients with isolated catheter tip contamination have no evidence of local inflammation. Although infected venous catheters usually grow *Staphylococcus*, infected arterial catheters grow gram-negative rods, enterococci, or *Can-*

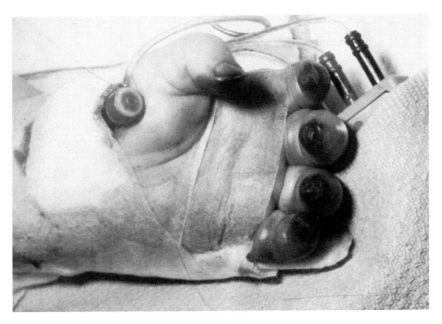

Figure 13-12 Ischemic necrosis of the fingertips developed in a patient with a radial arterial catheter. This complication occurred after an episode of profound cardiovascular collapse, which ultimately led to the patients demise. In order to prevent progression of ischemia, cannulated extremities should be inspected frequently, and if any signs of ischemia occur, the cannula must be removed immediately.

dida.[19] Preexisting bacteremias may colonize an arterial catheter and may not clear until the catheter is removed. If an arterial catheter is placed *after* a patient becomes septic and that patient fails to improve, the catheter should be removed because it may serve as a nidus for continued sepsis (Fig. 13-13).

Because of the increased risk of *Candida* infections associated with arterial catheters, the insertion site should be dressed with a povidone–iodine (PI$_2$) ointment rather than a polymyxin–neosporin bacitracin (PNB) ointment. Topical PNB ointment may be preferable for peripheral venous catheters because its use seems to decrease the rate of venous catheter-related infection more effectively.[19] Although no published studies involve arterial catheters, some evidence suggests that the risk of bacterial colonization of peripheral venous catheters is less with a gauze dressing that is changed every 24 hours than with a transparent polyurethane dressing.[20]

MISCELLANOUS

A variety of other complications have been reported. Median nerve neuropathy is associated with *radial* artery catheterization. Proposed mechanisms for this problem include stretching of the nerve during prolonged wrist hyperextension after catheter insertion, and nerve compression by blood in the carpal tunnel after several unsuccessful catheterization attempts.[21] Pseudoaneurysm of the radial artery usually is a delayed complication occurring up to 18 days after catheter removal.[22] Presumably, this complication may occur at any site. Intra-arterial drug injection sometimes causes skin necrosis and distal limb ischemia.

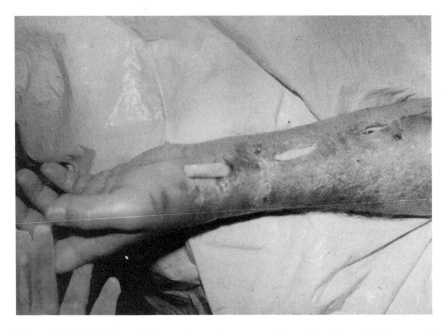

Figure 13-13 Cellulitis and abscess formation occurred throughout the entire forearm of this patient after radial artery catheterization. Although the catheter was removed as soon as signs of infection were noted, the infection spread wildly after removal and eventually required incision and drainage.

REFERENCES

1. Cohn J: Blood pressure measurement in shock: Mechanism of inaccuracy in auscultatory and palpatory methods. *JAMA* 1967; 199:972
2. Messerli F, Ventura H, Amodeo C: Osler's maneuver and pseudohypertension. *N Engl J Med* 1985; 312:1548
3. Youngberg J, Miller E: Evaluation of percutaneous cannulations of the dorsalis pedis artery. *Anesthesiology* 1976; 44:80
4. Bedford R: Long-term radial artery cannulation: Effects on subsequent vessel function. *Crit Care Med* 1978; 6:64
5. Greenhow D: Incorrect performance of Allen's test—Ulnar artery flow erroneously presumed inadequate. *Anesthesiology* 1972; 37:356
6. Clarke W, Freund P, Wasse L, et al: Assessment of adequacy of ulnar arterial flow prior to radial artery catheterization (abstr). *Anesthesiology* 1981; 55:A38
7. Little J, Zylstra P, West J, et al: Circulatory patterns in the normal hand. *Br J Surg* 1973; 60:652
8. Baker R: Severe ischemia of the hand following radial arterial catheterization. *Surgery* 1976; 80:449
9. Pyles S, Scher K, Vega E, et al: Cannulation of the dorsal radial artery: A new technique. *Anesth Analg* 1982; 61:876
10. Husum B, Eriksen T: Percutaneous cannulation of the dorsalis pedis artery. *Br J Anaesth* 1979; 51:1055
11. Barnes R, Foster E, Janssen A, et al: Safety of brachial artery catheters as monitors in the intensive care unit—Prospective evaluation with the Doppler ultrasonic velocity detector. *Anesthesiology* 1976; 44:260
12. Macon W, Futrell J: Median-nerve neuropathy after percutaneous puncture of the brachial artery in patients receiving anticoagulants. *N Engl J Med* 1973; 288:1396
13. Puri V, Carlson R, Bander J, et al: Complications of vascular catheterization in the critically ill. *Crit Care Med* 1980; 8:495
14. Downs JB, Chapman R, Hawkins I: Prolonged radial artery catheterization. *Arch Surg* 1974; 108:671
15. Bedford R: Wrist circumference predicts the risk of radial-arterial occlusion after cannulation. *Anesthesiology* 1978; 48:377
16. Bedford R, Wollman H: Complications of percutaneous radial artery cannulation. An objective prospective study in man. *Anesthesiology* 1973; 38:228

17. Bedford R, Ashford T: Aspirin pretreatment prevents post-cannulation radial artery thrombosis. *Anesthesiology* 1979; 51:176
18. Lowenstein E, Little J, Har H: Prevention of cerebral embolization from flushing radial artery cannulas. *N Engl J Med* 1971; 285:1414
19. Maki D, Band J: A comparative study of polyantibiotic and iodophor ointments in prevention of vascular catheter-related infection. *Am J Med* 1981; 70:739
20. Craven D, Lichtenberg D, Kunches L, et al: A randomized study comparing a transparent polyurethane dressing to a dry gauze dressing for peripheral intravenous catheter sites. *Infect Contr* 1985; 6:361
21. Gurman G, Kriemerman S: Cannulation of big arteries in critically ill patients. *Crit Care Med* 1985; 13:217
22. Wolf S, Mangano D: Pseudoaneurysm, a late complication of radial artery cannulation. *Anesthesiology* 1980; 52:80

CHAPTER FOURTEEN

HEMODYNAMIC MONITORING: PULMONARY ARTERY CATHETERS

Cheryl A. Clark
Eloise M. Harman

Flow-directed pulmonary artery (PA) catheterization was introduced in 1970.[1] As physicians gained expertise in the interpretation of data obtained from the technique, its use in critically ill patients became commonplace. The most frequent use of these catheters is to assess the intravascular volume status in hypotensive patients. Measurement of filling pressures and cardiac output and information gained from the calculation of systemic and pulmonary vascular resistances and other values (see Appendix) can be used to guide the administration of intravenous fluids, inotropes, and afterload reducing agents. Pulmonary artery catheters are crucial in the diagnosis and treatment of some cases of adult respiratory distress syndrome (ARDS).

IMMEDIATE CONCERNS

PRESSURE WAVEFORMS

Recognition of normal pressure waveforms is crucial for correct interpretation of information derived from the pulmonary artery catheter (Fig. 14-1). The a wave is due to atrial contraction and follows the P wave of the EKG. A small c wave occurs after the QRS complex as a result of tricuspid valve closure. Owing to atrial relaxation, atrial pressure continues to fall after the c wave, even though the atrium is filling with blood. After complete atrial relaxation occurs, at the nadir of the x descent, atrial pressure starts to increase as atrial filling continues. This rise in atrial pressure causes the v wave. When the tricuspid valve opens, the atrium empties passively into the right ventricle, resulting in the y descent. During catheterization the *mean* right atrial pressure and *peak* a and v wave pressures are measured.[2]

The diastolic phase of the right ventricular pressure waveform consists of a rapid filling period, during which 60% of right ventricular filling occurs, and a slow filling period, which accounts for 25% of ventricular filling. Atrial contraction causes an a wave and accounts for the remaining 15%. During catheterization, the *peak* systolic right ventricular pressure and the *end-diastolic* right ventricular pressure (following the atrial a wave) are measured.[2]

Right ventricular emptying, which occurs after the QRS complex on the EKG, results in the PA systolic pressure waveform (Fig. 14-2). Pulmonary artery pressure (PAP) falls when

Figure 14-1 Normal pressure waveforms measured through a PA catheter. (Reproduced from Braunwald E: *Heart Disease: A Textbook of Cardiovascular Medicine*. Philadelphia, WB Saunders, 1980)

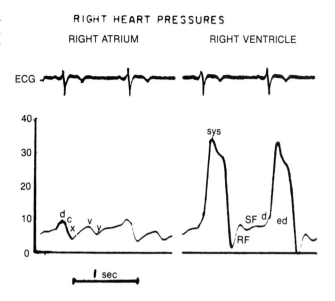

right ventricular systole ends. The pulmonary valve closes when right ventricular pressure falls below PA pressure, resulting in the incisura on the waveform. After closure of the pulmonary valve, pressure in the PA continues to fall to its nadir, the end-diastolic pulmonary artery pressure (PAD). The *peak* systolic and end-diastolic pressures are recorded.[2]

When the balloon at the tip of the catheter is inflated, a *branch* of the PA is occluded and *no blood flow* occurs from the tip of the catheter to the point where the pulmonary vein joins with another pulmonary vein draining a separate branch of the ipsilateral pulmonary artery (Fig. 14-3). Since pressure in the pulmonary vein is almost identical to left atrial pressure, the pressure transmitted to the catheter when the balloon is inflated (pul-

Figure 14-2 PA systolic, diastolic, and wedge *(PAO)* pressures (see text). (Reproduced with permission from Braunwald E: *Heart Disease: A Textbook of Cardiovascular Medicine*. Philadelphia, WB Saunders, 1980)

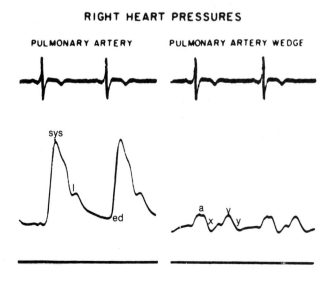

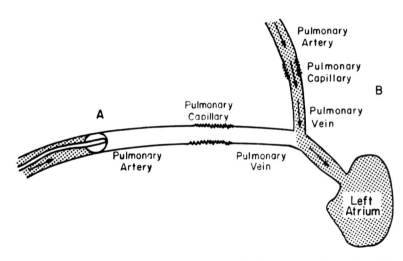

Figure 14-3 Inflation of the balloon at the tip of the PA catheter occludes the distal PA branch. The pressure transmitted to the catheter is equal to that of the pulmonary vein and left atrium.

monary artery occlusion pressure [PAOP]) is that of the left atrium (LAP), and hence the end-diastolic pressure of the left ventricle (LVEDP).

The PAOP waveform is similar to that of the right atrium. A good PAOP tracing reveals a and v waves and x and y descents but no c wave. Careful inspection of Figures 14-1 and 14-2 demonstrates that the a and v waves of the PAOP tracing occur later in relation to the EKG cycle and are more damped than the a and v waves of the right atrium, as a result of delayed transmission of these pressures from the left atrium through the pulmonary capillaries. (The PAOP tracing a wave *follows* the QRS, and the v wave *follows* the T wave of the EKG). The *peak* a and v pressures and the *mean* pressure are usually measured during catheterization, similar to those in the right atrium. Locations on the waveform where pressures normally are measured and the usual values obtained are shown in Figure 14-4 and Table 14-1.

If an air bubble enters the transducer dome, a clot forms on the catheter tip, or if excessive tubing is placed between the transducer and the PA catheter, the pressure tracing appears damped. Casual inspection can lead one to believe erroneously that the catheter is "wedged."[3] Correlation of the pressure tracing with the EKG should clarify the situation.

INSERTION SITES

The catheter can be inserted through the external jugular, internal jugular, subclavian, femoral, or antecubital veins. Each insertion site has its relative advantages and disadvantages (See also Chapter 12, "Vascular Cannulation").[4,5] The subclavian approach is most rapid; however, the incidence of pneumothorax is high (about 1–6%). Subclavian artery puncture is also a serious complication because bleeding cannot be controlled by local pressure. Sterility is difficult to maintain with neck insertion sites, and there is a risk of carotid artery puncture. The risk of pneumothorax, however, is low. The antecubital site *sometimes* requires a surgical cutdown but is probably the safest insertion site in throm-

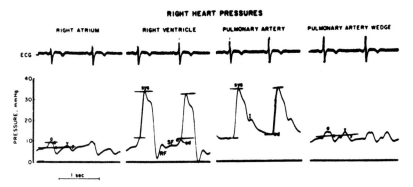

Figure 14-4 Location of PA waveforms where pressures normally are measured. (Reproduced with permission from Braunwald E: *Heart Disease: A Textbook of Cardiovascular Medicine.* Philadelphia, WB Saunders, 1980)

bocytopenic patients or in patients with a bleeding tendency. However, the catheter also is difficult to pass from the arm to the subclavian vein. Local complications such as phlebitis and venous stasis occur, and cutdowns increase the risk of infection. The femoral site carries the risk of deep venous thrombosis and pulmonary embolization.

"WEDGING" THE CATHETER

After initial insertion into the venous system, the catheter is advanced until the tip reaches an intrathoracic vein. (The inspiratory decrease in intrathoracic pressure in a spontaneously breathing patient or the inspiratory increase in intrathoracic pressure in a patient on mechanical ventilation is transmitted to the catheter when it enters the chest.) The right atrium should be reached about 50 cm from the left antecubital fossa; 40 cm from the right antecubital fossa; 55 cm from the femoral vein; 10 to 15 cm from the jugular vein; and 10 cm from the subclavian vein.[5] After the catheter enters the right atrium, the balloon should be inflated fully (1.0–1.5 ml of air) to prevent cardiac damage and ectopy from a protruding catheter tip. Catheter tip position can be determined by the waveform. The catheter is then advanced through the right ventricle and into the PA until a "wedge" (PAOP) tracing is obtained. The amount of air required for balloon inflation is always measured before insertion of the catheter. If less than 1.0 ml produces a PAOP tracing, the catheter is located too far

TABLE 14-1 RANGE OF NORMAL RESTING HEMODYNAMIC VALUES (mm/Hg)

Pressures	a Wave	v Wave	Mean	Systolic	End-Diastolic	Mean
Right atrium	2–10	2–10	0–8			
Right ventricle				1–30	0–8	
Pulmonary artery				5–30	3–12	9–16
Pulmonary artery wedge and left atrium		3–15	3–12	1–10		
Left ventricle				100–140	3–12	
Systemic arteries				100–140	60–90	70–105

distally in a peripheral vessel and should be pulled back a few centimeters. A protruding catheter tip can cause ventricular dysrhythmias or damage to the pulmonary artery unless the balloon is *completely* inflated with the recommended volume of air.[6]

Certain criteria are useful to verify a true wedge position.[5] Since blood flows from the PA to the left atrium, the *mean* PAOP must be less than the *mean* PA pressure. (Otherwise blood would flow from the left atrium to the PA.) The *mean* PAOP can be greater than the PAD pressure in mitral regurgitation. Blood withdrawn from the catheter when it is wedged should show a step-up in oxygenation, but withdrawal of 15 to 40 ml may be required before a true postcapillary blood sample can be obtained. Blood oxygen tension cannot be used as an absolute criterion for a wedge position because blood drawn from an area of the lung with a low $\dot{V}/\dot{Q}$ ratio will not show a step-up in oxygenation when the balloon is inflated.

RELATION BETWEEN PAOP AND LEFT VENTRICULAR VOLUME

Pulmonary artery diastolic pressure usually correlates with the PAOP but will *exceed* it in patients with tachycardia or pulmonary hypertension associated with acidosis, hypoxemia, pulmonary embolus, or pulmonary parenchymal disease.[3,5] The PAOP is a useful approximation of LVEDP because, during end-diastole, the PAO, pulmonary venous, left atrial, and left ventricular pressures equalize in normal patients. Left ventricular end-diastolic pressure usually correlates with left ventricular end-diastolic *volume* (LVEDV). However, this relationship may not hold in patients with left ventricular dysfunction or in patients receiving positive airway pressure (PEEP/CPAP).[3]

Myocardial ischemia and pericardial disease decrease ventricular compliance. The "stiff" ventricle causes LVEDP to be high, even if LVEDV is low or normal. A patient with a stiff ventricle may need an LVEDP of 20 mm Hg or more to achieve adequate ventricular filling volume. The best way to evaluate the need for a higher PAOP is to initiate a fluid challenge and measure systemic blood pressure, cardiac output, and wedge pressure. If the patient responds to the fluid challenge by a modest increase in PAOP (less than 3–4 mm Hg) and an increase in systemic blood pressure and cardiac output, more fluids and a higher PAOP are desirable. If the fluid challenge results in a large increase in PAOP and no change or a decrease in blood pressure or cardiac output, diuretics, inotropes, and possibly afterload reduction, individually or in combination, are indicated.[3] The PAOP exceeds LVEDP in patients with mitral stenosis, mitral insufficiency, or left atrial myxoma.[3] The fluid challenge poses a risk: if LVEDV is not increased the increase in PAOP only increases the likelihood of pulmonary edema.

EFFECTS OF POSITIVE AIRWAY PRESSURE ON PAOP

Positive airway pressure causes increased LVEDP even when LVEDV is low or normal. Accurate measurement of PAOP may not be possible because of [1] the increased airway pressure to the pulmonary microvasculature and [2] increased pleural pressure (Ppl). Physiologists divide the lung into zones based on the relationships among alveolar, pulmonary arterial, and pulmonary venous pressures (Fig. 14-5).[7] In zone 1 (upright position), no blood flow is present because alveolar pressure exceeds PAP. In zone 2, the amount of blood flow depends on the difference between PA and alveolar pressures, since pressure in the alveolus

Figure 14-5 Effect of "zoning" on PAOP. In zones 1 and 2 alveolar pressure (P_A) exceeds pulmonary venous pressure (P_V). Hence an alveolar artifact occurs during balloon occlusion. (Reproduced with permission from Marini J: *Respiratory Medicine and Intensive Care for the House Officer.* Baltimore, Williams & Wilkins, 1981)

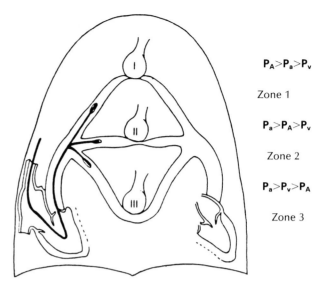

$P_A > P_a > P_v$

Zone 1

$P_a > P_A > P_v$

Zone 2

$P_a > P_v > P_A$

Zone 3

is less than arterial pressure but greater than pulmonary venous pressure. Blood flow in zone 3 depends on the pressure difference between the pulmonary artery and vein. These zones are *physiologically* defined and do *not* correspond to fixed anatomic divisions.[7]

Hypovolemia and PEEP/CPAP increase the proportion of zones 1 and 2 relative to zone 3.[3,7] If the catheter tip is located in a zone 1 or 2 area, the PAOP reading actually reflects alveolar pressure, not left atrial pressure.[8] An example of a tracing that "would not wedge" is seen in Figure 14-6. Careful inspection shows that the QRS complexes occur twice as fast as the "waveforms" and that they are not in phase with the pressure tracing. This catheter tip was placed in a zone 1 or 2 area. For the PAOP to reflect left atrial pressure, the catheter tip must be located in a zone 3 area. Because the catheter is flow-directed, it usually migrates to a zone 3 location during insertion. Catheters located *below* the level of the left atrium

Figure 14-6 "Failure to wedge." Large pressure deflections are respiratory in origin, not PA systolic: Note EKG rate, which is twice that of respiratory rate. (Reproduced with permission from Quinn K, Quebbeman E: Pulmonary artery pressure monitoring in the surgical intensive care unit. *Arch Surg* 1981; 116:872)

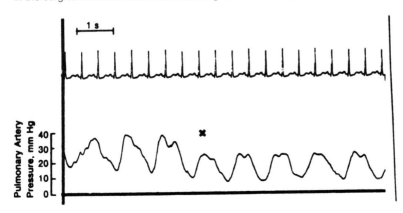

as viewed on *lateral* chest radiographs usually reflect LAP accurately at all levels of PEEP/ CPAP (zone 3 phenomenon), but catheters located *at* or *above* the level of the left atrium provide inaccurate readings, especially with PEEP/CPAP.[6,9] One should suspect that the catheter tip is located in a zone 1 or 2 area when an increase in the PAOP exceeds more than one half of an increment in PEEP/CPAP.[3]

Ventilation with positive airway pressure may increase the proportion of zones 1 and 2 in the normal lung, but in ARDS patients, the alveolar capillaries seem to be somewhat protected from the effects of increased airway pressure. In such cases, the PAOP measured in an area of injury corresponds to actual LAP better than if it was measured in a normal part of the lung. If the catheter tip migrates to a normal lung region, lateral placement of the patient with the "good" lung dependent will improve the correlation in measured PAOP and actual LAP.[10]

The flow of blood in the vascular system is related to the transmural pressure, which is determined by the difference between pressures inside and outside the vessel or heart. The major pressure surrounding the heart and intrathoracic vessels is the Ppl. When Ppl is increased, the increment is transmitted to the pulmonary vessels and the heart, resulting in an elevated measured PAOP even when intravascular volume is normal (Fig. 14-7). The *transmural* pressure, not the measured PAOP, reflects the patient's intravascular volume status in such cases.[3,5,7] During normal *spontaneous* breathing, the Ppl becomes negative (subambient) with inspiration but is near zero at the end of expiration. If the patient is mechanically ventilated without PEEP/CPAP, Ppl is positive during inspiration but returns toward zero at the end of expiration. Since the changes in Ppl are transmitted to the intrathoracic vessels, PA and PAO pressures should be measured when Ppl is zero, that is, at the end of expiration.[3,7]

If the patient is receiving PEEP/CPAP, Ppl may be positive during expiration. This pressure is transmitted to the intrathoracic vessels, resulting in an elevation in the measured PAOP, even if the transmural pressure is normal (see Fig. 14-7). Pleural pressure can be measured by placing a balloon in the distal esophagus or by placing a catheter in the pleural space and subtracting the measured pressure from the PAOP. Because it is difficult to obtain reliable Ppl in ICU patients, a more practical approach is to estimate this value and subtract it from the measured PAOP. In patients with very compliant lungs (emphysema) or very stiff

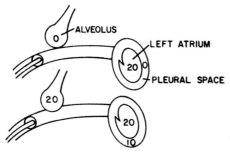

Figure 14-7 An increase in Ppl is transmitted to the PA, causing the measured pressure to increase although the transmural pressure is unchanged. (All pressures are in mm Hg.)

PEEP	PLEURAL PRESSURE	INTRACARDIAC PRESSURE	MEASURED PAWP	TRANSMURAL PRESSURE
0	0	20	20	20
20	10	20	30	20

chest walls (obesity, neuromuscular disease), a greater percentage of the airway pressure is transmitted to the pleural space than in patients with very stiff lungs (ARDS).[3,10,11]

Although PEEP increases Ppl, it also tends to decrease venous return to the heart. The net effect of PEEP on PAOP is determined by how much Ppl increases in comparison to how much the venous return decreases. Studies of patients with ARDS show that Ppl does not become positive at levels of PEEP below 10 cm H_2O. At levels greater than 10 cm H_2O, Ppl increases 2 to 3 cm H_2O for every 5 cm H_2O increase in PEEP above 10 cm H_2O. The following equation shows how this information can be used to *approximate* transmural pressure in patients with *ARDS:*[11]

$$\text{Transmural PAOP} = \text{measured PAOP} - 0.5\,(\text{PEEP} - 10)$$

If PEEP is less than 10 cm H_2O, the measured PAOP is equivalent to the transmural pressure.

Patients with normal lung compliance develop positive Ppl at lower levels of PEEP/CPAP.[12,34] A more accurate estimate of transmural pressure in such individuals is obtained by subtracting one half of the applied airway pressure from the measured PAOP.

$$\text{Transmural PAOP} = \text{measured PAOP} - 0.5(\text{PEEP})$$

Remember, however, that these equations only *estimate* the effects of PEEP/CPAP on pleural pressure. They are useful primarily because of the difficulties in measuring Ppl accurately.

Patients should not be temporarily disconnected from PEEP/CPAP to measure PA or PAOP. Hypoxemia may supervene and not be quickly reversed after resuming therapy. Removal of PEEP also can result in inaccurate hemodynamic data, since venous return to the heart will increase and the filling pressures rise. These elevated filling pressures could lead the clinician to incorrect conclusions concerning the patient's intravascular volume status.[5,7]

When possible, PAOP should be read from a strip recorder to allow correlation of measured pressures with the respiratory cycle. Most digital display modules scan a 3- to 4-second interval and report the highest and lowest pressures as "systolic" and "diastolic," respectively, without consideration of the effects of respiration on the pressure tracings (Fig. 14-8).[7] These monitors also display a "mean" value, which actually is a mathematical average of the highest and lowest pressures. Some newer monitors display PA and PAO pressures at end-expiration. If digital displays must be used, the best estimate of end-expiratory PAOP in *spontaneously* breathing patients is the systolic pressure shown on the digital display module. When patients are mechanically ventilated, the diastolic pressure correlates best.[7] However, the mathematical method used by the monitor to create the digital display must be determined. If a mean value determined by averaging 3 to 4 seconds of data is used, positive artifact from mechanical breaths and/or negative artifact from spontaneous breaths would be included in the numbers used to calculate the digital display. It may be more accurate to determine PAOP from a calibrated screen.

MEASUREMENT OF CARDIAC OUTPUT

Cardiac output can be measured with the thermodilution technique (see also Chapter 5, "Cardiac Output Measurement Technology"). A solution that is cooler than body temperature is injected into the right atrium and the resultant drop in blood temperature at the catheter tip is used to calculate cardiac output. The thermodilution technique is not accurate

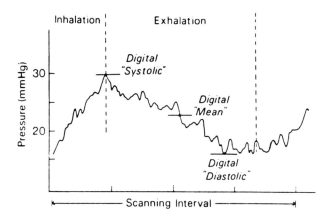

Figure 14-8 Effect of respiratory pressure variation on PAOP during mechanical ventilation. The digital readings represent 3- to 4-second scans during which highest and lowest pressures are displayed as "systolic" and "diastolic." (Reproduced from Marini J: *Respiratory Medicine and Intensive Care for the House Officer.* Baltimore, Williams & Wilkins, 1981)

in the presence of tricuspid regurgitation or any intracardiac shunt. Originally, 10 ml of ice-cold 5% dextrose solution was used as the injectate, but now 10 ml of room temperature injectate or 5 ml of ice-cold injectate gives results that are just as reproducible and accurate.[12–14] The accuracy of thermodilution cardiac output determinations in hypothermic patients may be improved by the use of ice-cold injectate.[15]

Customarily, the average value of three cardiac output measurements is recorded. Clinically significant variation in measurements obtained at different times during the respiratory cycle is often seen (probably as a result of variation in right and left ventricular outputs caused by respiratory-induced changes in intrathoracic pressure). The accuracy of thermodilution cardiac output can be improved by initiating the injection at evenly spaced intervals throughout the respiratory cycle;[16] however, the results are also less reproducible. If the bolus is injected at specific times during the respiratory cycle, reproducibility of the measured cardiac output increases, but significant differences in the average cardiac output will be seen compared to the random injection technique. Because changes in cardiac output owing to respiratory variation cannot be differentiated from those owing to alterations in cardiovascular function, we recommend measurement at end-expiration. This approach may overestimate or underestimate the true cardiac output, but it maximizes the *reproducibility* of the measurement.[17]

Automatic hand-held devices are available for injecting the thermal indicator. They are probably no more accurate than a carefully performed manual injection.[18] Usually, the thermal indicator is injected into the proximal port of the pulmonary catheter, but injection into the side port of the catheter introducer also provides accurate and reproducible cardiac output measurements.[19]

CLINICAL APPLICATION

In addition to those conditions for which pulmonary artery catheterization is commonly used (*e.g.*, ARDS, myocardial infarction, shock), several others may be more easily diagnosed if such monitoring is used.

CARDIAC TAMPONADE

Accumulation of fluid in the pericardium results in increased intrapericardial pressure. When the pericardial pressure equals the pressure in the right heart, cardiac tamponade occurs.

The increased pericardial pressure causes decreased cardiac filling and thus a decreased stroke volume. Cardiac output and blood pressure can be maintained initially by increasing the heart rate and systemic vascular resistance, but, as intrapericardial pressure continues to increase, the cardiac output falls and systemic hypotension occurs.[2]

Pressure tracings obtained during cardiac tamponade are shown in Figure 14-9. Chamber filling begins at the onset of diastole but stops when it is impaired by the elevated intrapericardial pressure. This limitation results in elevation and equalization of the diastolic pressures. A pressure tracing from the right atrium reveals a prominent x descent with an absent or attenuated y descent. The x descent normally occurs as a result of atrial relaxation after the right ventricle empties. It is preserved in cardiac tamponade because the decrease in intracardiac volume after right ventricular emptying allows the right atrial pressure to decrease. The y descent normally is caused by passive emptying of the right atrium into the right ventricle. It is absent or damped in cardiac tamponade because there is no decrease in intracardiac *volume* during this stage of the cardiac cycle and the elevated pericardial pressure prevents a fall in right atrial pressure.[2,20]

CONSTRICTIVE PERICARDITIS

Constrictive pericarditis also causes elevation and equalization of diastolic pressures. Right atrial pressure may increase with inspiration (Kussmaul's sign). The a and v waves are small and equal and are followed by prominent x and y descents, resulting in a typical "M" waveform (Fig. 14-10). The y descent is more prominent than the x descent, and the PAOP waveform resembles the right atrial pressure waveform. Unlike tamponade, the y descent is prominent because there is no restriction of early ventricular filling.[2,20] The "square root sign" is seen in both the right and left ventricular pressure curves because ventricular compliance is reduced, leading to a rapid rise in ventricular pressure during early diastolic filling. This sign is less obvious when the heart rate is increased. In pericardial constriction with a pericardial effusion ("effusive-constrictive disease"), the y descent of the right atrial pressure and PAOP tracings, and the square root sign of the ventricular pressure curves, are attenuated (see Fig. 14-10).

MITRAL REGURGITATION

Acute mitral regurgitation produces large v waves in the PAOP tracing because the left atrium fills with blood from the pulmonary veins during diastole and from regurgitant flow from the left ventricle during systole. If the v wave is mistaken for a pulmonary artery pressure tracing that "will not wedge," one may attempt to advance the catheter, thereby

Figure 14-9 Cardiac tamponade results in identical right atrial, right ventricular end-diastolic, PA diastolic, and wedge (PAO) pressures. (Reproduced from Weeks KR: Bedside hemodynamic monitoring. *J Thorac Cardiovasc Surg* 1976; 71:250)

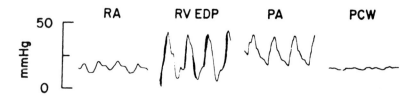

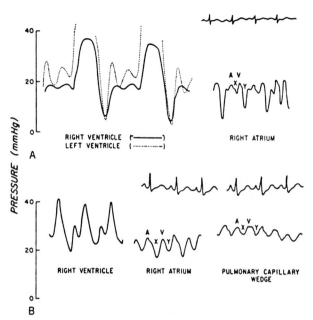

Figure 14-10 Pressure tracings in two patients with constrictive pericarditis. **A.** Early ventricular diastolic dip, early diastolic pressure plateau, and dominant Y descent in atrial pressure. **B.** Diastolic pressure plateau is present, but early ventricular diastolic pressure dip is not prominent and X descent dominates Y descent in atrium. These pressure characteristics occur in about one fourth of patients with constrictive pericarditis, particularly when effusion is present. (Reproduced with permission from Johnson RA, Haber E, Austen WG: *The Practice of Cardiology.* Boston, Little Brown, 1980)

dampening the v waves and missing the diagnosis of mitral regurgitation.[21] Subsequently, if the balloon is inflated when the catheter is located distally in a peripheral vessel, rupture of the pulmonary artery may occur. Pulmonary hypertension with normal pulmonary vascular resistance is seen in acute mitral regurgitation. In chronic mitral regurgitation, pulmonary vascular resistance is high.[21]

COMPLICATIONS

Complications associated with pulmonary artery catheterization are summarized in Table 14-2.

TABLE 14-2   COMPLICATIONS OF BALLOON FLOTATION RIGHT HEART CATHETERIZATION

Dysrhythmias	Endocardial damage
Premature ventricular contractions (PVCs)	Valve cusps
Ventricular tachycardia, fibrillation	Chordae tendineae
Atrial fibrillation, flutter	Papillary muscles
Right bundle branch block	Complications during insertion
Pulmonary infarction	Pneumothorax
Pulmonary artery rupture, right ventricular perforation	Arterial puncture
ration	Venous thrombosis, phlebitis
Catheter-related infections, sepsis	Air embolism
Balloon rupture	
Catheter knotting	

VENTRICULAR DYSRHYTHMIAS

Dysrhythmias occur in 12% to 67% of pulmonary arterial catheterizations but usually are self-limited PVCs when the catheter enters the right ventricle. Ventricular tachycardia and, less often, ventricular fibrillation occasionally occur. The most significant risk factors are hypoxemia (P_{O_2} < 60 mm Hg) and acidosis (pH < 7.0).[22] Prolonged catheterization times probably increase the incidence of ventricular dysrhythmias.[23] Full inflation of the balloon prevents the catheter tip from protruding into the right ventricular wall and may prevent ectopy. Prophylactic intravenous lidocaine during catheter insertion seems to prevent ventricular ectopy if the catheterization takes less than 20 minutes. Transient right bundle branch block may occur during catheter insertion.[22] Complete heart block can develop in patients with preexisting left bundle branch block. Prophylactic insertion of a pacemaker is indicated in patients with a left bundle branch block before pulmonary artery catheterization.

PULMONARY INFARCTION

A wedge-shaped infiltrate distal to the catheter tip suggests that pulmonary infarction has occurred. Avoidance of a peristent wedge position and the use of a continuous flush system with heparin reduced the incidence of pulmonary infarction from 7.2% in 1974 to 1.3% in 1983.[5] Even with these precautions, thrombus formation occurs in the right atrium of 91% of catheterized patients.[5] New heparin-bonded catheters *may* reduce this problem.[24]

PULMONARY ARTERY RUPTURE

Rupture of the pulmonary artery may occur during inflation of the balloon. Although this complication is rare (0.2% of catheterizations), it is often fatal.[25] Pulmonary hypertension, age over 60 years, anticoagulation, distal placement of the catheter, and overinflation of the balloon increase the risk of pulmonary artery rupture. Hypothermia, which occurs during cardiopulmonary bypass, seems to cause the catheter to stiffen and may also increase the risk of perforation. Hemoptysis is common, but the severity varies from scant, frothy, pink sputum (which can be mistaken for pulmonary edema) to massive, exsanguinating hemorrhage.[25,26]

Several mechanisms predispose to rupture. The pulmonary artery becomes noncompliant in patients with pulmonary hypertension, and balloon inflation may cause rupture. Balloon inflation may also be eccentric, causing the catheter tip to protrude. The eccentric balloon then forces the protruding catheter tip into the wall of the artery. An "overwedge" pattern (Fig. 14-11) suggests that eccentric balloon inflation, overdistension, or both, are occurring. If this pattern appears, the balloon must be deflated immediately and the catheter withdrawn until the pulmonary artery tracing returns. In fact, the overwedge tracing should *not* be seen on the screen. The person inflating the balloon must watch the monitor constantly as air is *slowly* injected. As soon as the tracing changes, inflation must be stopped. If the inflation volume is less than 1.0 ml (or ideally 1.29 ml), the catheter should be repositioned. Rupture of the artery can occur only if inflation is continued beyond the point at which the balloon occludes the pulmonary artery—rembember the terminology: pulmonary artery occlusion pressure.

If the catheter is advanced with the balloon deflated, it may migrate too far distally and perforate the pulmonary artery. Inflation should *always* precede advancement. When a loop forms in the right ventricle, the catheter must be withdrawn and reinserted so that no

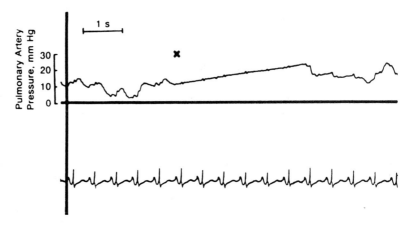

Figure 14-11 Overinflation of balloon after PAOP tracing (to left of X) is obtained. (Reproduced with permission from Quinn K, Quebbeman E: Pulmonary artery pressure monitoring in the surgical intensive care unit. *Arch Surg* 1981; 116:872)

slack is available for distal migration. Flushing the catheter while it is in a wedge position may cause hemoptysis.

Any hemoptysis in a patient with a pulmonary artery catheter should suggest the diagnosis of perforation or rupture. A chest radiograph often reveals a new infiltrate around the tip of the catheter if arterial rupture has occurred. When the amount of hemoptysis is small and the patient is hemodynamically stable, observation may be all that is needed; however, the catheter must not be wedged again. Tracheal suctioning and coughing should be minimized, and coagulation abnormalities, if present, must be corrected. Larger amounts of hemoptysis require placement of a double-lumen endotracheal tube and emergency lobectomy or pneumonectomy.[25] Hemoptysis from pulmonary artery rupture can be so massive that exsanguination occurs within a few minutes.

BALLOON RUPTURE

The balloon on the catheter tip loses elasticity with exposure to blood. The longer the catheter is in place, the greater is the risk of balloon rupture. When attempted balloon inflation is not met with the usual resistance, rupture should be suspected. If blood can be aspirated through the balloon lumen, it is ruptured. However, the inability to aspirate blood through the balloon lumen does not rule out a rupture. Attempts to inflate a ruptured balloon will release small air boluses into the pulmonary circulation. These may be harmless, but if air enters the systemic circulation the results can be devastating. Whenever a right-to-left cardiac shunt is suspected, the balloon should be inflated with carbon dioxide, not air, during measurement of the PAOP.

SEPSIS

Catheter-induced sepsis occurs in up to 2% of insertions. However, positive culture of catheter tip, blood and nonblood culture site negative and organism from the catheter tip and a nonblood source occur in 5% to 35% of catheterizations.[27–30] Catheter-related infections are more common when the catheter is left in place for more than 3 or 4 days and may be more common if a known source of infection existed before catheter insertion. Systems using a sterile sleeve around the part of the catheter that is proximal to the insertion site *may* reduce the incidence of infection. Pulmonary artery catheterization predisposes patients to right-sided endocarditis.[31]

AIR EMBOLISM

Venous air embolism (VAE) can occur during central line placement. When a vein is open to air, the subambient pressure generated by spontaneous inspiration results in the entry of air into the venous system. Subclavian and jugular venous catheter placement are the most commonly performed procedures associated with air embolism. The symptoms and signs of VAE include dyspnea, chest pain, tachycardia, tachypnea, expiratory wheezes, and focal neurologic deficits. Elevated right heart pressures, hypotension, hypoxemia, and hypercarbia are present. A mill-wheel cardiac murmur, although classic, is only occasionally heard. Radiographic manifestations of VAE include air in the main pulmonary artery, intracardiac air, air in the hepatic venous system, pulmonary edema, atelectasis, or focal oligemia. The chest radiograph also can be normal. Placement of the patient in the left lateral decubitus position allows the air that is obstructing the pulmonary outflow tract to float to the right ventricular apex, thus relieving the obstruction. Aspiration of the air through the central venous catheter and administration of 100% oxygen (which causes the size of the embolus to decrease) are also effective measures. Embolization can be prevented by placing the patient in the Trendelenburg position before central line placement and instructing him to hold his breath during introducer insertion.

KNOTTING

Intracardiac knotting of the catheter, seemingly a preventable complication, may occur during insertion. No more than 10 to 15 cm should be introduced after crossing the tricuspid valve (appearance of RV tracing) unless the pulmonary valve is traversed (PA tracing is seen). Commonly, the operator continues to advance the catheter, hoping the tip will float out the pulmonary valve. In reality, if it has missed the outflow tract, it can only curve back on itself, forming a loop and then a knot. Ventricular dysrhythmias, which occur while the right atrial pressure is recorded, suggest that knotting is present.[31] Insertion of a long guidewire into the catheter, followed by slow withdrawal of the catheter over the wire, may resolve the problem. If this maneuver fails, remove the guidewire, pull the catheter tightly against the introducer (to shrink the size of the knot), and withdraw it. If you cannot withdraw through the introducer, remove the introducer and pull the catheter out through the skin. Stone-retriever baskets introduced through the saphenous vein also can be used.

REFERENCES

1. Swan HJC, Ganz W, Forrester J, et al: Catheterization of the heart in man with use of a flow-directed balloon-tipped catheter. *N Engl J Med* 1970; 283:447
2. Braunwald E: *Heart Disease: A Textbook of Cardiovascular Medicine*, pp 288, 1530. Philadelphia, WB Saunders, 1980
3. O'Quinn R, Marini J: Pulmonary artery occlusion pressure: Clinical physiology, measurement and interpretation. *Am Rev Respir Dis* 1983; 128:319
4. Pierson D, Hudson L: Monitoring hemodynamics in the critically ill. *Med Clin North Am* 1983; 67:1343
5. Wiedemann H, Matthay M, Matthay R: Cardiovascular-pulmonary monitoring in the intensive care unit. *Chest* 1984; 85:537, 656

6. Shin B, Ayella R, McAslan G: Pitfalls of Swan-Ganz catheterization. *Crit Care Med* 1977; 5:125
7. Marini J: *Respiratory Medicine and Intensive Care for the House Officer*, pp 58, 161. Baltimore, Williams & Wilkins, 1981
8. Quinn K, Quebbeman E: Pulmonary artery pressure monitoring in the surgical intensive care unit. *Arch Surg* 1981; 116:872
9. Shasby D, Dauber I, Pfister S, et al: Swan-Ganz location and left atrial pressure determine the accuracy of the wedge pressure when positive end-expiratory pressure is used. *Chest* 1981; 80:666
10. Hasan F, Weiss W, Braman S, et al: Influence of lung injury on pulmonary wedge-left atrial pressure correlation during positive end-expiratory pressure ventilation. *Am Rev Respir Dis* 1985; 131:246
11. Jardin F, Farcot JC, Boisante L, et al: Influence of positive end-expiratory pressure on left ventricular performance. *N Engl J Med* 1981; 304:387
12. Elkayam U, Berkley R, Azen S, et al: Cardiac output by thermodilution technique. *Chest* 1984; 84:418
13. Nelson L, Anderson H: Patient selection for iced versus room temperature injectate for thermodilution cardiac output determinations. *Crit Care Med* 1985; 13:182
14. Vennix C, Nelson D, Pierpont G: Thermodilution cardiac output in critically ill patients: Comparison of room-temperature and iced injectate. *Heart Lung* 1984; 13:574
15. Stetz C, Miller R, Kelly G, et al: Reliability of the thermodilution method in the determination of cardiac output in clinical practice. *Am Rev Respir Dis* 1982; 126:1001
16. Snyder J, Powner D: Effects of mechanical ventilation on the measurement of cardiac output by thermodilution. *Crit Care Med* 1982; 10:682
17. Stevens J, Raffin T, Mihm F, et al: Thermodilution cardiac output measurement. *JAMA* 1985; 253:2240
18. Nelson L, Houtchens B: Automatic vs. manual injections for thermodilution cardiac output determinations. *Crit Care Med* 1982; 10:190
19. Lee D, Stevens G: Comparison of thermodilution cardiac output measurements by injection of the proximal lumen versus side port of the Swan-Ganz catheter. *Heart Lung* 1985; 14:126
20. Johnson RA, Haber E, Austen WG: *The Practice of Cardiology*, p 669. Boston, Little, Brown, 1980
21. Friedman A, Stein L: Pitfalls in bedside diagnosis of severe acute mitral regurgitation. *Chest* 1980; 78:436
22. Sprung C, Pozen R, Rozanski J, et al: Advanced ventricular arrhythmias during bedside pulmonary artery catheterization. *Am J Med* 1982; 72:203
23. Iberti T, Ernest B, Gruppi L, et al: Ventricular arrhythmias during pulmonary artery catheterization in the intensive care unit. *Am J Med* 1985; 78:451
24. Hoar P, Wilson R, Mangano D, et al: Heparin bonding reduces thrombogenicity of pulmonary artery catheters. *N Engl J Med* 1981; 305:993
25. McDaniel D, Stone J, Faltas A, et al: Catheter-induced pulmonary artery hemorrhage. *J Thorac Cardiovasc Surg* 1981; 82:1
26. Page D, Teres D, Hartshorn J: Fatal hemorrhage from Swan-Ganz catheter. *N Engl J Med* 1974; 291:260
27. Applefeld J, Caruthers T, Reno D, et al: Assessment of the sterility of long-term cardiac catheterization using the thermodilution Swan-Ganz catheter. *Chest* 1978; 74:377
28. Michel L, Marsh M, McMichan J, et al: Infection of pulmonary artery catheters in critically ill patients. *JAMA* 1981; 245:1032
29. Pinilla J, Ross D, Martin T, et al: Study of the incidence of intravascular catheter infection and associated septicemia in critically ill patients. *Crit Care Med* 1983; 11:21
30. Hudson-Civetta JA, Civetta JM, Martinez OV, et al: Risk and deletion of pulmonary artery catheter-related infection in septic surgical patients. *Crit Care Med* 1987; 15:29
31. Rowley K, Clubb KS, Smith GJ, et al: Right-sided endocarditis as a consequence of flow directed pulmonary artery catheterization. *N Engl J Med* 1984; 311:1152
32. Lipp H, O'Donoghue K, Resenkov L: Intracardiac knotting of a flow-directed balloon catheter. *N Engl J Med* 1971; 284:220
33. Voci G, Gazek F, Burris A, et al: Retrieval of entrapped and knotted balloon-tipped catheters from the right heart. *Ann Intern Med* 1980; 92:638

APPENDIX

EQUATIONS USEFUL IN HEMODYNAMIC MONITORING

Mean Arterial Pressure (MAP)

MAP = (systolic BP − diastolic BP) 1/3 + diastolic BP
(Normal = 85–95 mm Hg)

Systemic Vascular Resistance

$$SVR = \frac{MAP\ (mm\ Hg) - CVP\ (mm\ Hg)}{Cardiac\ output\ (liters/min)} \times 79.9$$

(Normal = 770–1500 dynes·sec·cm^{-5})

Pulmonary Vascular Resistance

$$PVR = \frac{Mean\ pulmonary\ artery\ pressure\ (mm\ Hg) - PAOP\ (mm\ Hg)}{Cardiac\ output\ (liters/min)} \times 79.9$$

(Normal = 20–120 dynes·sec·cm^{-5})

Arterial O$_2$ Content

$Ca_{O_2} = (Hgb \times 1.34)\ Sa_{O_2} + (Pa_{O_2} \times 0.0031)$
(Sa_{O_2} = percent saturation of arterial blood)

Mixed Venous O$_2$ Content

$C\bar{v}_{O_2} = (Hgb)\ (1.34)\ S\bar{v}_{O_2} + (P\bar{v}_{O_2} \times 0.0031)$
$S\bar{v}_{O_2}$ = percent saturation of mixed venous blood

Shunt Fraction

$$\frac{\dot{Q}s}{\dot{Q}t} = \frac{Cc'_{O_2} - Ca_{O_2}}{Cc'_{O_2} - C\bar{v}_{O_2}}$$

$C\dot{c}_{O_2} = (1.34)\ (Hgb)\ 100\%\ saturation + 0.0031\ Pa_{O_2}$

$$PA_{O_2} = (P_B - P_{H_2O})\ FI_{O_2} - \frac{P_{CO2}}{0.8}$$

(P_B = barometric pressure)
(P_{H_2O} = water vapor pressure)
(Normal shunt ≤ 0.05 [5%])

CHAPTER FIFTEEN

APPLICATION OF VENOUS SATURATION MONITORING

Loren D. Nelson

PHYSIOLOGY OF OXYGEN TRANSPORT

The process of oxygen transport includes not only loading oxygen into the red cells and delivering it to the tissue, but also utilization of the oxygen in the periphery and the return of desaturated blood to the right side of the heart.[1] Several terms must be defined to understand the components of oxygen transport (Table 15-1). Oxygen demand is the amount of oxygen *required* by the body tissues to function under conditions of aerobic metabolism. Because oxygen demand is determined at the tissue level, it is presently impossible to quantitate clinically. Oxygen consumption ($\dot{V}_{O_2}$), on the other hand, is the amount of oxygen *consumed* by the tissue as calculated by the Fick equation (CO times arterial–venous oxygen content difference). $\dot{V}_{O_2}$ is a mechanism by which the body "protects" the oxygen demand created at the tissue level.[2] Factors associated with increases in $\dot{V}_{O_2}$ are associated with increased survivorship,[3] whereas low $\dot{V}_{O_2}$ is associated with a mortality as high as 80%. $\dot{V}_{O_2}$ may increase by increasing CO or widening the arterial–venous oxygen content difference. In the normal state, both cardiac output and arterial–venous oxygen difference may increase by about threefold, providing a total increase of $\dot{V}_{O_2}$ during times of stress to about ninefold above the resting state. Normally $\dot{V}_{O_2}$ and oxygen demand are equal; however, in times of great oxygen demand or times in which either CO or arterial–venous oxygen content difference cannot increase to meet the oxygen demand of the cells, oxygen demand may exceed $\dot{V}_{O_2}$. When this occurs, anaerboic metabolism and lactic acidosis ensue.[2]

Oxygen uptake differs slightly from $\dot{V}_{O_2}$ in that the latter is a *calculated* value (from the Fick equation) and the former is the *measured* volume of oxygen taken up by the patient each minute. Oxygen uptake is measured by analyzing inspired and expired gas concentrations and inspired and expired volumes. Measurement of oxygen uptake may be useful for metabolic studies since it can be performed continuously for long periods of time to account for variation in $\dot{V}_{O_2}$ owing to activity and the like.

Oxygen delivery ($\dot{D}_{O_2}$) is the volume of oxygen delivered from the heart each minute and is calculated as the product of cardiac output and arterial oxygen content. Oxygen utilization or extraction ratio is the *fraction* of delivered oxygen that is consumed ($\dot{V}_{O_2}$ divided by $\dot{D}_{O_2}$). Therefore, the oxygen utilization coefficient defines the balance between

TABLE 15-1 OXYGEN TRANSPORT TERMINOLOGY

Oxygen demand = cellular oxygen requirement to avoid anaerobic metabolism

Oxygen consumption ($\dot{V}_{O_2}$) = calculated (Fick) volume of oxygen consumed each minute [C(a-v̄)O_2 × CO × 10]

Oxygen uptake = measured volume of oxygen extracted each minute

Oxygen delivery ($\dot{D}_{O_2}$) = volume of oxygen delivered from the left ventricle each minute [CO × Ca$_{O_2}$ × 10]

Oxygen utilization coefficient (extraction ratio) = fraction of delivered oxygen that is consumed [$\dot{V}_{O_2}/\dot{D}_{O_2}$] or [CO × C(a − v̄)$O_2$/CO × Ca]

Oxygen transport = processes contributing to oxygen delivery and oxygen consumption

---

oxygen supply (delivery) and demand (consumption). Clinically, oxygen utilization ratio may be calculated from the Fick equation substitution of CO × C (a − v̄) O_2 for $\dot{V}O_2$. When this is divided by oxygen delivery, the equation can be simplified by cancelling cardiac output from the numerator and denominator, leaving Ca − Cv̄/Ca. When arterial saturation is nearly 1.0, the mathematical formula approximates 1 − Cv̄, thus Sv̄ O_2 (which expresses the only variable in the equation for venous content, which changes significantly) is closely related mathematically to oxygen utilization ratio. In fact, it actually is the complement, thus explaining the excellent correlation seen clinically (See Fig. 15-4D).

ASSESSMENT OF OXYGEN TRANSPORT BALANCE

Oxygen transport balance may be assessed on several levels. First, examination of the patient may reveal signs of hypoperfusion, including altered mentation, cutaneous hypoperfusion, oliguria, tachycardia, and, when all compensatory systems have failed, hypotension. Although these clinical signs may be useful, they are unfortunately often late, nonspecific, and at times uninterpretable in critically ill patients. A more physiologic approach is to assess the determinants of oxygen transport balance individually by using the Fick equation. The arterial–venous oxygen content difference may be used to assess the relative balance between CO and $\dot{V}_{O_2}$. An increase in the arterial–venous oxygen content difference indicates that either flow is too low or consumption is too high.

Although oxygen demand cannot be measured, the relative balance between consumption and demand is best indicated by the presence of excess lactate in the blood. Lactic acidosis means that demand exceeds consumption and anaerobic metabolism is present.[2] The relative balance between oxygen supply and demand is best assessed by the oxygen utilization coefficient.[1] Calculation of this coefficient, however, requires the measurement of CO, Hgb, Sa$_{O_2}$, Pa$_{O_2}$, Sv̄$_{O_2}$, and mixed venous oxygen tension.

When the Fick equation is solved for Sv̄$_{O_2}$ (Table 15-2), it becomes apparent that there is an inverse linear relation between Sv̄$_{O_2}$ and oxygen utilization coefficient[4] as long as Sa$_{O_2}$ is maintained at a high level. Sv̄$_{O_2}$ measured continuously is, therefore, an on-line indicator of the adequacy of oxygen supply and of the demand in perfused tissues, and the determinants of Sv̄$_{O_2}$ are $\dot{V}_{O_2}$, Hgb, CO, Sa$_{O_2}$, and, to a very small degree, Pa$_{O_2}$ (Table 15-3).

Sv$_{O_2}$ represents the flow-weighted average of the venous oxygen saturations from all perfused tissues.[1] Therefore, tissues that have high blood flow but relatively low oxygen

TABLE 15-2 DERIVATION OF $S\bar{v}_{O_2}$ FROM FICK EQUATION

1. $\dot{V}_{O_2} = C(a\text{-}\bar{v})O_2 \times CO \times 10$	{Fick equation
2. $\dot{V}_{O_2}/(CO \times 10) = C(a\text{-}\bar{v})O_2$	{Divide by CO × 10
3. $\dot{V}_{O_2}/(CO \times 10) = Ca_{O_2} - C\bar{v}_{O_2}$	{Definition of $C(a\text{-}\bar{v})O_2$
4. $\dot{V}_{O_2}/(CO \times 10) - Ca_{O_2} = -C\bar{v}_{O_2}$	{Subtract Ca_{O_2}
5. $C\bar{v}_{O_2} = Ca_{O_2} - [\dot{V}_{O_2}/(CO \times 10)]$	{Multiply × −1
6. $C\bar{v}_{O_2}/Ca_{O_2} = 1 - [\dot{V}_{O_2}/(CO \times 10 \times Ca_{O_2})]$	{Divide by Ca_{O_2}
7. $C\bar{v}_{O_2}/Ca_{O_2} = 1 - \dot{V}_{O_2}/\dot{D}_{O_2}$	{Definition of $\dot{D}_{O_2}$
8. $S\bar{v}_{O_2} = 1 - \dot{V}_{O_2}/\dot{D}_{O_2}$	{Definition of $S\bar{v}_{O_2}$ if $Sa_{O_2} = 1.0$

extraction (kidney) will have a greater effect on $S\bar{v}_{O_2}$ than will tissues with low blood flow, even though the oxygen extraction of these tissues, may be quite high (myocardium). The interpretation of $S\bar{v}_{O_2}$ requires consistent and intact vasoregulation.[5] When vasoregulation is altered (such as in sepsis), oxygen uptake may be severely altered, causing a marked increase in $S\bar{v}_{O_2}$. This increase, however, should not be interpreted to mean that all tissues are being well perfused.

MONITORING OXYGEN TRANSPORT

Patients admitted to intensive care units may be grouped into three large categories.[6] Category 1 consists of patients requiring intensive observation or monitoring. These patients may have major risk factors or may be admitted because of the nature of their illness or the nature of the therapy they are receiving. Category 2 patients require intensive nursing care and often specialized technology and care facilities to direct therapy for major systemic illness. Category 3 patients need continuous physician intervention for hemodynamic and other instabilities. Continuous venous oximetry may have clinical applications in each of these broad classes of patients.

The three major objectives of monitoring critically ill patients are [1] to assure that the patient is, in fact, stable, [2] to provide an early warning system as to untoward events, and [3] to evaluate the efficiency and efficacy of interventions performed. The role of the three monitoring objectives differs in the three categories of patients being monitored.

In patients who undergo preoperative hemodynamic and oxygen transport monitoring only because of underlying risk factors, a normal and stable $S\bar{v}_{O_2}$ can be presumed to indicate that the balance between oxygen supply and demand is intact and the patients are stable. Further assessment of CO and arterial and mixed venous blood gas analysis that would be performed to reach that conclusion can be eliminated, and there is "safety in no (other) numbers."[7] If the patient becomes "unstable" as manifested by a decreasing $S\bar{v}_{O_2}$, the monitoring system will meet the second objective by providing an early warning[8] of the imbal-

TABLE 15-3 DETERMINANTS OF Sv_{O_2}

Cardiac output
Hemoblobin concentration
Arterial oxygen saturation
Oxygen consumption

ance in oxygen supply and demand. In this situation, although an alert has been given, the cause of the oxygen transport imbalance is not necessarily clear. The change in $S\bar{v}_{O_2}$ is sensitive but not specific. In this clinical situation it is necessary to measure CO, Sa_{O_2}, and Hgb. These numbers can be used to calculate $\dot{V}_{O_2}$ and the other components of oxygen transport balance. When the cause of the imbalance is identified, specific therapy may be instituted to restore the oxygen supply/demand balance. When therapy is instituted to correct an oxygen supply/demand imbalance, continuous venous oximetry demonstrates its greatest efficacy.[9] As interventions are instituted, the on-line assessment of supply/demand balance may be used to evaluate the efficacy of the intervention. Because the measurement is continuous, the evaluation of responses to therapy is instantaneous rather than delayed by blood gas analysis and measurement of CO. Patients may change from class to class as their condition improves or deteriorates. The precise use of continuous venous oximetry will vary with the patient's condition.

CLINICAL USEFULNESS OF CONTINUOUS SV$_{O_2}$ MONITORING

Reflectance spectrophotometry is the technology currently used for continuous venous oximetry today (Fig. 15-1). Transmitting and receiving fiberoptic bundles are located in the

Figure 15-1 Principle of reflectance spectrophotometry. (Courtesy of Oximetrix, Inc., Mountain View, California)

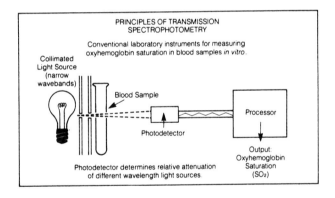

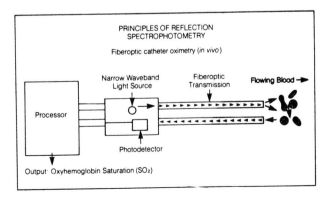

wall of the PA catheter. Light from the transmission bundle is emitted in two or three specific wavelengths that correspond to the maximum reflectance of oxyhemoglobin and deoxyhemoglobin. As red cells flow past the tip of the catheter, light is reflected from the cells to the receiving fiberoptic bundle. The microprocessor uses the relative reflectances (Fig. 15-2) to calculate the oxyhemoglobin and total hemoglobin, the fraction of which represents $S\bar{v}_{O_2}$.

As is the case with most monitoring devices, the continuous oximetry system must be calibrated before use. This may be done *in vitro* by positioning the catheter tip next to a target that will reflect the transmitted light in such a manner that the microprocessor can be calibrated.[10] When this is done (before insertion of the catheter), the oxygen saturation of the central venous system, right atrium, right ventricle, and pulmonary artery can be measured while the catheter is being floated into the proper position. Taking these measurements during the insertion of the catheter may be useful to rule out intracardiac left-to-right shunts.

Once the PA catheter is in proper position, blood may be sampled through the distal port to calibrate or to verify the calibration of the system. A mixed venous sample is withdrawn and analyzed by laboratory cooximetry. The value obtained by the microprocessor at the time the blood sample is drawn is retained by the memory of the system. This may be compared against the value obtained from the laboratory sample, and, if there is a significant (greater than 4%) difference, the instrument may be recalibrated to the laboratory cooximeter value.

The system should be calibrated before insertion of the catheter (Fig. 15-3) and the calibration verified at any time the optical module is disconnected from the catheter or whenever the measurement is suspected of being erroneous. The calibration of the system should also be checked every 24 hours to ensure stability of the system.[11]

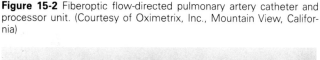

Figure 15-2 Fiberoptic flow-directed pulmonary artery catheter and processor unit. (Courtesy of Oximetrix, Inc., Mountain View, California)

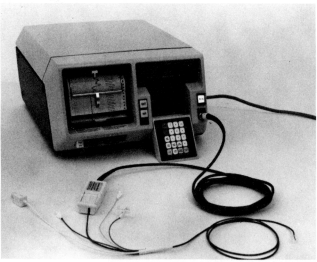

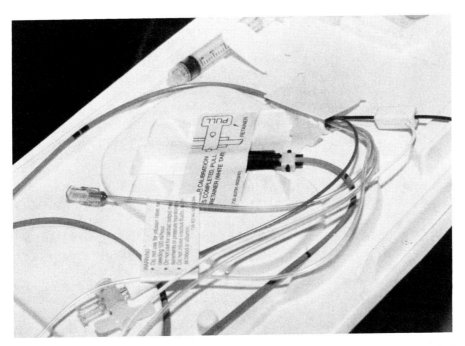

Figure 15-3 "In vitro" callibration of the oximetry lumen is performed by attaching the optical module to the fiberoptics while the tip of the catheter remains in its original position in the insertion kit. This should be done in order to verify function of the catheter and processor and so that the venous saturation can be monitored during insertion.

Because it is crucial that red cells be flowing past the tip of the catheter, proper positioning of the catheter in the pulmonary artery is necessary. Distal migration of the PA catheter tip is a common source of error. When the catheter tip advances into the distal segments of the pulmonary artery, a high or increased $S\bar{v}_{O_2}$, a decreased light intensity signal, or damping of the pulmonary artery tracing may become evident.[9] If these signs are encountered, the distal lumen of the catheter should be vigorously irrigated with flush solution because fibrin formation on the catheter tip may also cause these artifacts. If the pressure waveform is not restored to a proper PA tracing by irrigation, the catheter should be slowly withdrawn until the PA pressure tracing is restored. At this point the PA catheter balloon may be slowly inflated until an occlusion or wedge tracing is observed. If this tracing is not produced by inflation of the balloon to maximum volume (1.5 ml), the catheter should be slowly advanced until wedge pressure tracing is observed. At that point the balloon can be deflated again and then slowly reinflated until a wedge tracing occurs. The volume required to restore this tracing should be about 75% or more of the total capacity of the balloon. Using the maximum balloon volume to attain a wedge tracing ensures that the catheter is in the proximal section of the pulmonary artery and is in fact a "physiologic confirmation" of the catheter tip position.[12]

Not only does distal migration of the PA catheter cause an artifactually high oxygen saturation owing to highly saturated pulmonary capillary blood being analyzed, but also the catheter tip may be lodged against a vessel wall or bifurcation, causing an alteration in the light intensity received by the fiberoptic bundles. It is important that a low light intensity alarm be corrected before the venous saturation measurement is considered to be reliable or before the system is recalibrated.

The light intensity signal may decrease if there is an alteration of blood flow past the tip of the catheter, if there is fibrin deposition over the fiberoptic bundles, or if the catheter is lodged against a vessel wall. Large fluctuations in the light intensity signal may indicate that the catheter tip is malpositioned but also may indicate a condition of intravascular volume deficit that allows compression or collapse of the pulmonary vasculature (especially during positive pressure ventilation). The display of venous saturation is illustrated in Fig. 15-4.

INTERPRETATION OF VENOUS OXYGEN SATURATION

Mixed venous oxygen saturation values within the normal range (0.68–0.77) indicate a normal balance between oxygen supply and demand provided that vasoregulation is intact and there is a normal distribution of peripheral blood flow. Values of $S\bar{v}_{O_2}$ greater than 0.77 indicate an excess of $\dot{D}_{O_2}$ over $\dot{V}_{O_2}$ and are most commonly associated with syndromes of vasoderegulation such as cirrhosis and sepsis. High values are also seen in states of low V_{O_2} (hypothermia, muscular paralysis, sedation, coma, or a combination of these factors), hyperoxygenation, high CO, and, rarely, cyanide toxicity.

Figure 15-4 A commercially available display device (Oximetrix). Note that both the current value and a graphic representation of prior data are displayed. Other display options are also available.

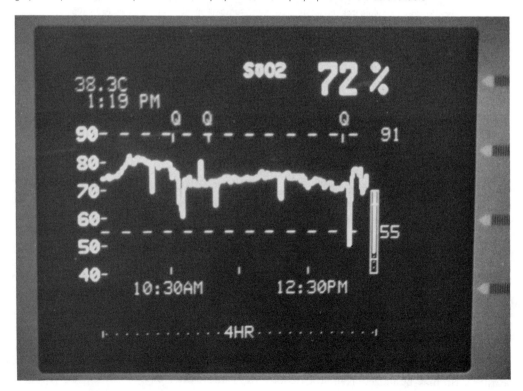

Uncompensated changes in any of the four determinants of $S\bar{v}_{O_2}$ may result in a decrease in the measured value, but in complex, critically ill patients the correlation between changes in $S\bar{v}_{O_2}$ and changes in any of the individual determining factors is low. In a study of the patients in a surgical intensive care unit,[4] there was no statistical correlation between changes in either Pa_{O_2} or Sa_{O_2} and $S\bar{v}_{O_2}$ (Fig. 15-5). Although there was a statistically significant correlation between changes in $S\bar{v}_{O_2}$ and CO and $\dot{D}_{O_2}$, the correlation was not sufficiently great to be clinically significant. Also, there was no statistical correlation between $S\bar{v}_{O_2}$ and either arterial–venous oxygen content difference or calculated $\dot{V}_{O_2}$. There was, however, using the Fick equation substitution for measured oxygen consumption, a highly significant inverse correlation between $S\bar{v}_{O_2}$ and oxygen utilization coefficient (Fig. 15-6). This inverse correlation represents graphically plotting one number against its complement as discussed in the section "Physiology of Oxygen Transport," above. This study emphasizes that the determinants of $S\bar{v}_{O_2}$ are multifactorial and, in critically ill patients, the degree of compensation for changes in one variable cannot be predicted.

It is, however, useful to appreciate the magnitude of change in $S\bar{v}_{O_2}$ that would occur with an isolated change in any of the individual determinants. If there are no compensatory changes in either $\dot{V}_{O_2}$ or CO, even very large fluctuations in Hgb produce a surprisingly

Figure 15-5 Relation between arterial oxygenation and Sv_{O_2}. There is no statistically significant correlation between either Pa_{O_2} **(Panel A)** or Sa_{O_2} **(Panel B)** and Sv_{O_2}. (Reproduced with permission from *Ann Surg* 1986; 203:329)

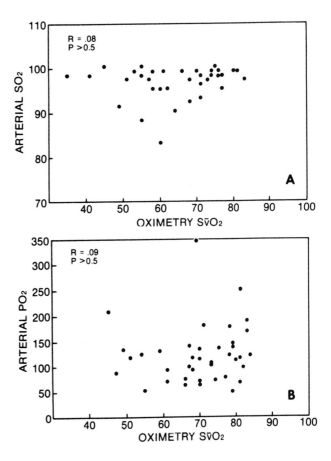

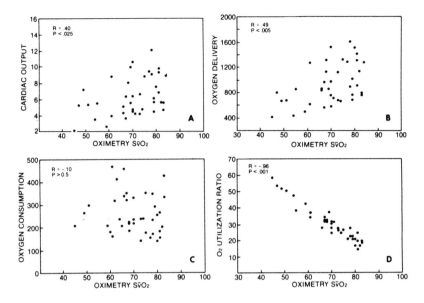

Figure 15-6 Correlation between oxygen transport variables and Sv_{O_2}. There is no statistically significant correlation between oxygen consumption and Sv_{O_2} **(Panel B)**, and a very low correlation between either cardiac output **(Panel A)** or oxygen delivery **(Panel C)** and Sv_{O_2}. There is a highly significant inverse correlation between oxygen utilization ratio **(Panel D)** and Sv_{O_2}. This is the mathematical representation of plotting the derived oxygen utilization ratio (from the substitution of CO × C (a − v̄)O_2 for its Fick equivalent, $\dot{V}O_2$). $S\bar{v}O_2$ thus represents the complement of oxygen utilization ratio and is expressed graphically as the line with a negative shape. (Reproduced with permission from *Ann Surg* 1986; 203:329)

small change in $S\bar{v}_{O_2}$ until the Hgb reaches extremely low levels (Table 15-4). Although these changes are small in this mathematical model, in actuality the changes would be even smaller because of an almost certain increase in CO that would be caused by the acute anemia. For example, a patient who has a slowly decreasing Hgb, in general, will increase CO to maintain $\dot{D}_{O_2}$. However, if CO is fixed because of underlying cardiovascular disease, a decrease in Hgb will be reflected by a decrease in $S\bar{v}_{O_2}$.

The effect of arterial oxygen tension on $S\bar{v}_{O_2}$ in the absence of other compensatory changes is demonstrated in Table 15-5. As long as Sa_{O_2} is maintained in a relatively normal range, the direct effect on $S\bar{v}_{O_2}$ is minimal. However, when there is sufficient arterial hypoxemia to produce arterial desaturation, the $S\bar{v}_{O_2}$ falls in direct proportion to the change in Sa_{O_2}. Similarly, changes in CO (Table 15-6) and $\dot{V}_{O_2}$ (Table 15-7) may be shown to affect

TABLE 15-4   EFFECT OF CHANGES IN HEMOGLOBIN CONCENTRATION ON $S\bar{v}_{O_2}$

HEMOGLOBIN	13	10	7.5	5
Ca_{O_2}	18	14	10.5	7
$C\bar{v}_{O_2}$	14	10	6.5	3
$S\bar{v}_{O_2}$	0.77	0.71	0.61	0.42

[Calculated change in $S\bar{v}_{O_2}$ caused by a change in Hgb (g/dl), assuming no compensatory changes in other determinants of $S\bar{v}_{O_2}$; Pa_{O_2} = 100 mm Hg, Sa_{O_2} = 0.98, C(a-v̄)O_2 = 4.0 ml/dl, and $\dot{V}_{O_2}$ and CO are not changed.]

TABLE 15-5   EFFECT OF VARIATION IN Pa_{O_2} ON $S\bar{v}_{O_2}$

Pa_{O_2}	600	200	100	80	60	40
Sa_{O_2}	1.0	1.0	0.98	0.95	0.90	0.75
Ca_{O_2}	19.8	18.6	17.9	17.3	16.3	13.6
$C\bar{v}_{O_2}$	15.9	14.6	13.9	13.3	12.3	9.6
$S\bar{v}_{O_2}$	0.87	0.81	0.77	0.73	0.68	0.53

[Calculated change in $S\bar{v}_{O_2}$ caused by an uncompensated change in Pa_{O_2} (mm Hg), assuming Hgb = 13 g/dl, $C(a-\bar{v})O_2$ = 4.0 ml/dl, and $\dot{V}_{O_2}$ and CO are unchanged.]

directly $S\bar{v}_{O_2}$, although the magnitude of changes in any of these individual parameters does not predict the magnitude of change in $S\bar{v}_{O_2}$ because compensatory factors are usually involved.

A decrease in $S\bar{v}_{O_2}$ greater than 0.10 is likely to be of clinical significance regardless of the initial value.[1] A change from 0.70 to 0.60 may be associated with a large fractional change in CO (assuming, for argument, that other factors did not change). On the other hand, although a change from 0.60 to 0.50 is associated with a much smaller fractional change in CO, it occurs at a time of greatly limited oxygen transport reserve. While $S\bar{v}_{O_2}$ is a sensitive indicator in oxygen transport balance, it cannot specifically determine the actual change of any of the individual components of $\dot{D}_{O_2}$ or $\dot{V}_{O_2}$. Therefore, because a sustained decrease in $S\bar{v}_{O_2}$ of greater than 0.10 does not explain the cause for the imbalance in oxygen supply and demand, this change should alert the clinician to the need for further evaluation of the the individual factors likely to affect oxygen transport balance. The first step in this evaluation should be to rule out artifact in the measurement owing to the catheter positioning, low light intensity, or miscalibration of the microprocessor. When a change in $S\bar{v}_{O_2}$ is determined to be both clinically significant and valid, measurement of Sa_{O_2}, Hgb, and CO, used in conjunction with the $S\bar{v}_{O_2}$ measurement, will provide the database necessary to evaluate the etiology for the change in $S\bar{v}_{O_2}$. When the derived cardiopulmonary parameters of arterial–venous oxygen content difference, $\dot{V}_{O_2}$, intrapulmonary shunt fraction (venous admixture), and oxygen extraction or utilization coefficient are calculated, the clinician should be able to interpret the oxygen transport imbalance identified by continuous venous oximetry and institute immediate therapy.

PITFALLS IN CONTINUOUS VENOUS OXIMETRY

The most common sources of error in the continuous measurement of $S\bar{v}_{O_2}$ are calibration and catheter malposition. Before instituting major therapeutic changes, it is prudent to

TABLE 15-6   EFFECT OF CARDIAC OUTPUT ON $S\bar{v}_{O_2}$

CO	10	7.5	5.0	4.0	3.0	2.0
$C(a-\bar{v})_{O_2}$	2.5	3.3	5.0	6.3	8.3	12.5
Ca_{O_2}	18.3	18.3	18.3	18.3	18.3	18.3
$C\bar{v}_{O_2}$	15.8	15.0	13.3	12.0	10.0	5.8
$S\bar{v}_{O_2}$	0.87	0.83	0.73	0.66	0.55	0.31

[Calculated effect of uncompensated changes in CO (liters/min) on $S\bar{v}_{O_2}$, assuming Hgb = 13 g/dl, Pa_{O_2} = 100 mm Hg, Sa_{O_2} = 0.98, and $\dot{V}_{O_2}$ is fixed at 250 ml/min.]

TABLE 15-7   EFFECT OF OXYGEN CONSUMPTION ON $S\bar{v}_{O_2}$

$\dot{V}_{O_2}$	150	200	250	300	400	500
$C(a-\bar{v})_{O_2}$	3.0	4.0	5.0	6.0	8.0	10.0
Ca_{O_2}	18.3	18.3	18.3	18.3	18.3	18.3
$C\bar{v}_{O_2}$	15.3	14.3	13.3	12.3	10.3	8.3
$S\bar{v}_{O_2}$	0.85	0.79	0.74	0.68	0.57	0.46

[Effect of uncompensated changes in $\dot{V}_{O_2}$ (ml/min) on $S\bar{v}_{O_2}$, assuming Hgb = 13 g/dl, Pa_{O_2} = 100 mm Hg, Sa_{O_2} = 0.98, and CO is fixed at 5.0 liters/min.]

confirm that the $S\bar{v}_{O_2}$ value displayed is actually correct by performing cooximetry on a mixed venous blood sample and comparing the value with that from the on-line instrument. Calibration should be done only after correcting any light intensity alerts.[10] The finding of a normal or high $S\bar{v}_{O_2}$ when the light intensity alert is present should be viewed with skepticism.[9]

Although there are no differences in insertion techniques between fiberoptic and other PA catheters,[13] the fiberoptic catheters may require more frequent repositioning (unreported data). This may be due to differences in the handling characteristics of the catheters or may be related to the fact that alarms caused by distal migration of the catheter tip alert the clinical team as to the need for repositioning. Finally, there are no differences in complications reported between traditional and fiberoptic catheters.[13]

COST-EFFECTIVENESS

The increased cost of the fiberoptic catheter over other types of flow-directed PA catheters must be justified in today's cost-minded medical care. It is difficult to prove cost-effectiveness of any new technology in terms of time to recovery or improved mortality. However, if savings can be shown in other areas because of the use of the new technology, it may be cost effective. With continuous venous oximetry, the potential for cost savings lies in decreased use of other modes for assessing oxygen transport balance (*i.e.*, CO measurements and blood gas analyses). We found that the number of venous blood gas analyses in our surgical ICU were reduced by 4.9 during a 72-hour study period, resulting in a charge reduction of $245 per patient. In this same population we were able to decrease the number of CO measurements by 2.5 in the same 72-hour period, resulting in a estimated cost reduction to the hospital (for venous blood gas analysis alone) of $104 per catheter and an estimated charge savings to the patient of $278 per catheter. Other studies have confirmed similar savings,[14] and one study has demonstrated savings of arterial blood gas analyses also.[15]

CONCLUSION

Continuous venous oximetry offers a cost-effective, on-line assessment of the relative balance between oxygen consumption and delivery. Although the properly measured values represent a flow-weighted average of blood from only perfused vascular beds, the value may be used in a variety of clinical circumstances to improve the efficiency of the delivery of care in critically ill patients with oxygen transport imbalance.

REFERENCES

1. Nelson LD: Venous oximetry. In Snyder JV (ed): *Oxygen Transport in the Critically Ill Patient.* Chicago, Yearbook Medical Publishers, 1986
2. Kandek G, Aberman A: Mixed venous oxygen saturation: Its role in the assessment of the critically ill patient. *Arch Intern Med* 1983; 143:1400
3. Wilson RF, Christensen C, LeBlanc LP: Oxygen consumption in critically ill surgical patients. *Ann Surg* 1972; 276:801
4. Nelson LD: Continuous venous oximetry in critically ill surgical patients. *Ann Surg* 1986; 203:329
5. Snyder JV, Carroll GC: Tissue oxygenation: A physiologic approach to a clinical problem. *Curr Probl Surg* 1982; 19:650
6. Cullen DG, Civetta JM, Briggs BA, et al: Therapeutic intervention scoring system: A method for quantitative comparisons of patient care. *Crit Care Med* 1974; 2:57
7. Civetta JM: Continuous mixed venous saturation: Neither too little nor too much (panel). Chicago, Society of Critical Care Medicine, May 1985
8. Watson CB: The PA catheter as an early warning system. *Anesthesiol Rev* 1983; 10:34
9. Nelson LD: Continuous venous oximetry: Part 1. Physiology and technical considerations. *Curr Rev Respir Ther* 1986; 8:99
10. Oximetrix, Inc: *Shaw Catheter Oximetry System Instruction Manual.* Mountain View, California, Oximetrix, 1981
11. Baele PL, McMichan JC, Marsh HM, et al: Continuous monitoring of mixed venous oxygen saturation in critically ill patients. *Anesth Analg* 1982; 61:513
12. Nelson LD, Snyder JV: Technical problems with data acquistion. In Snyder JV (ed) *Oxygen Transport in the Critically Ill Patient.* Chicago, Yearbook Medical Publishers 1986
13. McMichan JC, Baele PL, Wignes MW: Insertion of pulmonary artery catheters—A comparison of fiberoptic and nonfiberoptic catheters. *Crit Care Med* 1984; 12:517
14. Orlando R: Continuous mixed venous oximetry in critcally ill surgical patients: "High-tech" cost-effectiveness. *Arch Surg* 1986; 121:470
15. Fahey PJ, Harris K, Vanderwarf C: Clinical experience with continuous monitoring of mixed venous oxygen saturation in respiratory failure. *Chest* 1984; 86:748

APPENDIX

NORMAL RANGE, UNITS, AND DERIVATION FOR COMMON OXYGEN TRANSPORT TERMS

PARAMETER	NORMAL RANGE	UNITS	DERIVATION
Pa_{O_2}	(varies with $F_{I_{O_2}}$)	mm Hg	Measured
Sa_{O_2}	>0.92	(fraction)	Measured
Ca_{O_2}	16–22	ml/dl	$(Sa_{O_2} \times Hgb \times 1.38) + Pa_{O_2} \times 0.0031)$
$P\bar{v}_{O_2}$	35–45	mm Hg	Measured
$S\bar{v}_{O_2}$	0.68–0.77	(fraction)	Measured
$C\bar{v}_{O_2}$	12–17	ml/dl	$(S\bar{v}_{O_2} \times Hgb \times 1.38) + (P\bar{v}_{O_2} \times 0.0031)$
$C(a\text{-}\bar{v})O_2$	3.5–5.5	ml/dl	$Ca_{O_2} - C\bar{v}_{O_2}$
$\dot{V}_{O_2}$	180–280	ml/min	$C(a\text{-}\bar{v})O_2 \times CO \times 10$
$\dot{D}_{O_2}$	700–1400	ml/min	$Ca_{O_2} \times CO \times 10$
OUC	0.23–0.32	(fraction)	$\dot{V}_{O_2}/\dot{D}_{O_2}$

[Normal ranges are approximate and may vary between laboratories. Pa_{O_2} = arterial oxygen tension; Sa_{O_2} = arterial oxygen saturation; Ca_{O_2} = arterical oxygen content; $P\bar{v}_{O_2}$ = mixed venous oxygen tension; $S\bar{v}_{O_2}$ = mixed venous oxygen saturation; $C\bar{v}_{O_2}$ = mixed venous oxygen content; $C(a\text{-}\bar{v})O_2$ = arterial–venous oxygen content difference; $\dot{V}_{O_2}$ = oxygen consumption; $\dot{D}_{O_2}$ = oxygen delivery; OUC = oxygen utilization coefficient (extraction ratio).

CHAPTER SIXTEEN

CONTINUOUS EVALUATION OF OXYGENATION AND VENTILATION

Alan R. Patterson
Andrew F. Stasic

NONINVASIVE TECHNIQUES

PULSE OXIMETRY

Oxyhemoglobin (HbO_2) is red and reduced hemoglobin (Hb) is blue. At a given wavelength, each has a different absorption of light. Measurement of Sa_{O_2} depends on changes in light transmittance that occur with each arterial pulse of blood through the tissues. Because the ratio of transmittance at each of two wavelengths (660 nm, red; 940 nm, infrared) varies according to the percentage of HbO_2, pulse oximeters can be programmed to calculate and display the percentage of oxygen saturation at each pulse.[1]

Hemoglobin saturation depends on the types of hemoglobin that are present. The normal oxygen saturation (Sa_{O_2}) at sea level while one breathes room air is 95%.[2] Hemoglobin may be unbound, bound to oxygen and carbon monoxide, or functionally inert. A separate wavelength is required to measure each type. Hence, to detect oxyhemoglobin, reduced hemoglobin, carboxyhemoglobin, and methemoglobin, a pulse oximeter must emit four separate wavelengths. Commercially available pulse oximeters detect only oxyhemoglobin and reduced hemoglobin, measuring only hemoglobin involved in oxygen transport, termed *functional hemoglobin saturation:*

$$\% \text{ Sat} = \frac{HbO_2}{HbO_2 + Hb} \times 100$$

This value may be higher than that measured by cooximetry, which would also detect nonfunctional hemoglobin, resulting in a larger denominator with the same numerator. Thus, cooximetry results in a lower quotient than the functional saturation measured by pulse oximetry.

The microprocessor of a pulse oximeter contains several hardware and software components. The transducer comprises a photodiode and two light-emitting diodes (LEDs) in the visible red spectrum (660 nm) and in the infrared spectrum (940 nm). These components are mounted in a probe (finger, ear, nasal septum). Transillumination of the tissue by the LEDs allows the photodiode to receive a combination of transmitted and backscattered light from the vascular bed. Each LED alternates its on/off status with the other so that the photodiode detects the light from only one LED at a time. Because the transducer phase is not temperature-dependent, heating and temperature sensing elements are not required. The microprocessor is programmed to distinguish arterial pulse waveforms, minimize the effects of ambient light, patient motion, and electrocautery, and vary the intensity of transmitted light required to obtain the waveforms.

The major technical problem with pulse oximetry is to differentiate between the absorption caused by HbO_2, Hb, and all tissue constituents. Light transmitted through a tissue site is partially absorbed by each component. Elimination of the error caused by light absorption of venous blood and tissue is accomplished by sampling the pulsating arterial bed, which during expansion and contraction modifies the amount of light absorbed and transmitted. At a given site, absorption is constant except during the entry of arterial blood with each systolic pulsation. The change in absorption from the nonflow baseline is translated into a plethysmographic waveform at both the 660 nm and 940 nm wavelengths by the microprocessor. Saturation is directly related to the amplitude of these plethysmographic waveforms and thus is calculated using the ratio of the two wave amplitudes (Fig. 16-1, 16-2). In Figure 16-1, the plethysmographic waveform amplitudes are approximately equal when the Sa_{O_2} is 85%.[2] Pulsatile waves are collected for a period of 3 to 10 seconds, and the average saturation of the last 5 to 7 values is displayed. Heart rate is calculated from the time-interval between pulse waves.

Pulse oximetry is used in a variety of clinical settings[3-7] and helps to reduce the number of arterial blood gas determinations and to provide rapid feedback on therapeutic interventions. The advantages and limitations of pulse oximetry are summarized in Tables 16-1 and 16-2, respectively.

Pulse oximetry and venous oximetry form a valuable monitoring pair for patients with combined respiratory and cardiac insufficiency. The bedside display of both parameters can be used to evaluate oxygenation and cardiac function. This is especially valuable during augmentation and weaning from ventilatory support (including selecting PEEP levels) and when using vasoactive drugs (Fig. 16-3).

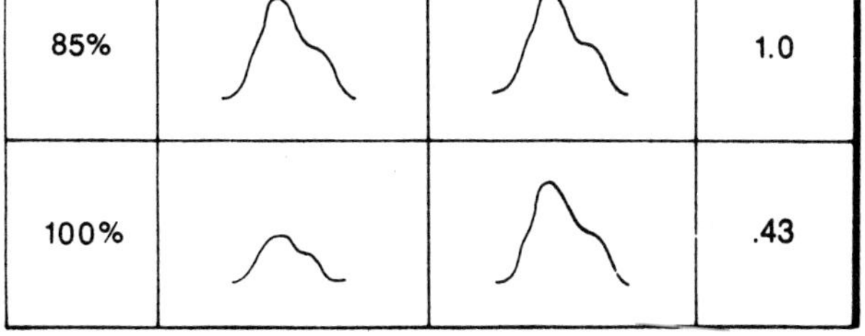

Figure 16-1 Relative pulse signal amplitudes at equal transmittance intensities for red *(R)* and infrared *(IR)* light at three different percentage oxygen saturation levels. (Courtesy of Ohmeda, BOC Health Care, 1986)

SaO_2	660nm (RED)	940nm (IR)	$\dfrac{R}{IR}$
0%			≈3.4
85%			1.0
100%			.43

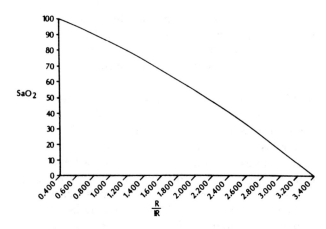

Figure 16-2 Oxygen saturation of hemoglobin (Sa$_{O_2}$) is compared with the ratio of the plethysmographic amplitudes for red *(R)* and infrared *(IR)* light (R/IR), assuming equal intensity for each wavelength. (Courtesy of Ohmeda, BOC Health Care, 1986)

TRANSCUTANEOUS MONITORING OF RESPIRATORY GASES

Transcutaneous gas monitoring was developed about 15 years ago, primarily for use in the neonatal ICU.[8] Subsequently, it was applied in the adult ICU, the operating room, and in exercise-stress-test laboratories. Because both oxygen and carbon dioxide diffuse through the skin, they can be detected by means of electrochemical sensors applied to the skin surface (Fig. 16-4).

Oxygen

Oxygen is delivered from the capillary bed to the tissues, where it is used for metabolism. Some oxygen molecules slowly diffuse through the stratum corneum (outermost layer of skin) to the skin surface. A nonheated surface electrode normally measures 0 to 3 mm Hg of oxygen. To facilitate the diffusion of oxygen, the skin and underlying tissue beds are heated to promote active vasodilation of the cutaneous vessels. Heat is supplied by a heating element in the sensor unit. Oxygen molecules diffuse from the "arterialized" capillary bed to the surface and through a 25-μm polyethylene sensor membrane, after which they are consumed in an electrochemical reaction. An electrical current is induced through the cathode of a modified Clark-type polarographic electrode. The cathode and anode are electrically connected by a thin electrolyte layer. An amplifier connected to the cathode measures the current flow and converts it into a value proportional to the oxygen tension at the electrode/membrane interface. The signal is displayed on a recorder or digital display (transcutaneous P$_{O_2}$, or Ptc$_{O_2}$).

Heating by the oxygen electrode produces three major effects: [1] vasodilation of the cutaneous blood vessels beneath the electrode; [2] increased temperature of blood flowing under the electrode, resulting in a rightward shift of the oxyhemoglobin dissociation curve

---

TABLE 16-1 ADVANTAGES OF PULSE OXIMETRY

1. Noninvasive
2. Continuous real-time information
3. No calibration
4. No skin heating
5. May be left in place for many hours
6. Rapid response time (5–7 seconds)
7. Minimal saturation error (1–2%) over the range of 60% to 90% saturation[3]
8. Unaffected by skin pigmentation

TABLE 16-2   LIMITATIONS OF PULSE OXIMETRY

1. Loss of adequate pulsations
   a. Significant hypothermia
   b. Significant hypotension (*i.e.*, mean arterial pressure less than 50 mm Hg)
   c. Infusion of vasoconstrictive drugs (*e.g.*, norepinephrine)
   d. Direct arterial compression
2. Inadequate hemoglobin (*e.g.*, anemia, hemodilution)
3. Intravascular dyes (*e.g.*, indocyanine green, methylene blue, or indigo carmine red)
4. Extraneous movement (*e.g.*, shivering, exercise)
5. Pulsating venous blood (tricuspid regurgitation, cor pulmonale, or hepatic congestion)
6. Dysfunctional hemoglobins (*i.e.*, hemoglobins that are not available for reversible binding to oxygen
   a. Carboxyhemoglobin (COHb), which results in a HIGHER saturation reading, the ratio of which is approximately 1:1. For example, if the pulse oximeter reads 100% and the percentage of COHb is 7%, then the true oxyhemoglobin fraction is 93% (100% - 7%)
   b. Methemoglobinemia (MetHb), which results in a LOWER saturation reading, the ratio of which is approximately 1:1
7. Fetal hemoglobin (HbF), which results in a lower saturation reading. To obtain the accurate fractional oxyhemoglobin, a correction formula is required[4]
8. Overestimation of Sa_{O_2} below 65% saturation[5,6]

Figure 16-3 Continuous venous oximetry and pulse oximetry units "stacked" at the bedside. Since hemoglobin saturation accounts for most of the oxygen content of both arterial and venous blood, these units provide information relative to continuous arterial venous oxygen content difference, which is related to oxygen consumption and cardiac output through the Fick principle. When arterial saturation is below 0.99, changes in arterial oxygen tension will be reflected by changes in arterial oxygen saturation.

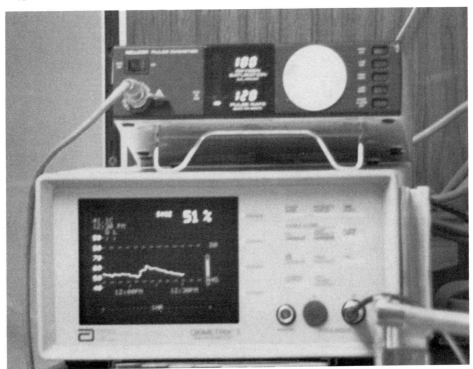

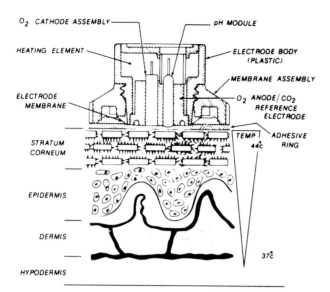

O₂ CATHODE ASSEMBLY

pH MODULE

HEATING ELEMENT

ELECTRODE BODY
(PLASTIC)

MEMBRANE ASSEMBLY

ELECTRODE
MEMBRANE

O₂ ANODE/CO₂
REFERENCE
ELECTRODE

STRATUM
CORNEUM

TEMP
44°C

ADHESIVE
RING

EPIDERMIS

DERMIS

37°C

HYPODERMIS

Figure 16-4 Cross-section of combined O_2/CO_2 transcutaneous electrode and underlying skin. (Figure adapted from and courtesy of Novametrix Medical Systems, Inc., 1986)

and an increase in the partial pressure of oxygen under the electrode site; and [3] altered lipid structure of the stratum corneum, allowing more rapid diffusion of oxygen.

Electrode temperature is varied depending on the age and size of the patient and skin thickness. The electrode temperature required for neonatal patients is between 43°C and 44°C and for children and adults, up to 45°C.

Carbon Dioxide

The transcutaneous carbon dioxide (TC_{CO_2}) electrode is based on the Stow–Severinghaus principle.[9] The skin is separated from a bicarbonate solution by a thin hydrophobic (Mylar, Silastic, or Teflon) membrane that is permeable to carbon dioxide but not to charged ions. Carbon dioxide molecules diffuse through the membrane and react with water in the electrolyte to form carbonic acid (H_2CO_3), which immediately dissociates into H^+ and HCO_3^-. This reaction alters the pH of the electrolyte solution, which in turn changes the voltage across a conventional pH-sensitive glass electrode and silver/silver chloride reference electrode. A special amplifier measures this voltage change and converts it into a value corresponding to the PTC_{CO_2}, which is displayed on the monitor.

Carbon dioxide is produced in the tissues and diffuses fairly rapidly through the skin. It is possible, therefore, to measure carbon dioxide on the skin surface with a nonheated electrode. However, electrode heating causes the skin surface values to respond more quickly to changes in Pa_{CO_2} and produces several related effects: [1] altered structure of the stratum corneum, allowing faster diffusion of carbon dioxide molecules to the skin surface, thus facilitating faster electrode response; [2] decreased solubility of carbon dioxide, leading to increased carbon dioxide partial pressure; and [3] increased local metabolism of the tissue beneath the electrode, thereby causing increased carbon dioxide production.[10]

The combination of these three heating effects causes transcutaneous readings to be 1.2 to 2 times greater than corresponding arterial values. However, the linearity between arterial and transcutaneous values is consistent, as long as adequate perfusion is maintained.

TABLE 16-3   CONTRAINDICATIONS TO TRANSCUTANEOUS GAS MONITORING

1. Excessive skin edema (creates a barrier to gas diffusion)
2. Deep hypothermia (peripheral vasoconstriction decreases cutaneous perfusion)
3. Volatile anesthetic such as halothane (diffuses through the sensor membrane, and is reduced at the cathode, resulting in inaccurately high P_{TCO_2} values)
4. Nitrous oxide (results in inaccurately high reading as it diffuses across the electrode membrane)

The optimal operating temperature for monitoring $P_{TC_{CO_2}}$ with a heated electrode is 44°C for both neonatal and adult patients.[11] Contraindications to transcutaneous gas monitoring are summarized in Table 16-3.

In hemodynamically stable patients, such monitors can follow trends in Pa_{O_2} and changes in mechanical ventilation. When cardiac output and systemic perfusion are severely reduced, P_{TCO_2} and $P_{TC_{CO_2}}$ values deviate from their relationship with arterial partial pressures and become flow-dependent, thereby providing qualitative information on blood flow.[12] As the circulatory condition improves, P_{TCO_2} changes back toward its baseline values.[13]

The disadvantages of transcutaneous gas monitoring are listed in Table 16-4. Risks of transcutaneous gas monitoring include burns from the heated electrode if the electrode site is not changed every 2 to 6 hours and skin irritation from the adhesive ring. The latter problem is especially prevalent in premature neonates.

CAPNOGRAPHY

Measurement of end-tidal carbon dioxide (ET_{CO_2}) provides insight into several normal and pathologic processes. Its multiple uses are well documented.[16] Mainstream and sidestream infrared capnometers are commercially available. A mainstream capnometer connects directly to the endotracheal tube, thus providing real-time, breath-by-breath analysis. The infrared sensor is connected directly to the capnometer, where the result is displayed or

TABLE 16-4   DISADVANTAGES OF TRANSCUTANEOUS GAS MONITORING

1. More mechanical adjustment is required compared to other monitors
   a. Preparation time (*i.e.*, cleaning electrode surface, changing electrode and membrane) can require up to 60 minutes
   b. Stabilization time (*i.e.*, on patient's skin) requires 10 to 20 minutes
   c. Electrode site must be changed every 2 to 6 hours to prevent burns
   d. Calibration required every 2 to 6 hours or each time the electrode is repositioned
   e. Electrode site must be carefully chosen to provide reliable results (*i.e.*, upper chest versus bony prominences that constrict blood flow beneath electrode)[14]
   f. Pressure on electrode (*e.g.*, patient lying on probe) reduces signal.[14]
2. Arterial blood gas calibration always required

3. Values do not reflect "true" arterial values
   a. In most studies, the P_{TCO_2} is about 80% of the Pa_{O_2} in hemodynamically stable patients
   b. The $P_{TC_{CO_2}}$ value is about 1.2 to 2 times the arterial value
   c. In individual patients, however, the linearity of the relationships is consistent provided that the patient remains hemodynamically stable during the monitoring period.
4. Hemodynamically unstable patients often do not demonstrate a correlation between arterial values
   a. P_{TCO_2} values do not correlate well if cardiac index < 1.5 liters/min/m².[15]

recorded, or both. The major disadvantage of this system is its size and bulk and the fact that it cannot be used in nonintubated patients.

Sidestream capnometers aspirate gas at the sample site, from whence it is carried through nylon sample tubing to the infrared analyzer located in the capnometer. The principal advantages of this system are that it reduces the mechanical dead space and can be used in nonintubated patients. The major disadvantage is that the result is affected by several mechanical factors.[17] The response time, or total transit time, is equal to the transit time plus the rise time:

$$\text{Total transit time (TTT)} = \text{transit time (TT)} + \text{rise time (RT)},$$

where transit time is the time required for a sample of respiratory gas to travel from the sampling port to the infrared analyzer, and the rise time is the measured 10% to 90% interval on the carbon dioxide curve from the baseline value to peak concentration. Other factors of importance include the sample aspiration flow rate, the length of sample tubing, and the respiratory cycle time.

Capnometers used for respiratory gas analysis employ a double-beam-in-space arrangement.[18] Two infrared beams are focused through a sample cell and a reference cell. The beams are transmitted intermittently by means of a "chopper disk," a spinning circular disk divided into four equal "pie-slice" sections, two of which have been removed, leaving a "bow-tie" shaped disk. The chopper disk rotates at a speed of about 60 revolutions per second, thus intermittently occluding the infrared beams. When not occluded, the two infrared beams fall onto each half of a balanced condenser microphone detector that is specific for the infrared wavelengths of carbon dioxide. The beams pass through two identical chambers (i.e., cells) that are separated by a thin, flexible metal diaphragm. The reference cell usually is filled with an inert gas such as nitrogen. The sample cell is filled with either the aspirated sample (sidestream capnometer) or a portion of the total gas flow (mainstream capnometer).

Infrared respiratory gas analysis is based on the fact that gases and vapors absorb specific wavelengths of infrared radiation. The main absorption bands arise from vibrational energy changes in the sample molecules. Rotational energy changes occur; therefore, each vibrational energy level is associated with a series of rotational levels.

Cross-sensitivity or interference can occur when other gases or vapors have overlapping absorption bands (e.g., carbon dioxide and nitrous oxide). To eliminate this problem, filter cells filled with 100% of the interfering gas are placed between the infrared beam and the sample cell. In this manner, any wavelength that can be absorbed by the interfering substance is completely absorbed in the filter cell before it can fall on the detector. Assuming that carbon dioxide is present in the sample, absorption of infrared energy occurs. Therefore, the sample beam falling on the detector will be of lower intensity than the reference beam. This asymmetric warming of the detector will cause the metal diaphragm to vibrate toward the sample half of the detector. The diaphragm forms one half of a parallel plate capacitor, which is supplied with a constant electric charge. The resulting voltage changes are amplified, rectified, and sent to a meter, digital display, or strip recorder. The meter or recorder typically is calibrated in terms of concentration percentage or millimeters of mercury.

End-tidal carbon dioxide measurement provides information on cardiovascular status (primarily cardiac output), respiratory gas exchange, metabolic carbon dioxide production, and patient management errors or problems.[19,20]

TABLE 16-5   CAUSES OF DECREASED ET$_{CO_2}$

1. Hypothermia
2. General anesthesia
3. Decreased metabolic rate (*e.g.*, hypothyroidism)
4. Decreased cardiac output
   a. Acute heart failure (*e.g.*, myocardial infarction, cardiac arrest)
   b. Hypovolemia with peripheral vasoconstriction
5. Decreased pulmonary perfusion
   a. Thromboembolism
   b. Amniotic fluid
   c. Methylmethacrylate (*e.g.*, hip surgery)
   d. Air (*e.g.*, neurosurgery)
6. Acute changes in respiratory gas exchange resulting in a gradual decrease in ET$_{CO_2}$
   a. Atelectasis
   b. Endobronchial intubation
   c. Pneumothorax
   d. Pulmonary edema or congestion
7. Mechanical problems
   a. Inadvertent esophageal intubation[19]
   b. Inadvertent extubation
   c. Obstructed endotracheal tube (*e.g.*, kinking, mucus plug)
   d. Disconnections (*e.g.*, anesthetic or ventilator circuits)

Because carbon dioxide production is directly dependent on metabolic rate, lower values for ET$_{CO_2}$ result in conditions listed in Table 16-5. Increases generally are due to hypermetabolic states,[21] examples of which are listed in Table 16-6. Advantages and disadvantages of capnography are summarized in Table 16-7.

The most common use of ET$_{CO_2}$ is to evaluate the adequacy of ventilation. Inadvertent esophageal intubation, tracheal extubations, and endotracheal tube obstruction can be detected.[19,20] In the ICU setting, these monitors are useful in weaning patients from mechanical ventilatory support and reduce the number of arterial blood gas determinations obtained. Capnometers are portable, relatively inexpensive, and reliable under various clinical settings.[22–24] They improve patient safety and, in my view, are cost effective.

MASS SPECTROMETRY

Mass spectrometry only recently has become available for the operating room and the ICU. It allows measurement of all respiratory (carbon dioxide, oxygen, and nitrogen) and anesthetic (isoflurane, halothane, enflurane, nitrous oxide) gases on a breath-by-breath basis. Analysis of inspired and expired respiratory gases by mass spectrometry is accurate (to 0.1% of the measured value) and rapid. The gas sample enters an ionization chamber and is bombarded by an electronic beam that fragments each gas into characteristic ion fragments. The ion fragments travel through a window in a magnetic field, which causes each to spin in a unique arc. Less spin deviation is imposed on heavier ions, whereas more spin deviation occurs with a higher charge. The ion fragments strike the walls of the chamber at different sites as a function of their mass and charge. Detector plates are placed at appropriate sites within the chamber to detect ion fragments from the gases which are to be analyzed. Each

TABLE 16-6   CONDITIONS THAT INCREASE ET$_{CO_2}$

1. Multiple trauma
2. Burns
3. Hyperthyroidism
4. Malignant hyperthermia[21]
5. Carbon dioxide insufflation (*e.g.*, laparoscopy)[22]

TABLE 16-7 ADVANTAGES AND DISADVANTAGES OF CAPNOGRAPHY

Advantages	Disadvantages
1. Continuous "devoted" real-time monitor in contrast to "shared" mass spectrometer	1. Relatively expensive (up to $6500 per monitoring station)
2. Noninvasive	2. Prone to mechanical influences (*i.e.*, respiratory cycle time < total transit time)
3. Detection of air or carbon dioxide embolism[23]	3. Not useful in neonates and small children because of the high sampling flow rate (about 200–400 ml/min).
4. Determination of proper endotracheal tube position[24]	
5. Life-threatening intraoperative complications (air embolism, malignant hyperthermia, ETT obstruction)	

ion detector plate generates an electric current proportional to the number of ion fragments that strike it in a specified time.[25]

The value of mass spectrometry during anesthesia was limited until recently because the deflection spectra (*i.e.*, ion fragments) of several anesthetic gases and vapors overlap those of respiratory gases. For example, nitrous oxide and carbon dioxide have the same molecular weight, 44, and both are deflected by mass spectrometry at this mass number. Halothane, with a molecular weight of 197.4, is fragmented to produce charged particles, some of which generate signals at mass numbers close to those of both oxygen and carbon dioxide. Thus, the spectral signals overlap.

The overlap problem is now resolved by a deflection system overlap eraser, which allows quantitative measurement of individual gases in a mixture when several contribute to the signal detected at one or more of the mass numbers. The principle of this modification is that nitrous oxide and volatile anesthetics ionize into fragments that occur in fixed proportion to one another within the mass spectrometer. Provided that at least one fragment is detectable as the sole output at a particular mass number or detection point, the proportion of the parent compound in the original gas mixture can be determined, as can the contribution made by the parent substance to the outputs detected at the mass numbers of the respiratory gases. Subtraction circuits are used to eliminate these unwanted signals so that the output voltages detected at mass numbers 28, 32, and 44 are proportional to the fractional concentrations in the original sample.[26]

As the number of monitoring stations increases, so does the time between analysis and respiratory gas samples. The interval between samples at a particular location depends on four factors: [1] the distance from the mass spectrometer; [2] the number of stations being

TABLE 16-8 DELAYS IN MASS SPECTROMETER (MS) ANALYSIS

Number of Rooms in Use	Time Between Samples Seconds	Minutes
6	48–60	1
10	80–100	1.5
20	160–200	3
30	240–300	5

(Assumes one sample/room/cycle and 100 feet to MS).

TABLE 16-9 MASS SPECTROMETRY USES FOR OPERATING ROOM AND INTENSIVE CARE UNIT

1. Monitoring $F_{I_{O_2}}$
   a. Detect hypoxic gas mixture
   b. Ensures delivery of desired $F_{I_{O_2}}$
   c. Estimation of oxygen consumption
   d. Backup oxygen analyzer
2. Monitoring $F_{I_{CO_2}}$ and $F_{E_{CO_2}}$
   a. Adequacy of ventilation
   b. Cardiovascular status
   c. Early detection of esophageal intubation, inadvertent extubation, and endotracheal tube obstructions[29]

3. Monitoring of $F_{I_{N_2}}$ and $F_{E_{N_2}}$
   a. Assure adequate denitrogenation before anesthetic induction (*i.e.*, if the $F_{E_{N_2}} \leq 5\%$)
   b. Sensitive monitor for detection of circulatory air from air embolism (*i.e.*, 0.1 ml/kg)[30]
   c. Detection of disconnects, anesthetic system leaks, air leaks in ventilators, hose connections, and so forth
   d. Detection of a leak in the endotracheal tube cuff
4. Monitoring F_I(agent) and F_E(agent)
   a. Detection of vaporizer malfunction
   b. Assures delivery of desired agent
   c. Safe use of low-flow anesthetic techniques

sampled; [3] the number of breaths sampled (1–3); and [4] the station priority settings and distance from the mass spectrometer.

Jameson[27] determined the sampling interval between respiratory gas measurements using a shared mass spectrometer with a variety of sampling stations of equal priority (*i.e.*, each room is sampled once per cycle of locations) (Table 16-8). These data indicate that shared mass spectrometer systems require 8 to 10 seconds per sampling location before a subsequent cycle of determinations is made. In order to provide the most recent respiratory gas determinations, all monitoring stations are sampled continuously (*i.e.*, common draw) at a flow rate equal to one half of the nylon catheter's natural flow rate. The natural flow rate is an intrinsic property of each individual catheter. Typically, this flow rate is 200 to 280 ml/min; therefore, the common draw flow rate is between 100 and 140 ml/min.

The common draw flow rate continuously aspirates respiratory gas samples into a constant pressure vacuum line in preparation for analysis. Despite the common draw flow rate, data analyzed by the mass spectrometer are not real-time but are delayed anywhere from 9 to 22 seconds.[28] This delay results from the aspirated sample's having to traverse 150 feet of the catheter before reaching the mass spectrometer. At a common draw flow rate of 100 to 140 ml/min, 10 to 14 seconds are required for transit and, at minimum, another 7 seconds to analyze the sample. In a system with more than ten monitoring stations, updated sample determinations may be delayed for more than 2 minutes (Table 16-8).

TABLE 16-10 ADVANTAGES OF THE MASS SPECTROMETER

1. Shared cost of sampling (many patients monitored by single instrument)
2. Small sample for analysis
3. Single sampling port
4. Rapid response time (*i.e.*, usually gives updated results within 90 seconds; time is dependent upon the number of sampling stations)
5. Single analyzer that can measure several respiratory and anesthetic gases

TABLE 16-11 DISADVANTAGES OF THE MASS SPECTROMETER

1. Relative high cost (about $35,000/10 stations)
   a. At present, only 10% of U.S. ORs have a mass spectrometer; unknown number of ICUs
   b. Maintenance fees and disposable equipment costs additional
2. Multiple site or "shared" mass spectrometers provide sample data too infrequently to prevent serious injury to the patient
   a. False sense of security
   b. Patient safety dictates the use of an oxygen analyzer, low pressure alarm, and low flow alarm, unless sampling can occur once per minute. (Firms producing mass spectrometers now provide infrared O_2 and CO_2 sensors at each station to provide continuous breath-by-breath analysis to counter this deficiency.)

A mass spectrometer evaluates the carbon dioxide partial pressure curve in order to determine inspired and expired gas values. When the value is minimal (not necessarily zero), the inspired fractions (FI) will be determined. Maximum carbon dioxide values determine the time of the expired gas fractions (FE) measurements. If the carbon dioxide waveform does not conform to software programmed guidelines, the mass spectrometer continues to sample a given location for up to 30 seconds if only one station is active or 15 seconds if more than one station is active in order to collect two consecutive breaths (carbon dioxide waveforms). If two consecutive carbon dioxide waveforms in the allotted period of time are not detected, a "no breath" alarm will sound, and the mass spectrometer proceeds to analyze gas from the next monitoring station. Uses for mass spectrometry in the operating room and ICU are listed in Table 16-9. Advantages and disadvantages of mass spectrometry are enumerated in Tables 16-10 and 16-11.

OXYGEN ANALYSIS

Paramagnetic, polarographic, and fuel cell oxygen analyzers are commercially available today. The paramagnetic method takes advantage of the fact that oxygen molecules experience a force proportional to their concentration when they are introduced into a nonhomogeneous magnetic field (provided the temperature remains constant). A quartz suspension is used to mount two small hollow glass spheres filled with nitrogen into a dumbbell-like shape between the poles of a powerful magnet. These pole pieces are shaped so as to render

TABLE 16-12 ADVANTAGES OF IN-LINE OXYGEN ANALYZERS

1. Detection of hypoxic gas mixtures
2. Detection of inaccurate or leaking flowmeters
3. Detection of rebreathing (low gas flows or disconnections)
4. Backup protection for failure of systems designed to ensure a safe oxygen–nitrous oxide mixture
5. Backup protection for failure of machines equipped with oxygen failure safety valve
6. Secondary check against inadvertent, improper connection of the oxygen, air, or nitrous oxide lines at the central hospital supply
7. Prevention against hyperoxia in situations in which inadvertent increases in oxygen concentration could lead to tissue damage to the eyes (neonates) or lungs (bleomycin chemotherapy)

TABLE 16-13 PROBELMS WITH OXYGEN ANALYZERS

1. Failure of personnel to install, activate, and provide timely maintenance to these instruments
2. Sensitivity to effects of nitrous oxide, humidity, or volatile anesthetics[32]
   a. Distortion secondary to humidity in the circuit (*e.g.,* paramagnetic and certain polarographic analyzers)
   b. Failure to provide accurate and reliable data when nitrous oxide is used and batteries are weak (IL 402; all models produced before November 1976)[33]

the magnetic field nonhomogeneous. When gas containing oxygen molecules flows between the spheres, the oxygen molecules experience a force that causes them to move along a field gradient, displacing the dumbbell. Displacement of the dumbbell is proportional to the partial pressure of oxygen. The quartz suspension contains a tiny mirror from which a beam of light is reflected onto a point of fixation. The deflection of the light from its neutral position is opposed and nullified by means of a current passed through a coil attached to the dumbbell (the so-called null-balance method). A pontentiometer controls the intensity of the movement-nullifying current and is calibrated in terms of oxygen concentration. Typical accuracy of these instruments is about 0.1% over the range from 0 to 100%. Ninety percent response time is less than 8 seconds for changes in oxygen concentration, and 99% response time is within 1 minute. Thus, this type of analyzer is not sufficiently rapid to follow oxygen changes in a single breath and can tolerate only low sampling rates.[18]

Polarographic and fuel cell analyzers are similar in appearance. They are small, compact, and battery-powered. Polarographic analyzers employ the ubiquitous Clark electrode.[18] These analyzers contain a charged platinum electrode (cathode) and a silver/silver chloride reference electrode (anode), both of which are surrounded by an electrolyte solution and covered by a polyethylene membrane. A voltage $(-0.67\ V)$ is supplied to the cathode to facilitate the reduction of oxygen. The reduction of oxygen produces a current that is proportional to the concentration of oxygen outside the membrane.

Fuel cell analyzers differ only with respect to the choice of metals used for the anode and cathode, the nature of the electrolyte gel, and the fact that no external polarizing voltage is needed. Metals for the cathode and anode are sufficiently electromagnetic so that when placed in the electrolyte solution, they supply the chemical energy needed to establish the reduction of oxygen at the surface of the cathode. Silver often is used for the cathode and lead for the anode. Fuel cell analyzers may read about 6 mm Hg higher than conventional polarographic electrode oxygen analyzers over the range of 0 to 100%.[31]

Advantages and disadvantages of in-line oxygen analyzers are listed in Tables 16-12 and 16-13, respectively. Most of the disadvantages are nonexistent in the ICU. However, both testing and calibration of every oxygen analyzer installed into a ventilator circuit are essential.

REFERENCES

1. Yelderman M, Corenmen J: Real time oximetry. In *Computing in Anesthesia and Intensive Care*, p 328. Boston, Martinus Nijoff Publishers, 1983

2. Petty TL: *Clinical Pulse Oximetry*, p 1. Boulder, Colorado, Ohmeda Corporation, Division of BOC Group, 1986
3. Yelderman M, New W: Evaluation of pulse oximetry. *Anesthesiology* 1983; 59:349
4. Cornelissen PJH, van Woensel CLM, van Oel WC, et al: Correction factors for hemoglobin derivatives in fetal blood, as measured with the IL 282 co-oximeter. *Clin Chem* 1981; 29:1555
5. Scheller MS, Unger RJ, Kelner MJ: Effects of intravenously administered dyes on pulse oximetry readings. *Anesthesiology* 1986; 65:550
6. Mihm FG, Halperin BD: Noninvasive detection of profound arterial desaturations using a pulse oximetry device. *Anesthesiology* 1985; 62:85
7. Hay WW: *Application of Pulse Oximetry in Neonatal Medicine.* Boulder, Colorado, Ohmeda, Division of BOC Group, 1986
8. Finer NN: Newer trends in continuous monitoring of critically ill infants and children. *Pediatr Clin North Am* 1980; 27:553
9. Severinghaus JW, Stafford M, Bradley AF: TcPCO$_2$ electrode design, calibration and temperature gradient problems. *Acta Anaesthesiol Scand [Suppl]* 1978; 68:118
10. Monaco F, Nickerson BG, McQuitty JC: Continuous transcutaneous oxygen and carbon dioxide monitoring in the pediatric ICU. *Crit Care Med* 1982; 10:765
11. Rithalia SVS, Booth S: Factors influencing transcutaneous oxygen tension. *Intens Care World*, p 126, December 1985
12. Tremper KK, Shoemaker WC, Shippy CR, et al: Transcutaneous PCO$_2$ monitoring on adult patients in the ICU and the operating room. *Crit Care Med* 1981; 9:752
13. Shoemaker WC, Vidyasagar D: Physiological and clinical significance of PtC$_{O_2}$ and PtC$_{CO_2}$ measurements. *Crit Care Med* 1981; 9:689
14. Cassady G: Transcutaneous monitoring in the newborn infant. *J Pediatr* 1983; 103:837
15. Tremper KK, Shoemaker WC: Transcutaneous oxygen monitoring of critically ill adults, with and without low flow shock. *Crit Care Med* 1981; 9:706
16. Smalhout B, Kalenda Z: *An Atlas of Capnography*, vol 1, 2nd ed, p 20. Zerckebosch-Zeist, The Netherlands, 1981
17. Schena J, Thompson J, Crone RK: Mechanical influences on the capnogram. *Crit Care Med* 1984; 12:672
18. Hill DW: Methods of analysis in the gaseous and vapor phase. In Scurr C, Feldman S (eds): *Scientific Foundations of Anesthesia*, 3rd ed, p 84. London, Heinemann Medical Books, 1982
19. Linko K, Paloheimo M, Tammisto T: Capnography for detection of accidental oesophageal intubation. *Acta Anaesthesiol Scand* 1983; 27:199
20. Hazerian TE, McGowan MS, Buckle FG: Continuous bedside CO$_2$ monitoring in the diagnosis of acute airway obstruction. *Crit Care Med* 1986; 13:449
21. Triner L, Sherman J: Potential value of expiratory carbon dioxide measurement in patients considered to be susceptible to malignant hyperthermia. *Anesthesiology* 1981; 55:482
22. Shulman D, Aronson HB: Capnography in the early diagnosis of carbon dioxide embolism during laparoscopy. *Can Anaesth Soc J* 1984; 31:455.
23. Symons NLP, Leaver HK: Air embolism during craniotomy in the seated position: A comparison of methods for detection. *CASJ* 1985; 32:174
24. Linko K, Paloheimo M: Capnography facilitates blind nasotracheal intubation. *Acta Anaesthesiol Belg* 1983; 34:117
25. Eger EI: Monitoring the depth of anesthesia. In Saidman LJ, Smith NT (eds): *Monitoring in Anesthesia*, 2nd ed, p 10. Boston, Butterworths Publishers, 1984
26. Davis WOM, Spence AA: A modification of the MGA 200 mass spectrometer to enable measurement of anaesthetic gas mixtures. *Br J Anaesth* 1979; 51:987
27. Jameson LC: Applications of mass spectrometry in clinical anesthesia. In *ASA Annual Refresher Course Lectures*, no 226. American Society of Anesthesiologists, 1986
28. Ozanne GM, Young WG, Mazzei WJ, et al: Multipatient anesthetic mass spectrometry: Rapid analysis of data stored in long catheters. *Anesthesiology* 1981; 55:62
29. Lichtiger M: Recent advances in clinical monitoring: Mass spectrometry. *Curr Rev Clin Anesth* 1985; 5:114
30. Matjaskoj-Petrozza P, Mackenzie CF: Sensitivity of end-tidal nitrogen in venous air embolism in dogs. *Anesthesiology* 1985; 63:418
31. Folwaczny H, Finsterer U: Blood oxygen analyzer BOA 802. *Anaesthetist* 1976; 25:402
32. Westenskow DR, Jordan WS, Jordan R, et al: Evaluation of oxygen monitors for use during anesthesia. *Anesth Analg* 1981; 60:53
33. Piernan S, Roizen MF, Severinghaus JW: Oxygen analyzer dangerous-senses nitrous oxide as battery fails. *Anesthesiology* 1979; 50:146

CHAPTER SEVENTEEN

AIRWAY MANAGEMENT

Gary W. Gammage

INTRODUCTION

The importance of tracheal intubation in the management of critically ill patients is obvious. This chapter presents the options available in airway management to enable an educated choice that will lead to minimal complications.

INDICATIONS

Critically ill patients require tracheal intubation for a variety of reasons. Often, multiple indications exist (Table 17-1). In a conscious, cooperative patient, CPAP can be applied to the airway by means of a tight-fitting mask, thus avoiding the need for tracheal intubation on occasion. When a patient is conscious, nasotracheal suction may be attempted before tracheal intubation. Insertion of the suction catheter through a nasal airway makes the technique more tolerable.

EMERGENCY TRACHEAL INTUBATION

Orotracheal intubation under direct vision is the procedure of choice in an emergency. In true emergencies, anesthesia and muscle relaxants usually are not necessary because apneic and hypoxemic patients offer little resistance. If adequate visualization of the larynx is not achieved initially, you should ventilate the patient with oxygen by mask and reassess factors such as proper head positioning (Fig. 17-1). Digital pressure applied to the cricoid cartilage (Sellick maneuver) not only aids laryngoscopy, but also helps prevent aspiration of gastric contents.

If orotracheal intubation is not possible, then the cricothyroid membrane provides the most appropriate alternate entrance to the airway. Cricothyrotomy (Fig. 17-2), either with a catheter[1] or a scalpel,[2] eliminates the indication for a "slash tracheostomy" and markedly decreases the incidence and severity of complications.[1-3] Successful oxygenation and ventilation after cricothyrotomy entail the steps in Table 17-2.

ELECTIVE TRACHEAL INTUBATION

Patients who require urgent but not emergent airway support can be dealt with in a number of ways. Factors to consider are the urgency of the situation, coexistent patient disease

TABLE 17-1   INDICATIONS FOR TRACHEAL INTUBATION

Open an obstructed airway
Provide airway pressure support to treat hypoxemia
  $Pa_{O_2} < 60$ with $F_{IO_2} > 0.5$
  Alveolar to arterial oxygen gradient > 300 mm Hg
  Intrapulmonary shunt $> 15\%$ to 20%
Provide mechanical ventilation
  Respiratory acidosis
  Inadequate respiratory mechanics
    Respiratory rate > 30/min
    FVC < 10 ml/kg
    PNP > -20 cm H_2O
    Deadspace $> 60\%$
Facilitate suctioning
Prevent aspiration
  Gag and swallow reflexes absent

(elevated intracranial pressure or coronary artery insufficiency), and your own skills. A number of questions should be considered before embarking on this often hazardous course (Table 17-3).

Frequently, you will be required to change an endotracheal tube in a patient who is already intubated because of a cuff leak, the need for a larger tube to enable fiberoptic bronchoscopy, or to switch from nasal to oral techniques (and *vice versa*). Usually, such changes can be made under direct vision. After administering the appropriate sedative (and perhaps muscle relaxant), you can perform direct laryngoscopy to visualize the vocal cords and the *in situ* endotracheal tube. With suction available, the old tube is removed and the new one inserted. Be prepared to ventilate the patient by mask if visualization is lost after removal of the old tube. This problem is particularly likely in traumatized and edematous patients.

If you cannot visualize the cords, consider using the fiberoptic bronchoscope as a stylet. The bronchoscope with the new tube mounted on it can be inserted beside[5] or through the old endotracheal tube. If you choose to insert the fiberoptic bronchoscope through the endotracheal tube, the old tube must be cut off as it is removed from the airway.[6] The new tube is then advanced through the glottis. Insertion of the bronchoscope through the glottis and into the trachea beside the old endotracheal tube[6] avoids cutting the old tube and allows nearly continuous control of the airway.

Changing an endotracheal tube blindly over a stylet is also recommended.[7] A *rigid*, commercially available tube changer (stylet) is inserted down the old tube, which is then removed, leaving the tube changer in the trachea. The new tube is subsequently inserted. This technique avoids laryngeal visualization but does not ensure success. Difficulty passing the new tube over the changer has been reported because the top of the tube catches on the posterior commissure. Rotation of the tube 180° changes its orientation and may allow passage. The stylet must be rigid; soft, pliable nasogastric tubes are unacceptable and often fail.[8]

Initial elective tracheal intubation in a critically ill patient is a more complicated problem. In choosing among the available options, you must consider the difficulty of the airway, risk of aspiration of gastric contents, and the presence of complicating medical conditions such as cardiac disease, increased intracranial pressure, and intravascular volume depletion.

The Difficult Airway

Most difficult airways can be anticipated from the patient's history and a current physical examination (Table 17-4).[9] Remember that extensive peripheral edema strongly suggests that airway edema and distortion are present. Tumor and upper airway trauma, including frac-

Figure 17-1 Proper head position is important for successful orotracheal intubation. **A.** The oral *(OA)*, pharyngeal *(PA)*, and laryngeal *(LA)* axes must be aligned for direct laryngoscopy. **B.** Elevate the head 10 cm above the shoulders with a folded towel to align the pharyngeal and laryngeal axes. **C.** Extend the atlanto-occipital joint to achieve the straightest possible line from the incisors to the glottis. (Adapted from Stoelting RK: Endotracheal intubation. In Miller RD [ed]: *Anesthesia,* 2nd ed, vol 1, p. 525. New York, Churchill Livingstone, 1986)

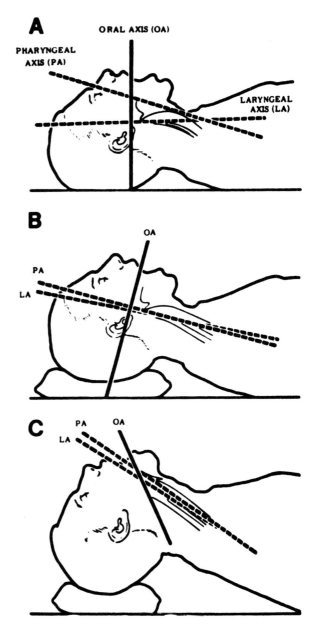

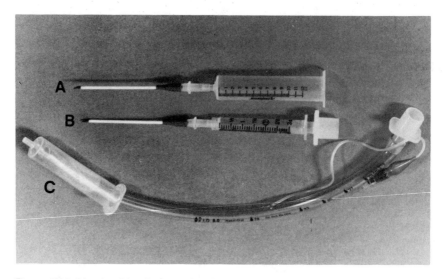

Figure 17-2 Cricothyroid catheter equipment. An emergency cricothyroid catheter can be easily attached to a conventional breathing apparatus with readily available equipment. Once introduced into the trachea, the intravenous cannula is connected to **(A)** a 12-ml or **(B)** a 3-ml syringe barrel with the plunger removed. The stylet may be removed from the catheter to prevent damage to the posterior trachea or left in place to prevent kinking of the catheter. The syringe barrel is connected to the breathing circuit by means of **(B)** a 7-mm endotracheal tube adapter with the 3-ml syringe barrel or **(C)** an endotracheal tube inserted into the 12-ml syringe with cuff inflated.

tures of the mandible, maxilla, or larynx, can make transglottic intubation impossible, even by the most skillful laryngoscopist.

Aspiration

Pulmonary aspiration of acid gastric contents often results in fatal pneumonitis.[10] The important time-interval in determining the risk of a full stomach is the time from ingestion to injury or illness, at which time gastric emptying slows or stops—not from ingestion to intubation. If in doubt, assume the patient has a full stomach, and take precautions to avoid

TABLE 17-2   OXYGENATION AND VENTILATION AFTER EMERGENCY CRICOTHYROTOMY

1. Insert a large-bore intravenous catheter (14 gauge) through the cricothyroid membrane. (Aspiration of air indicates proper location in the airway.)

2. Remove the needle; attach the barrel of a 12-ml syringe (plunger removed) to the catheter.

3. Insert an endotracheal tube into the syringe barrel; inflate cuff, and attach the endotracheal tube to oxygen.[3,4]

4. If the glottic opening is patent, deliver high flows of oxygen (promotes elimination of carbon dioxide).

5. If the glottis is not patent, deliver low flows of oxygen to maintain oxygenation while a tracheostomy is performed.

6. Alternatively, open the cricothyroid membrane widely with a scalpel and insert an endotracheal tube through the wound (allows more adequate ventilation but risks more complications).

TABLE 17-3 QUESTIONS TO ANSWER BEFORE TRACHEAL INTUBATION

1. Is intubation indicated?
   Are there alternatives to intubation such as the CPAP mask?
2. How urgent is the situation?
3. What skills and equipment do I have?
4. What modifying factors exist?
   Is the patient breathing spontaneously?
   Is the airway anatomy abnormal?
   What medical problems complicate the problem?
   Full stomach?
   Hypovolemia?
   Congestive heart failure?
   Coronary artery disease?
   Elevated intracranial pressure?

aspiration. Aspiration is minimized by the maintenance of airway protective reflexes and the Sellick maneuver.

Unfortunately, the precautions necessary to prevent aspiration may produce other complications. Although awake intubation of an unanesthetized trachea may prevent aspiration, it can induce severe tachycardia, hypertension, and increases in ICP and is often an unpleasant event for the patient. Intravenous sedation or anesthesia blunts the hemodynamic and ICP effects of intubation but also compromises airway protective reflexes. Cricoid pressure followed by a rapid sequence induction with intravenous sodium thiopental (2–4 mg/kg) and an intubating dose of succinylcholine (1–2 mg/kg) is a frequently used compromise. This technique is known as a "crash induction," which describes what can happen to the blood pressure of a hypovolemic patient. Crash also is an appropriate summation of what happens to the patient if the airway cannot be secured after paralysis with succinylcholine.

Other options involve topical anesthesia of various parts of the airway and "conscious" intravenous sedation. The choice depends on the severity of the coexisting problems, the amount of time available for preparation, and the skills of the physician.

TABLE 17-4 THE DIFFICULT AIRWAY

1. Edema
2. Upper airway trauma
3. Short thick neck
4. Protruding maxillary incisors
5. Temporomandibular joint range of motion less than 40 mm (2 finger breadths)
6. Cervical range of motion from flexion to extension less than 90° to 165°, respectively
7. High-arched palate with narrow mouth
8. High anterior larynx (mandible to thyroid notch less than 3 finger breadths)
9. Base of tongue large enough to obscure view of the uvula and tonsillar pillars[10]
10. Trachea shifted away from the midline, or fixed and immobile
11. Tumor of the airway
12. History of difficult intubation
13. Previous tracheostomy or prolonged intubation

Complicating Medical Conditions

Laryngoscopy and intubation are associated with severe increases of ICP if intracranial compliance is decreased by head injury or brain tumors. The rise in heart rate and blood pressure accompanying intubation increases myocardial oxygen demand, leading potentially to myocardial ischemia in patients with coronary artery disease. This increase can be blunted by intravenous lidocaine (1.5 mg/kg) before laryngoscopy and by fentanyl (8 µg/kg) or sodium nitroprusside (1–2 µg/kg) but *not* by topical lidocaine.[9,11]

In hypovolemic patients who are dependent on sympathetic stimulation for maintenance of blood pressure, intravenous sedation or anesthesia can produce life-threatening hemodynamic depression. Once the patient is intubated, positive-pressure ventilation exacerbates the compromise of venous return and cardiac output. Such patients can be intubated awake or anesthetized with *small* doses of ketamine, which supports the blood pressure by causing a release of endogenous catecholamines. Remember, however, that the myocardium is depressed by ketamine if the sympathetic nervous system already is maximally active. Fluid resuscitation before intubation should always be used if the situation allows.

Preparation

Before an elective intubation, be sure to select the technique (oral, nasal, or tracheostomy), the type and amount of sedation or anesthesia, and alternate plans of action for unforeseen difficulties. To minimize such complications, you should have all equipment available before beginning the procedure, including [1] a means to ventilate the patient manually, (bag-valve-mask); [2] oxygen; [3] EKG and blood pressure monitors; [4] suction apparatus; [5] an adjustable bed; [6] an assortment of laryngoscope blades and endotracheal tubes; and [7] an assistant to watch vital signs and provide cricoid pressure. Advantages and disadvantages are associated with both nasal and oral routes of intubation (Table 17-5). Nasal tubes generally are believed to be more secure and more comfortable for the patient; however, they often cause sinusitis and occasionally otitis media, problems that do not occur with oral intubation. Oral intubation is indicated in patients with coagulopathies and potential nasal bleeding. The timing of a tracheostomy is debated, but most authorities agree that

TABLE 17-5   ORAL VERSUS NASAL INTUBATION

Variables	Oral	Nasal
Ease of procedure	Apneic patient	Awake breathing patient
Nasal bleeding	No	Yes
Sinusitus	No	Yes
Patient comfort	Less	More
Need for bite block	Yes	No
Oral hygiene	Difficult	Easy
Accidental extubation	More likely	Less likely
Tube size	Larger, shorter	Smaller, longer
Suctioning	Easier	More difficult
Laryngeal damage	More	Less
Contraindications	Mandibular fractures	Coagulopathies
		Nasal CSF leak
		Nasal sinusitus
		Nasal fracture

translaryngeal intubation should be performed in the intensive care unit, followed by elective tracheostomy in the operating room.[12]

Anesthesia

The airway can be topically anesthetized or the patient given intravenous drugs in sedative or anesthetic doses, with or without muscle relaxants, before intubation. Topical anesthesia preserves spontaneous ventilation and hemodynamic stability and is particularly advantageous when the patient has a compromised or distorted airway. However, an awake intubation usually is unpleasant for the patient, and intravenous or topical local anesthetics can cause toxic reactions. Loss of protective airway reflexes predisposes the patient with a full stomach to aspiration of acid gastric contents.

Properly performed topical anesthesia of the airway requires time, skill, and experience. Cotton pledgets soaked in 4% cocaine solution can be inserted into the nostril to provide anesthesia and vasoconstriction. The same result can be obtained with a combination of lidocaine ointment and phenylephrine nose drops. If direct laryngoscopy is performed, the base of the tongue can be anesthetized with lidocaine ointment applied with a tongue blade.

The oral pharynx down to the superior surface of the epiglottis is anesthetized by a regional block of the glossopharyngeal nerve. To block this nerve, you should have the patient open his mouth and protrude his tongue: Grasp the tongue with gauze and insert a small needle 1.0 cm deep into the mucosa just posterior to the palatopharyngeal fold midway between the tongue and the roof of the mouth. After careful aspiration to avoid injection into the nearby carotid artery, inject 5 ml of 1% lidocaine.[13]

The inferior surface of the epiglottis and the superior surface of the glottis are anesthetized by blockade of the superior laryngeal nerve as it passes the greater cornu of the hyoid bone. Inject 1 to 3 ml of 1% lidocaine beneath the right and left greater cornu.[14] To anesthetize the tracheal mucosa, puncture the cricothyroid membrane with a 25-gauge needle, aspirate air, and inject 4 ml of 4% lidocaine.

The upper airway and trachea may be anesthetized less traumatically by instructing the patient to inhale aerosolized 4% lidocaine (4–5 ml) from a disposable hand-held nebulizer. One milliliter of 1% phenylephrine can be added for vasoconstriction before nasal intubation, in which case the aerosol must be delivered by face mask rather than a mouthpiece.

Patient cooperation during intubation with topical or regional anesthesia may be enhanced with intravenous sedative drugs. Such agents, the dose of which cannot always be predicted in advance, can produce unconsciousness in critically ill patients, as opposed to only mild sedation in healthy patients. Careful intravenous titration in such cases will prevent overdose. Advantages to intubation under general anesthesia include rapidity of the technique, comfort, and blunting of the rise in ICP, pulse, and blood pressure. General anesthesia predisposes to potential complications, including apnea, aspiration of stomach contents, and hemodynamic depression (especially in hypovolemic patients). Muscle relaxants allow intubation with less anesthesia but are associated with complete loss of spontaneous ventilation and airway integrity. An anesthesiologist should be summoned if general anesthesia and muscle relaxation are advisable for elective intubations in the intensive care unit.

Techniques

Generally, sicker patients require less anesthesia for oral intubation. Sometimes, however, apparently obtunded patients "come alive" when the laryngoscope is inserted, and alternate plans must be considered. If direct laryngoscopy is not possible or is contraindicated (cervical fractures), visualization with a fiberoptic bronchoscope or a blind technique with a light wand may be helpful.[16] A light wand is a plastic stylet with a battery-powered light at the tip. The wand is inserted into the tube, the light turned on, and the tube inserted blindly into the trachea. When the tube enters the glottis, the light can be seen through the skin in the neck at the suprasternal notch if the room lights are dimmed. It cannot be seen if the tube passes posteriorly into the esophagus.

Elective blind nasal intubation can be performed in an awake patient. Frequently only the nasal mucosa must be anesthetized, thus preserving airway reflexes. Use a topical vasoconstrictor, such as phenylephrine, and gently dilate the nasal passage with a nasal airway liberally coated with lidocaine ointment to minimize nasal bleeding. Position the patient's head with the occiput elevated 10 cm above the scapulae and the neck in neutral position. Insert the endotracheal tube through the nostril into the oropharynx and listen for breath sounds. Advance the tube until breath sounds are maximal, at which time the tube will be just above the glottis. Wait for an inspiration and quickly advance the tube through the open cords. If the tube enters the trachea, the patient will cough unless the trachea has been anesthetized. If breath sounds disappear, the tube has entered one of the pyriform sinuses or the esophagus. Usually, it can be externally palpated lateral to the thyroid cartilage if it has passed into a pyriform sinus. Try again by withdrawing the tube until breath sounds are heard, then reinsert it. Twist the proximal end. Slight neck extension may help direct the tube forward, out of the esophagus and into the trachea.

If blind intubation is unsuccessful, visualize the vocal cords with a fiberoptic scope or a laryngoscope. Under direct visualization, the tube can usually be directed through the cords by twisting the proximal end and changing head position. Occasionally, it must be guided through the cords with Magill forceps.

The fiberoptic laryngoscope and bronchoscope provide a safe, effective technique for tracheal intubation of critically ill patients. They have relegated retrograde intubation to the category of historical interest. The latter technique involves puncture of the cricothyroid membrane with a hollow needle and passage of a guidewire through the needle retrograde up through the glottis and into the mouth. The wire is grasped in the mouth and an endotracheal tube threaded over it, through the cords, and into the trachea.[17] It should be used as a last resort only when the larynx cannot be visualized directly or by fiberoptic techniques.

TRACHEOSTOMY: ROLE AND TIMING

Factors of importance in translaryngeal intubation and tracheostomy are summarized in Table 17-6. Insertion of a tracheostomy involves a surgical procedure with a reported mortality as high as 5%[12] and potentially lethal complications such as erosion of the brachiocephalic artery. The rationale commonly cited for tracheostomy use, such as improved suctioning, decreased work of breathing, decreased deadspace, and improved patient comfort, has not been substantiated in the literature.[18] Despite serious potential complications, tracheostomy is used because, under optimal conditions with an experienced surgeon, it can be a safe procedure. Laryngeal complications of intubation can be reduced,[19] and a tracheostomy tube in a mature tracheostomy site is definitely easier to reinsert and care for than is an endotracheal tube.

TABLE 17-6 ENDOTRACHEAL INTUBATION VERSUS TRACHEOSTOMY

Variables	Tracheostomy	Endotracheal
Surgical procedure required	Yes	No
Permanent airway	Yes	No
Reintubation requirements, skilled personnel		
First 24 to 48 hours	Yes	Yes
After 48 hours	No	Yes
Sedation, relaxants		
1st 24 to 47 hours	Yes	Yes
After 48 hours	No	Yes
Accidental extubation	Less	More
Upper airway trauma	Less	More
Laryngeal damage	Less	More
Sinusitus	No	Yes (with nasal tube)
Oral hygiene	Easy	Difficult (with oral tube)
Tube size	Wider, shorter	Narrower, longer
Flow resistance	Less	More
Suctioning	Easy	More difficult
Massive hemorrhage	Yes, rare	No
Mainstem intubation	Uncommon	Common
Stomal complications	Yes	No
Airway infections	Perhaps more	Perhaps less
Patient comfort	Perhaps better	Perhaps less
Speech	Possible	Impossible

The role of tracheostomy in airway management of a critically ill patient remains controversial. Current opinion favors insertion of a translaryngeal tracheal tube initially, followed by elective tracheostomy under optimal surgical conditions.[3,12] There is general agreement that tracheostomy should be performed if long-term tracheal intubation is needed, but the period of time before tracheostomy is not rigidly delineated.[20] There is no rigid time period after which tracheostomy must be performed.

The definition of prolonged intubation has increased over time owing to improvements in tube and cuff design and improvements in management techniques. Intubation of a patient for 39 hours was first reported in 1880. Prolonged intubation usually is defined in terms of days and weeks; however, translaryngeal intubations lasting 2 to 6 months have been reported.[20,21] Recommendations in the current literature depend on the authors' experience and area of specialization. Dayal and Masri, who are otolaryngologists, stress the laryngeal complications of translaryngeal intubation and the decreased complications of tracheostomy when performed under optimal conditions by properly trained surgeons. They urge consideration of tracheostomy after 5 days.[19] A recent review by Berlauk, an anesthesiologist, emphasizes the safety of translaryngeal intubation maintained for up to 3 weeks.[22] My preference is to implement translaryngeal intubation for 2 to 3 weeks, as long as there is a reasonable chance for extubation during that period. After 2 to 3 weeks, a tracheostomy is performed because it is more secure and much easier to reinsert once the stoma is mature. If there is little or no hope for extubation within 2 weeks, I encourage early tracheostomy.

COMPLICATIONS OF AIRWAY MANAGEMENT

Some problems are common to all modes of tracheal intubation, whereas other problems are specific. The complications can also be classified according to time of onset (*i.e.*, during intubation, during maintenance, or after extubation) (see Table 17-6).[23]

Problems common to tracheostomy or tracheal intubation include tracheal mucosal damage from the tube cuff, humidity deficit, infection, inability to talk, tube obstruction, malposition, and unplanned extubation.

TRACHEAL MUCOSAL DAMAGE

The pressure of an inflated cuff against the tracheal mucosa causes damage whether the cuff is on a tracheostomy tube or an endotracheal tube.[24] Severity of the lesion is dependent on the pressure in the cuff, the duration of exposure, and the presence of severe respiratory failure or infected secretions.[15] Low-volume, high-pressure cuffs used in the past caused severe tracheal damage. This damage is now minimized by use of high-volume cuffs that allow sealing of the airway at a lower pressure. If the cuff pressure is below the perfusion pressure in the capillaries of the tracheal mucosa (about 25–30 mm Hg), blood flow to the mucosa continues and ischemic mucosal damage is minimized. Cuff pressure is kept to a minimum by inserting just enough air to prevent leakage at peak inspiratory pressure (minimum occlusive volume technique). The increased compliance of high-volume, low-pressure cuffs makes them safer because the addition of a small amount of air more than the minimally occlusive volume will not cause pressure to rise as much as in low-volume, high-pressure cuffs. However, when patients with markedly decreased compliance need both mechanical ventilation and positive end-expiratory pressures at high levels, it will not be possible to keep intact pressures below 30 mm Hg. In addition, a "minimal leak" technique is difficult to impossible to use because high peak inspired pressures compress the air in the balloon, resulting in movement of the tube and a greater air leak. In fact, if intracuff pressure is kept below 30 mmHg, ventilation with adequate total volumes will not be possible.* Wall thickness is also important. Thin-walled cuffs prevent the formation of large ridges on the surface, which can lead to channels for aspiration and to uneven pressure on the trachea.[26]

Although mucosal damage increases with time, it begins early. Acute tracheal mucosal damage contributes to the postintubation sore throat experienced by many patients. After only 2 hours, superficial loss of ciliated epithelium can be seen. Ulceration and inflammation then extend to involve the perichondrion and, ultimately, the tracheal cartilage. Because the ciliated epithelium is lost, mucociliary clearance is inhibited. Extensive tracheal damage leads to tracheomalacia if the cartilage is destroyed or to tracheal stenosis if the inflammation results in a contracted scar. Tracheal stenosis is particularly dangerous because it may not present until long after extubation when the patient is no longer in an ICU, when no one remembers that the patient had been intubated, and when the wheezing is almost always considered to be "asthma" despite a negatve history. Symptoms do not occur until the diameter of the lumen is narrowed to about 5 mm. An asymptomatic lesion can suddenly become symptomatic with a small amount of airway edema from an acute respiratory tract infection.

---

* Kirby, RR, Banner, MJ, unpublished observations.

TABLE 17-7 FACTORS IN TRACHEAL DAMAGE

Cuff pressure

Respiratory failure with high airway pressures

Infection

Duration of intubation

Cuff design
  Uneven cuff pressure
  Tube tip not centered

Tube and cuff material
  A problem before modern disposable tubes

A number of valves have been designed to regulate pressure inside tracheal tube cuffs. Attempts to decrease tracheal damage by intermittent cuff deflation have been unsuccessful and predispose to aspiration. Table 17-7 summarizes the adverse tracheal effects of intubation and cuff inflation.

HUMIDITY

When an artificial airway is inserted, humidification provided by the upper airway is lost. The tracheal tube allows direct access of cold, dry gases to the lower airways, which leads to mucosal damage and inspissation of secretions. Airway obstruction may result because ciliary clearance is inhibited. In the past, tracheostomy tubes had to be removed and cleaned regularly to prevent obstruction by inspissated secretions; however, this procedure is unnecessary if inspired gases are adequately humidified.[27]

INFECTION

An artificial airway also bypasses the antibacterial defense mechanisms of the upper airway. Bacteria normally are absent below the glottis, but insertion of a tracheal tube ensures contamination of the lower airways. Bacterial contamination of the lower airways may be as much as eight times more common with tracheostomy.[28] Because contamination of the lower airway is so common, differentiating between contamination and infection is a significant problem.

INABILITY TO TALK

Inability to communicate verbally causes a severe psychological strain for an intubated, critically ill patient. Attempts to talk with an endotracheal tube between the vocal cords increases laryngeal trauma[20] and should be discouraged. Other attempts at communication, such as writing and pointing to letters or pictures on a communication board, are often less than adequate. Talking tracheostomy tubes are commercially available. A separate cannula attached to the tracheostomy tube can be attached to a gas source and a constant flow of gas directed up through the cords, enabling vocalization. Attempts to develop talking endotracheal tubes have been reported.[29] The artificial larynx, a box held against the throat that transmits a buzzing sound to the oral pharynx, is another possible solution, but, to date, satisfactory verbal communication in intubated patients remains an elusive goal.

MALPOSITION AND UNPLANNED EXTUBATION

One final common, potentially lethal problem relevant to all types of tracheal intubation is malposition of the tube and unplanned extubation. Endotracheal tubes can be malpositioned into a mainstem bronchus, usually the right, or into the esophagus. Fresh tracheostomy tubes may be removed from the trachea and end up in the pretracheal fascia. Immediately after insertion, tube position should be verified by auscultation of bilateral breath sounds (best done in the axillae to minimize transmitted breath sounds) and by a chest radiograph. To ensure proper endotracheal tube position, watch the tube tip pass between the cords and advance it until the top of the cuff is 1 or 2 cm below the cords. In this position, it is possible to palpate cuff inflation at the suprasternal notch. If indirect visualization is not optimal, the distance marks on the endotracheal tube can be used as a rough guide to the proper depth of insertion. The tube is numbered in centimeters from the tip. In most adults, the distance from the teeth to midtrachea is 18 to 24 cm (Fig. 17-3).[30] The 20- or 22-cm mark should be at the teeth if the tube is at the proper depth. For nasal intubation, add 4 or 5 cm so that the 25- or 26-cm mark shows at the entrance of the tube into the nostril. If the 30-cm mark is at the teeth following oral intubation, a right mainstem intubation is likely. If the 22-cm mark is outside the nostril following nasal intubation, the cuff probably is at or above the cords. *Helpful hint:* After oral intubation with an uncut tube, you should be able to hold the protruding portion in your clenched fist.

An initially properly inserted tube subsequently can migrate above the cords or into a mainstem bronchus as a result of improper taping, weight and traction of the ventilator circuit, patient motion, and changes in head position. With flexion or extension of the neck,

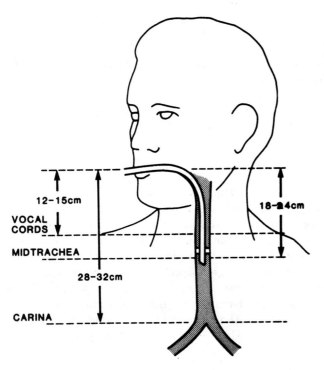

Figure 17-3 Malposition of the endotracheal tube can be suspected from the depth of insertion. In an average adult, the 18- to 24-cm mark will show at the incisors when the tip of the tube is midway between the vocal cords and the carina. (Distances from Natanson et al[30])

12–15cm

VOCAL CORDS

MIDTRACHEA

18–24cm

28–32cm

CARINA

the tip of the tube moves toward or away from the carina, respectively. The tube also moves away from the carina with lateral motion of the neck. As a general rule, remember that the tip of the tube follows movement of the chin (Fig. 17-4). In a radiographic study of intubated patients, the tube tip moved an average of 3.8 cm from full extension to full flexion. In some patients, movement was as much as 6.4 cm.[31] In evaluating tube and neck positions on a chest radiograph, remember that the head and neck are in neutral position if the chin is over C5 or C6. They are extended if the chin is above C4 and flexed if it is below C7. Optimal tube position radiographically is with the tip at the T2 level when the head and neck are in neutral position. It is thus midway between the cords at C5 or C6 and the carina at T6.[31]

Between 8.5% and 13% of intubated, critically ill patients sustain unplanned (accidental) extubation.[18,32] Replacement of an endotracheal tube requires skilled personnel to be readily at hand. Replacement of a fresh tracheostomy tube may be extremely difficult but is easier if the surgeon has left retraction sutures in the trachea.[33] If difficulty is encountered, quickly intubate the patient translaryngeally, allowing subsequent time for gentle, controlled exploration of the wound. Once a tracheostomy stoma has matured, replacement of the tube is simple and is a primary advantage of tracheostomy. Accidental extubation can be minimized by careful nursing practices, including secure taping, routine use of hand restraints, and care in turning and moving intubated patients. Endotracheal tubes are most secure when taped circumferentially around the upper neck using benzoin to improve adhesiveness of the tape to the skin and tube. Tracheostomy tubes should be secured with umbilical tape placed circumferentially around the neck and tied tightly enough to allow one finger beneath the tape.

SPECIFIC PROBLEMS

Problems specific to translaryngeal intubation result from trauma to the upper airway and larynx, whereas problems specific to tracheostomy result mostly from the surgical procedure and the stoma. Almost every structure above the diaphragm has been injured during endotracheal tube insertion.[23]

Figure 17-4 A. The tip of the endotracheal tube follows the chin and moves away from the carina with extension of the neck **(B)** and toward the carina with flexion **(C)** of the neck. (Conrardy PA et al: Alteration of endotracheal tube position: Flexion and extension of the neck. *Crit Care Med* 1976; 4:8. Copyright © 1976 by Williams & Wilkins)

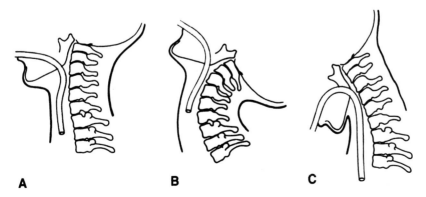

A   **B**   **C**

Bleeding is common and can be excessive during and after nasal intubation. Thus this technique should be avoided in patients with coagulopathies. Bleeding can be minimized with vasoconstrictors and small, gently inserted, well-lubricated tubes. Extensive bleeding may be controlled by withdrawing the endotracheal tube to the bleeding site and inflating the cuff to tamponade the bleeding, followed by oral intubation. Nasal intubation induces a transient bacteremia,[34] a factor to be considered in patients needing antibiotic prophylaxis for subacute bacterial endocarditis. The nasal turbinates can be damaged during insertion of a nasal tube, and adenoidal tissue fragments may obstruct the tube. *Gentle* pressure during tube insertion is important. If undue pressure is necessary and no breath sounds are heard, the tube may be dissecting submucosally along the posterior oropharynx.[9]

Oral insertion of an endotracheal tube is associated with damage of the lips, teeth, gums, tongue, oral pharynx, esophagus, and larynx.[23] Careful technique and patient cooperation (pharmacologically induced if necessary) minimize such trauma. If teeth are avulsed or chipped, the pieces should be removed before they are aspirated, or retrieved with a bronchoscope if aspiration occurs.

During tube insertion, the arytenoid cartilages can be dislocated and the vocal cords traumatized. After the tube is in place, ulceration and inflammation of the cords and subglottic area often occur. Ulceration is worse with larger tubes, in women (because of smaller glottic openings), and with friction caused by movement of the larynx along the tube. This movement results not only from traction or torsion of ventilator tubing and neck movement, but also from attempts to talk, and even from normal movement of the larynx during respiration.[20] Subsequent granuloma formation leading to chronic hoarseness after extubation may occur. Granuloma formation is not related to the duration of intubation but does appear to be related to tube material; the incidence is less than 1% after intubation with polyvinylchloride tubes.

Other causes of chronic hoarseness include severe ulceration of the vocal cords leading to a persistent glottic chink, vocal cord fibrosis, recurrent laryngeal nerve damage, cricoarytenoid arthritis, fracture dislocation of the arytenoid cartilages, and vocal cord polyps. Hoarseness after extubation is present in 71% to 86% of patients intubated for 5 days but is persistent beyond 3 months in only 0.7%. Chronic hoarseness appears to be related to the duration of intubation.[20]

Additional laryngeal complications occur after the tube has been removed. Acute partial to complete airway obstruction caused by glottic or subglottic edema is common and is unrelated to the duration of intubation. Glottic protective mechanisms are incompetent in the immediate postextubation period.[35] To protect against aspiration, the patient should be maintained in NPO status for at least 8 and possibly as long as 24 hours after extubation.[20,31] Laryngeal or subglottic stenosis may become evident 5 months or more after intubation. Scar tissue formation, as the ulcerated and inflamed tissues heal, may lead to fusion of the cords or circumferential narrowing of the subglottic area.[20,36] Factors of importance in laryngeal damage are summarized in Table 17-8.

Should you insert an endotracheal tube orally or nasally (see Table 17-5)? Advantages claimed for the nasal tube include patient comfort, secure fixation, and less laryngeal damage owing to the smaller size tube and a lesser angle of curvature through the glottis.[20] Disadvantages include nasal bleeding and trauma, transient bacteremia, cuff rupture on the turbinates during insertion, submucosal dissection, and sinusitis or otitis media from obstructed sinus openings or eustachian tubes. Sinusitis and otitis media should be considered sources of infection in critically ill patients who are nasally intubated.[37]

TABLE 17-8   FACTORS IN LARYNGEAL DAMAGE

Trauma
  During insertion
  During maintenance owing to tube movement
    Gross movements of ventilator circuit or patient
      Attempts to vocalize
      Respiratory movements
  During accidental extubation with cuff inflated

Route of intubation
  Less with nasal than oral

Duration of intubation

Infected secretions

Tube characteristics
  More damage with larger tubes
  Tube material (before single-use disposable tubes)

Complications of tracheostomy include mortality (0.9–5%),[12] with significantly better results in the controlled elective situation.[19] Pneumothorax, pneumomediastinum, subcutaneous emphysema, hemorrhage, and airway obstruction may complicate the procedure. After tracheostomy, a 0.5% to 4.5% incidence of massive hemorrhage from erosion of the tube into nearby major arteries (usually the innominate) has been reported.[38] This frequently fatal complication is heralded by hemoptysis, although a pulsating tracheostomy tube often provides an early warning.[12] Minor stomal bleeding is common and stomal infection practially ubiquitous, leading to an increased incidence of lower airway contamination and infection compared to translaryngeal intubation.[28] Tracheoesophageal fistula results acutely from a surgical incision through the back wall of the trachea into the esophagus. More commonly, however, it results from posterior erosion of the tube through the trachea and into the esophagus,[12] which usually presents 2 to 4 weeks after tracheostomy and is seen in about 0.5% of patients.

After decannulation, tracheal stenosis may occur either at the cuff site (similar to an endotracheal tube) or, more frequently, at the stomal site. A 40% to 60% decrease in diameter occurs in about one fourth of the patients, but clinical symptoms appear in only 1% to 2% (perhaps as high as 8%).[20] Tracheal stenosis at the stoma may be delayed in presentation but sudden in onset, similar to stenosis at the cuff site. It is more common when a portion of the trachea is excised.

In a prospectively randomized study comparing tracheostomy and prolonged translaryngeal tracheal intubation, investigators concluded that the early complications of tracheostomy were more severe, that patient discomfort and suctioning were rarely a problem with translaryngeal intubation, and that long-term laryngeal damage was rare.[18] Because some patients tolerated intubation for 22 days without serious complications, they recommended that tracheostomy not be routinely performed after a certain arbitrary period. Of interest, 13% of their intubated patients extubated themselves. Of those translaryngeally intubated patients who died and were autopsied, nearly all had posterior glottic ulcers, and laryngeal damage was more severe in tracheostomy patients with prior prolonged translaryngeal intubations.

FIBEROPTIC BRONCHOSCOPY IN THE ICU

The fiberoptic bronchoscope is a useful tool to avoid in elective intubation. When used with topical anesthesia and light intravenous sedation, it promotes elective intubation under visual control and allows spontaneous ventilation. If important guidelines are followed, success is easily achieved (Table 17-9).[9,36]

HUMIDIFICATION OF THE AIRWAY

Airway humidity is critical to the normal function and integrity of the respiratory epithelium. Humidity refers to the amount of water in the gaseous phase and is temperature dependent. Absolute humidity is expressed as mg H_2O/liter, whereas relative humidity is the ratio of the absolute humidity to the maximum possible humidity if the gas were saturated (expressed as a percentage). "Average" room air at 21°C has a relative humidity of 50% and an absolute humidity of 9 mg H_2O/liter. Alveolar air at 37°C, has a relative humidity of 100%, and has an absolute humidity of 44 mg H_2O/liter.[27] Because medical gases are anhydrous, 44 mg of water must be added to each liter to achieve full saturation of body temperature.

When the upper airway functions properly, ambient air (21°C and 50% relative humidity) is warmed to 34°C and the relative humidity increased to 80% to 90% as it passes through the nose.[27] When inspired gas reaches the carina or slightly beyond, it is 100% humidified, and its temperature is 37°C. If ambient air enters the oral pharynx from the mouth instead of the nose, its temperature and relative humidity are 21°C and 60%, respectively, but by the time it passes the carina it is fully saturated and warmed to body temperature. If the entire upper airway is bypassed by an endotracheal or tracheostomy tube and anhydrous medical gases are delivered directly to the trachea, the respiratory mucosa is quickly damaged. The normal watery mucus blanket becomes dried and viscous, eventually leading to inspissated secretions and airway obstruction. Ciliary function is impaired early, inhibiting the normal cephalad movement of the mucus blanket. The end-result is decreased bacterial clearance, atelectasis, and possibly pneumonia. When dry medical gases are administered, water vapor must be added before the gas reaches the patient. This goal is

TABLE 17-9 GUIDELINES FOR SUCCESSFUL FIBEROPTIC ENDOSCOPY AND INTUBATION

1. Secretions and blood obscure vision. Time taken to administer an anticholinergic premedication and to vasoconstrict the nose adequately will be well spent.
2. Careful topical anesthesia of the airway and judicious intravenous sedation should be considered.
3. The epiglottis appears higher, the pyriform sinuses are not stretched as in direct laryngoscopy, and the vocal cords appear much deeper. (The true cords are not seen until the false cords are passed.) Maintain the scope in the midline to avoid entering the unstretched pyriform sinuses, which resemble the entrance to the glottis.
4. The oral airway intubator is a modified oral airway that allows insertion of the tube and bronchoscope into the mouth in the midline, protecting it from the teeth, and directing it in proximity to the larynx. The anesthesia mask with diaphragm allows controlled ventilation of an anesthetized patient while the fiberoptic bronchoscope is inserted through the diaphragm in the mask and manipulated into the trachea.
5. Fiberoptic bronchoscopy is not indicated in an emergency situation in which the patient is apneic and cyanotic because the technique is not rapid enough.

accomplished with a humidifier, which delivers water vapor, or an aerosol generator, which delivers small particles of water suspended in the gas.

HUMIDIFIERS

Humidifiers depend on a gas water interface to generate water vapor. This interface can result from the flow of the gas over or through the water. Increasing the surface area of water exposed to the gas results in more water vapor formation. Heating the water also increases the vapor output from the humidifier.

Bubbling gas through a room temperature water bath results in the addition of 9 mg/ liter of water vapor. This conditioning is sufficient if the gas is delivered through a nasal cannula, since it will be further heated and humidified by the upper airway. If the patient is intubated, however, the humidification functions of the nose must be replaced. A variety of artificial noses in the form of heat and moisture exchangers and hydroscopic condensers are designed to conserve heat and moisture present in exhaled gas so that it can be added to inspired gases. The devices are placed in the breathing circuit at the airway connection where gas passes back and forth. These devices do not increase humidity within the respiratory tract but decrease the amount lost in expired gases. Advantages include simplicity and lack of added water or heating elements. Disadvantages include increased deadspace and airway resistance, and bacterial contamination. Although artificial noses have documented success at low fresh gas-flow rates, they are much less effective with the high fresh gas flows in commonly used IMV or CPAP circuits.

The simplest humidifier present on older Emerson ventilators consists of two pans welded together and placed on a hot plate. Fresh gas flows over the heated water, picking up water vapor. In a laboratory study by Poulton and Downs,[39] this humidifier delivered 30 mg/liter or less of water vapor even at low flows. The surface area, and thus the efficiency of flow-over humidifiers, is increased by incorporating a wick in the humidifier. In bubble-through humidifiers, the surface area is greatly increased by producing smaller bubbles with a cascade device incorporating a porous grid. Unfortunately, the casade also increases the resistance to flow through the humidifier at high flow rates, a significant impediment to spontaneous breathing by debilitated patients.

Recently manufactured humidifiers incorporate high and low temperature alarms and large external fluid reservoirs to minimize fluctuations of the water level in the humidifier. In the Conchatherm, temperature and humidity of the humidifier output increase when the fluid level drops because more of the wick is exposed. In the Bennett cascade, humidity and temperature decrease as the water level drops. Knowledge of the performance characteristics of the specific humidifiers in your institution is important (see also Chapter 9, "Oxygen Therapy").

NEBULIZERS (AEROSOL GENERATORS)

An aerosol is a suspension of liquid particles in the gaseous phase. Besides humidifying inspired gases, aerosol therapy improves clearance of secretions. Systemic hydration and humidification of inspired gases are important in preventing desiccation of the mucus blanket; however, particulate water must be added to aid clearance of dried secretions. Fifty milligrams per liter of aerosolized water at room temperature provides adequate humidification of inspired gases, but up to 100 mg/liter of particulate water is necessary when secretions are desiccated.[27] Aerosol therapy must be combined with instruction in deep breathing, proper coughing, and postural drainage to be maximally effective. It is frequently used to deliver medications, especially bronchodilators, to the respiratory tract.

Optimum particle size is important. Medical aerosols are made up of particles less than 3μm in diameter. Particles of 1 to 3 μm are most efficient. Nebulizers are pneumatic or electronic. Pneumatic nebulizers produce an aerosol by directing a stream of gas at the surface of a liquid. Mainstream types increase the water content of large volumes of gas and are used in ventilator circuits. Side-stream nebulizers are used to nebulize smaller volumes of liquid, primarily for the delivery of medications.

Electronic nebulizers use ultrasonic vibration to break apart the surface of the liquid, creating small particles in high concentrations without the addition of heat. Ultrasonic nebulizers can deliver 100 mg/liter of water particles with 90% of the particles in the appropriate therapeutic range. Most jet nebulizers deliver only 50 mg/liter of water particles, only 55% of which are in the proper size range.[27]

Delivery of an aerosol depends on more than the performance of the nebulizer. Aerosol particles may increase airway resistance, distilled water more so than normal saline. However, this resistance is more easily reversed with bronchodilators when distilled water is used. The optimum compromise seems to be 0.25% to 0.45% saline solutions, which produce diminished and reversible increases in airway resistance.[27] Aerosol delivery is also improved if the particles are inhaled through the mouth rather than through the nose, since many of the particles are filtered out nasally. Slow deep respirations from functional residual capacity to near vital capacity held for 5 to 10 seconds are most efficient for aerosol deposition.

COMPLICATIONS

Improperly functioning equipment or improper use can result in failure to attain therapeutic goals: inspired gas will not be properly humified or medication not delivered. Conversely, continuous use of highly efficient ultrasonic nebulizers in infants results in fluid overload. Heated humidification has resulted in airway burns and "hot-pot tracheitis," neither of which should occur with modern devices and functioning temperature alarms. Infection from contaminated nebulizers is a potential problem.

Ventilator circuit connections are more likely to become disconnected when wet than dry. Adhesive tape cannot be used to secure connections between wet circuit elements. Therefore, a "disconnect" (low pressure) alarm should be part of every ventilator and circuit. Even correct use of properly functioning equipment can result in unforeseen patient complications. Aerosol treatment may precipitate bronchospasm, and the moisture added to inspissated hydrophilic secretions may cause them to swell, thus obstructing the airways.[27]

TRACHEAL SUCTION

Airway secretions are cleared by coughing and by mucociliary action, in which cephalad flow at 10 mm/min occurs regardless of patient position. During a normal cough, high airway pressures are created behind a closed glottis, followed by glottic opening and a high flow of exhaled gases. The efficient mucociliary escalator and coughing are decreased by tracheal intubation and some disease conditions. During a cough, pressure cannot build up behind a closed glottis, resulting in a flow that begins sooner with a lower velocity and is decreased further by tube-induced flow resistance. Critically ill patients frequently have increased secretions, but, even with normal secretions, tracheal suctioning is periodically necessary. Before the importance of humidification of inspired gases was recognized, routine suctioning was performed to prevent airway obstruction. However, suctioning traumatizes the tracheal mucosa, and the resulting irritation increases secretions. Hence, suctioning should not be done routinely, but only for specific indications.

COMPLICATIONS

Suctioning leads to serious complications if not performed correctly and can result in significant hypoxemia. One of the earliest observations in respiratory therapy was that many cardiac arrests occur in critically ill patients during suctioning.[27] If the suction catheter is smaller than one-half the diameter of the tracheal tube, oxygen-enriched gas is suctioned from the airway and replaced by room air entrained around the suction catheter. If the catheter is too large to allow entrainment of room air, alveolar collapse and a decrease in lung volume result. Either situation leads to hypoxemia, which can be prevented by manual hyperinflations with 100% oxygen or by increasing the FI_{O_2} of the ventilator before suctioning. Suction adaptors (PEEP savers) are available that allow entrainment of oxygen-enriched gas and minimize airway pressure loss. Hypoxemia is less likely if suctioning is intermittent and limited to 10 to 15 seconds.

Suctioning is associated with dysrhythmias related to hypoxemia or tracheal stimulation, or both.[27] Tachydysrhythmias and premature ventricular complexes are common, but severe bradycardia may occur owing to a reflex vagal response. These responses can be minimized by prevention of hypoxemia and by intratracheal or intravenous injection of lidocaine.

Even with careful attention to proper technique, suctioning results in mucosal damage that may predispose to infection. To minimize damage, gently insert the cathether without suction, then apply intermittent suction during withdrawal while rotating the suction catheter between the thumb and index finger. Vacuum pressure should be limited to -80 to -120 mm Hg,[27] and the catheter should have a soft rounded end with side ports proximal to the tip. Tracheal damage results from the mucosa being sucked into the catheter, producing a hemorrhagic lesion. Ring-tipped catheters are designed to limit contact between the mucosa and the suction ports.

Suctioning may lead to nosocomial pulmonary infections, which can be prevented by careful adherence to sterile technique. A fresh, sterile disposable catheter should be used for each suction procedure. It should be handled with a sterile glove and rinsed in sterile solution. The nose and mouth may be suctioned with the same catheter *after* the trachea has been suctioned. Recently, an in-line catheter with protective sleeves (similar to the pulmonary artery catheters) has been introduced. It remains in place for 24 hours and obviates the flagrant problems of contamination that occur with repeated suctions. However, there have been no outcome data to document a decrease in nosocomial infection. Given the increased need for the caregiver to be protected from patients' secretions, the device seems worthy of further study.

A rise in ICP during suctioning may be significant in a patient with decreased intracranial compliance. This rise is due to tracheal stimulation rather than to increased carbon dioxide tension resulting from interrupted ventilation. To restrict the increase in ICP, inject lidocaine (1.5 mg/kg) either intravenously or into the tracheal tube before suctioning.

Occasionally, secretions will be localized and difficult to reach with the suction catheter, especially in the left bronchus. The fiberoptic bronchoscope can be used for selective

TABLE 17-10   PROPER SUCTIONING TECHNIQUE

1. Preoxygenate the patient with 100% oxygen. Continuously monitor the patient with EKG (and pulse oximetry, if available).
2. Suction the trachea:
    a. Use careful sterile technique and a suction catheter less than or equal to one-half the diameter of the tracheal tube.
    b. Insert the catheter without suction past the tracheal tube until obstruction is met, then withdraw slightly.
    c. Withdraw the catheter using intermittent suction and by rotating the catheter.
    d. Limit suction to 10 to 15 seconds and to -80 to -120 mm Hg suction pressure
    e. Limit interruption of ventilation to 20 seconds.
3. Reoxygenate the patient with 100% oxygen delivered by manual inflations, and wait until vital signs have returned to normal.
4. Repeat steps 1 through 3 until the secretions are cleared.
5. Suction the mouth and nose, and dispose of the suction catheter.

suctioning of specific bronchi. Alternatively, the left bronchus can be entered blindly. This maneuver reportedly is easier with a tracheostomy tube rather than with an endotracheal tube, when the head is turned to the right, and when a curved tip or coudé catheter is used. A summary of proper tracheal suctioning technique is presented in Table 17-10.[27]

DIAGNOSIS OF LOWER AIRWAY INFECTION

Diagnosis of lower airway infection in a critically ill patient with an artificial airway is difficult for several reasons. Although normally sterile, the respiratory tract below the glottis is contaminated with bacteria within 24 hours after tracheal intubation. Contamination denotes the presence of bacteria where they do not normally exist, whereas colonization denotes the presence of bacteria without an inflammatory host reaction. Normal flora colonize the mouth but so does *Pseudomonas* in patients in the intensive care unit. Infection occurs when the patient develops an inflammatory reaction involving phagocytic white cells that ingest and destroy the bacteria. Tracheal intubation (translaryngeal and tracheostomy) predisposes to aspiration of bacteria-laden oral secretions. The aspirated bacteria are not cleared efficiently because of mucociliary depression and cough suppression.

Diagnosis is imperative in a debilitated, immunocompromised patient in the intensive care unit who is continuously exposed to a variety of gram-negative organisms. Routine use of prophylactic antibiotics in this setting only leads to selection of more resistant organisms, excessive cost, and drug toxicity. Treatment should not be started solely on the basis of a radiographic chest infiltrate, because critically ill patients may have several noninfectious reasons for infiltrates (atelectasis, aspiration of acid gastric contents, cardiogenic and noncardiogenic pulmonary edema, or pulmonary emboli).

Unfortunately, no single laboratory test, including a sputum culture, establishes the diagnosis of pneumonia. Pneumonia remains a clinical diagnosis that should be made from a combination of clinical findings and laboratory data. Treatment should be started only when a combination of findings exist (Table 17-11).

Because sputum examination plays such an important part in the diagnosis of pneumonia, techniques of collection and interpretation must be emphasized. When collecting

TABLE 17-11   CRITERIA FOR DIAGNOSIS OF NOSOCOMIAL PNEUMONIA

1. Clinical deterioration is associated with physical and radiographic evidence of pneumonia. Fever and leukocytosis are helpful if present but may be absent in an immunocompromised patient. Attempts should be made to rule out noninfectious explanations for the findings.
2. Gram stain of sputum reveals white blood cells with intracellular bacteria. This is an important criterion because it helps to differentiate contamination from infection. Contamination should repeatedly be evaluated. Only infection should be treated with antibiotics.
3. Positive blood cultures or the appearance of a new cavitary lesion on chest radiograph requires immediate antibiotic therapy. Elastic fibers may be visible on microsopic examinaton of the sputum if the cavitary lesion represents necrotizing pneumonia.

sputum, be sure to avoid contamination with oral secretions. Such contamination is unavoidable in sputum collected by expectoration or nasotracheal suction. Transtracheal aspiration of sputum through the cricothyroid membrane is only a partial solution, since debilitated patients are prone to silent aspiration. Sputum aspirated from endotracheal or tracheostomy tubes often is contaminated with organisms from the upper airway. To circumvent these problems, use a protected specimen brush with the fiberoptic bronchoscope. If sputum examination is not diagnostic, a lung biopsy may be necessary for peripheral lesions. It can be obtained transbronchially through a bronchoscope, percutaneously by aspiration through a needle, or through an open surgical incision.

Proper interpretation of sputum samples necessitates microscopic examination, in addition to culture. Abundant squamous epithelial cells are a sure sign of contamination by oral secretions. Ciliated bronchial epithelial cells are an indication of a good specimen. The presence of organisms but no white cells signifies contamination, whereas white cells containing bacteria indicate active infection.

When to sample sputum is controversial. Some clinicians obtain routine surveillance cultures. Using this approach, the identification and sensitivies of predominant organisms are already known should clinical signs indicate the need for antibiotic treatment. The cost-effectiveness is questionable, since all intubated patients have positive cultures.

REFERENCES

1. Scuderi PE, McLeskey CH, Comer PB: Emergency percutaneous transtracheal ventilation during anesthesia using readily available equipment. *Anesth Analg* 1982; 61:867
2. Boyd AD, Romita MC, Conlan AA, et al: A clinical evaluation of cricothyrotomy. *Surg Gynecol Obstet* 1979; 149:365
3. Orringer MB: Endotracheal intubation and tracheostomy. Indications, techniques, and complications. *Surg Clin North Am* 1980; 60:1447
4. Gildar JS: A simple system for transtracheal ventilation. *Anesthesiology* 183; 58:106
5. Haleban P, Shires GT: A method for replacement of the endotracheal tube with continuous control of the airway. *Surg Gynecol Obstet* 1985; 161:285
6. Hudes ET, Fisher JA, Guslitz B: Difficult endotracheal reintubations: A simple technique. *Anesthesiology* 1986; 64:515
7. Millen JE, Glauser FL: A rapid, simple technique for changing endotracheal tubes. *Anesth Analg* 1978; 57:735
8. Rosenbaum SH, Rosenbaum LM, Cole RP, et al: Use of the flexible fiberoptic bronchoscope to change endotracheal tubes in critically ill patients. *Anesthesiology* 1981; 54:169
9. Stoelting RK: Endotracheal intubation. In Miller RD (ed): *Anesthesia.* New York, Churchill Livingstone, 1986
10. Patterson AR: Pulmonary aspiration syndromes. In Kirby RR, Taylor RW (eds): *Respiratory Failure,* pp 245–259. Chicago, Year Book Medical Publishers, 1986

11. Hamill JF, Bedford RF, Weaver DC, et al: Lidocaine before endotracheal intubation: Intravenous or laryngotracheal? *Anesthesiology* 1981; 55:578

12. Selecky PA: Tracheostomy: A review of present day indications, complications, and care. *Heart Lung* 1974; 3:272

13. Barton S, Williams JD: Glossopharyngeal nerve block. *Arch Otolaryngol* 1971; 93:186

14. Calcaterra TC, House J: Local anesthesia for suspension microlaryngoscopy. *Ann Otol* 1976; 85:71

15. Bourke DL, Katz J, Tonneson A: Nebulized anesthesia for awake endotracheal intubation. *Anesthesiology* 1985; 63:690

16. Ducrow M: Throwing light on blind intubation. *Anaesthesia* 1978; 33:827

17. Bourke D, Levesque PR: Modification of retrograde guide for endotracheal intubation. *Anesth Analg* 1974; 53:1013

18. Stauffer JL, Olson DE, Petty TL: Complications and consequences of endotracheal intubation and tracheostomy: A prospective study of 150 critically ill adult patients. *Am J Med* 1981; 70:65

19. Dayal VS, El Masri W: Tracheostomy in intensive care setting. *Laryngoscope* 1986; 96:58

20. Bishop MJ, Weymuller ER, Fink BR: Laryngeal effects of prolonged intubation. *Anesth Analg* 1984; 63:335

21. Via-Reque E, Rattenborg CC: Prolonged oro- or nasotracheal intubation. *Crit Care Med* 1981; 9:637

22. Berlauk JF: Prolonged endotracheal intubation vs. tracheostomy. *Crit Care Med* 1986; 14:742

23. Blanc VF, Tremblay NAG: The complications of tracheal intubation: A new classification with a review of the literature. *Anesth Analg* 1974; 53:202

24. Lindholm CE, Grenvik Å: Tracheal tube and cuff problems. *Int Anesthesiol Clin* 1982; 20:103

25. Kastanos N, Miro RE, Perez AM, et al: Laryngotracheal injury due to endotracheal intubation: Incidence, evolution, and predisposing factors. A prospective long-term study. *Crit Care Med* 1983; 11:362

26. Bernhard WN, Cottrell JE, Sivakumaran C, et al: Adjustment of intracuff pressure to prevent aspiration. *Anesthesiology* 1979; 50:363

27. Shapiro BA, Harrison RA, Kacmarek RM, et al: *Clinical Application of Respiratory Care,* 3rd ed. Chicago, Year Book Medical Publishers, 1985

28. El-Naggar M, Sadagopan S, Levine H, et al: Factors influencing choice between tracheostomy and prolonged translaryngeal intubation in acute respiratory failure: A prospective study. *Anesth Analg* 1976; 55:195

29. Walsh JJ, Rho DS: A speaking endotracheal tube. *Anesthesiology* 1985; 63:703

30. Natanson C, Shelhamer JH, Parrillo JE: Intubation of the trachea in the critical care setting. *JAMA* 1985; 253:1160

31. Conrardy PA, Goodman LR, Lainge F, et al: Alteration of endotracheal tube position: Flexion and extension of the neck. *Crit Care Med* 1976; 4:8

32. Zwillich CW, Pierson DJ, Creagh CE, et al: Complications of assisted ventilation. *Am J Med* 1974; 57:161

33. Chew JY, Cantrell RW: Tracheostomy: Complications and their management. *Arch Otolaryngol* 1972; 96:538

34. Berry FA, Blankenbaker WL, Ball CG: A comparison of bacteremia occurring with nasotracheal and orotracheal intubation. *Anesth Analg* 1973; 52:873

35. Burgess GE III, Cooper JR, Marino RJ, et al: Laryngeal competence after tracheal extubation. *Anesthesiology* 1979; 51:73

36. Hawkins DB: Glottic and subglottic stenosis from endotracheal intubation. *Laryngoscope* 1977; 87:339

37. Deutschman CS, Wilton P, Sinow J, et al: Paranasal sinusitis associated with nasotracheal intubation: A frequently unrecognized and treatable source of sepsis. *Crit Care Med* 1986; 14:111

38. Timmis HH: Tracheostomy: An overview of implications, management and morbidity. *Adv Surg* 1973; 7:199

39. Poulton JJ, Downs JB: Humidification of rapidly flowing gas. *Crit Care Med* 1981; 9:59

CHAPTER EIGHTEEN

IMPORTANT PROCEDURES IN THE INTENSIVE CARE UNIT

Neil S. Yeston
Joan M. Niehoff

Discussed herein are the numerous diagnostic and therapeutic procedures commonly performed in the intensive care unit setting. In general, attention to anatomic detail and sterile technique yields favorable results with a minimum of complications. Although there are numerous variations on a theme, the following methods for thoracentesis, tube thorarcostomy, peritoneal lavage, paracentesis, cardioversion and defibrillation, venous cutdown, and transtracheal aspiration have been shown to be safe and effective in the intensive care unit.

THORACENTESIS

The pleural cavity is normally a potential space and responds to the adjacent disease process with an outpouring of fluid, resulting in a pleural effusion.

The diagnosis of pleural fluid can be made on physical examination. Percussion dullness, reduced or absent breath sounds, and reduced transmission of whispered voice are usual findings. Grocco's triangle, or the presence of a triangle of dullness on the contralateral hemithorax, is caused by the bulging of fluid in the posterior mediastinal pleura and is considered pathognomonic of pleural effusion.[1] Characteristic radiographic findings include a partial or complete opacification of the hemithorax, which usually layers out on lateral decubitus projections. Computed tomography scanning and ultrasonography are often helpful in diagnosing and localizing free or loculated pleural effusions.

Thoracentesis is indicated when a sample of pleural fluid would be helpful in elucidating or confirming a diagnosis. Therapeutic thoracentesis may be useful when drainage of a restrictive effusion relieves respiratory compromise.

PROCEDURE

The patient is placed in the sitting position with the arms supported on a bedside table (Fig. 18-1). If unable to sit upright, the patient is placed supine and the head of the bed elevated as close to a 90° angle as possible.

The level of thoracentesis should be one or two interspaces below the percussed fluid

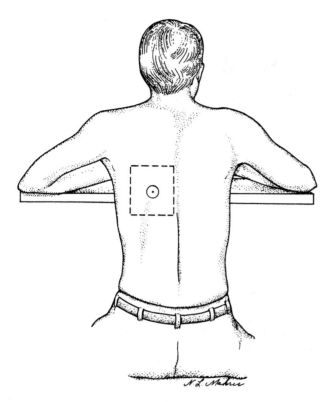

Figure 18-1 The patient is placed in the sitting position with the arms supported on a bedside table.

level but not lower than the eighth intercostal space. Count the ribs downward from the 2nd rib anteriorly and upward from the 12th rib posteriorly. Prepare the skin with povidine–iodine (Betadine) and create a sterile field with drapes.

Administer local anesthesia with a 25-gauge needle and 1% lidocaine, creating a skin wheal and then penetrating into the subcutaneous tissues. Use a 20-gauge needle to anesthetize the deeper tissues. Inject the local anesthetic over the middle of the rib. "Walk" up the rib over the superior margin of the rib to avoid the intercostal bundle. Aspirate frequently to avoid venous or arterial infusion of lidocaine. Infiltrate generously through the pleura (a "pop" may be felt when the pleura has been entered). At this point the patient may complain of some discomfort. Aspirate to confirm the presence of fluid. Mark the needle depth with a clamp and withdraw the needle (Fig. 18-2).

A pleural effusion can be drained by thoracentesis using several different methods. One method uses a catheter within a needle (*i.e.*, Deseret Intracath, 14-gauge needle, 16-gauge/8-in catheter) (Fig. 18-3).[2] Place a 10-ml non-Luer lock syringe on an Intracath needle. Mark the needle depth with a second clamp to prevent excess penetration. Insert the needle, with the bevel downward. Remove the syringe, occlude the needle with a finger to avoid creating a pneumothorax, and insert the cannula into the needle. During expiration, advance

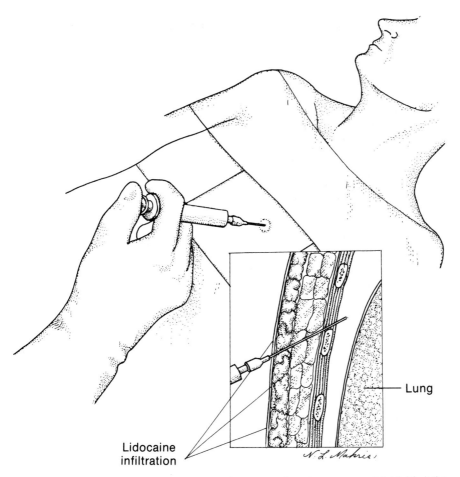

Lung

Lidocaine
infiltration

Figure 18-2 Inject the local anesthetic and aspirate to confirm the presence of fluid. Mark the needle depth with a Kelly clamp.

the cannula into the pleural space and slide the needle back over the cannula. Never pull the cannula back through the needle because this may shear the catheter. A three-way stopcock may be attached[3] so that the pleural fluid can be withdrawn into the syringe and then injected into IV tubing connected to a sterile container (Fig. 18-4). Alternatively a vacuum bottle can be used for a rapid, efficient method of collection (Fig. 18-5) by connecting the cannula to clamped intravenous tubing attached to a vacuum bottle and then opening the tubing clamp.

An 18- or 20-gauge Angiocath can also be used (needle within the catheter) to perform thoracentesis. Attach the syringe to the hub of the needle, which is advanced as previously discussed. When fluid is returned, advance the catheter over the needle. Withdraw the needle

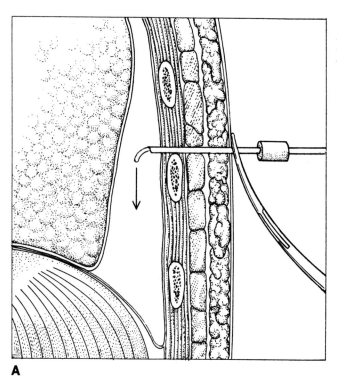

A

Figure 18-3 A. Insert the thoracentesis needle. Advance the cannula into the pleural space during expiration. **B.** Slide the needle back over the catheter.

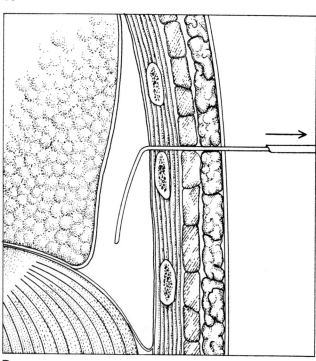

B

Figure 18-4 A three-way stopcock may be attached so the pleural fluid can be withdrawn into the syringe. The fluid is then injected into IV tubing connected to a sterile container.

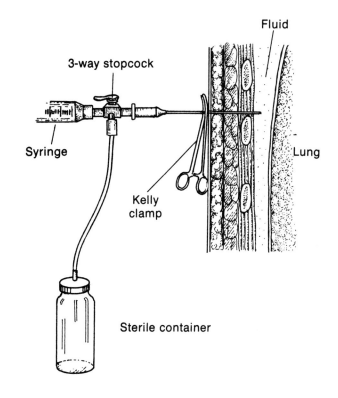

Figure 18-5 A vacuum bottle can be used for rapid and efficient collection.

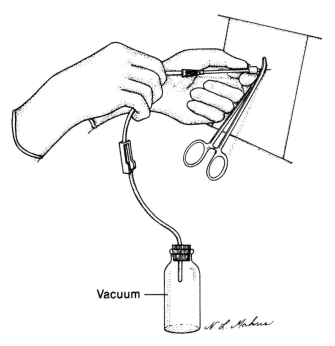

and place a finger over the hub of the catheter. Then evacuate the pleural effusion using the three-way stopcock or vacuum system as described above.

Obtain a chest radiograph after completion of the procedure. Fluid should be sent for cell count, Gram stain, TB and fungal smears, culture (aerobic, anaerobic, fungal, and *Mycobacterium*), cytology and cell block, protein, sugar, pH, LDH, and amylase. Obtain samples for pH anaerobically and place them on ice.

COMPLICATIONS

Complications of thoracentesis include pneumothorax, bleeding from lacerated intercostal vessels, and hepatic or splenic punctures.

Guidelines for examination of pleural fluid for infection, although somewhat variable, have been extensively evaluated. Most empyemas develop in patients with bacterial pneumonia. Up to 40% of patients with pneumonia have been noted to have a pleural effusion during the course of their illness.[4] A parapneumonic process should be considered in all patients with bacterial pneumonia in whom the posterior costophrenic angle is obliterated on chest radiograph.[5] If an effusion is documented on the lateral decubitus film, perform a diagnostic thoracentesis. The effusion is considered an exudate if the pleural LDH/serum LDH ratio is >0.6,[6] and the pleural protein/serum protein ratio is >0.5. Diagnostic criteria of an empyema generally include the presence of gross pus, organisms present on Gram stain,[5] and pleural fluid glucose <40 mg/dl or pleural fluid pH <7.20, or both.[7] The pleural fluid pH generally falls before the pleural glucose.[8,9] Patients with tuberculosis, rheumatoid, or malignant effusions may have a low pleural fluid pH.[8] Thus pH alone is unreliable in determining the presence of empyema in these patients. Early initiation of tube thoracostomy is recommended for therapy of an empyema, since the empyema becomes more loculated with time.[5,10]

TUBE THORACOSTOMY

Closed tube thoracostomy, or chest tube drainage, was first described by Hewett in 1876[11] but did not become commonplace until World War II.[12] Although variations have developed in technique and indications, the basic principles remain the same.

Indications for tube thoracostomy include the need to remove air or liquid (blood, exudate, chyle) from the pleural space or to instill chemotherapeutic agents after removal of malignant pleural effusions. Prophylactic chest tubes are inserted in patients with penetrating thoracic injuries before nonthoracic surgery, even without evidence of pneumothorax.

PROCEDURE

Place the patient in the supine position with the arm abducted to 90°. The preferred site for placement of the chest tube is the fourth or fifth intercostal space in the anterior axillary line. An alternate site for thoracostomy is the second or third intercostal space in the midclavicular line, but this is useful only when pneumothorax alone is present (Fig. 18-6). Prepare the skin with 10% povodine–iodine solution (Betadine) and create a sterile field with drapes. Measure the chest tube from the lateral chest wall to the apex and mark it with a suture tied at the estimated intrathoracic distance. Local anesthesia with 1% lidocaine

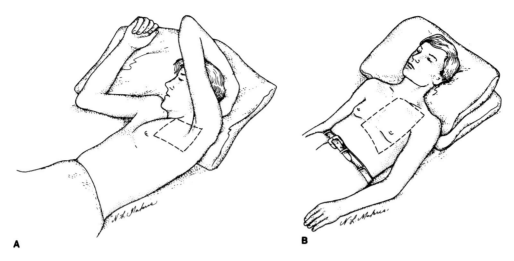

A   **B**

Figure 18-6 A. The preferred site for placement of the chest tube is the fourth or fifth intercostal space in the anterior axillary line. **B.** The second or third intercostal space is an alternate site for thoracostomy when pneumothorax alone is present.

using a 25-gauge needle should include the skin, subcutaneous tissue, intercostal muscles, periosteum, and the pleura (Fig. 18-7).

Make a 2-cm incision in the anterior axillary line in the midportion of the rib just inferior to the interspace that the tube will traverse. Do not enter the space from mid axillary to posterior axillary line because the patient will lie on the tube, causing discomfort and kinking of the tube.

Fashion a subcutaneous tunnel with blunt and sharp dissection using a Kelly clamp. (The trochar method is not recommended.) The entrance point into the pleural space should

Figure 18-7 Local anesthesia should include the skin, subcutaneous tissue, intercostal muscles, periosteum, and pleura.

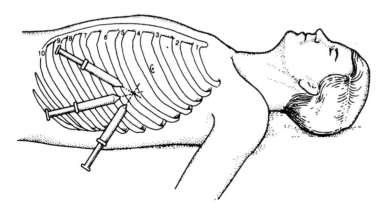

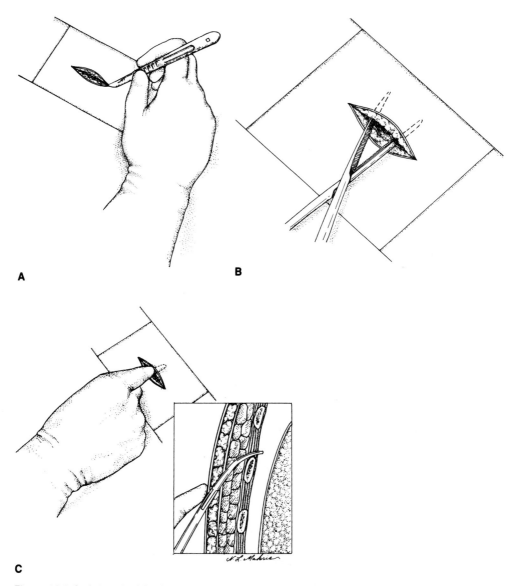

A

B

C

Figure 18-8 A. A 2-cm incision is made in the anterior axillary line, just inferior to the rib that the tube will traverse. **B.** A subcutaneous tunnel is fashioned with a Kelly clamp. **C.** The entrance point into the pleural space should be just over the superior margin of the upper rib.

be just over the superior margin of the lower rib to avoid injury to the neurovascular bundle (Fig. 18-8). Slipping over the superior margin of that rib, bluntly perforate the pleura with a Kelly clamp (Fig. 18-9). Once the instrument has entered the pleural cavity, open the pleura about 1 cm by spreading the handles of the Kelly clamp. As the pleura is spread, a "gush" of air may be heard leaving the pleural space, if a tension pneumothorax was present.

Figure 18-9 The pleural space is then entered using a Kelly clamp.

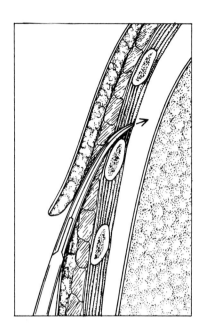

Place a gloved finger into the pleural space to confirm thoracic penetration. Palpate the lung medially (Fig. 18-10). If unable to confirm thoracic penetration, consider intra-abdominal penetration. Using the gloved finger, sweep away any intrapleural adhesions, which opens the intrapleural space and allows for safe entrance of the chest tube.

Grasp the tip of the thoracostomy tube with a Kelly clamp and direct it into the pleural

Figure 18-10 A gloved finger is placed into the pleural space confirming thoracic penetration.

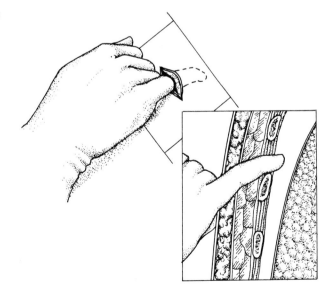

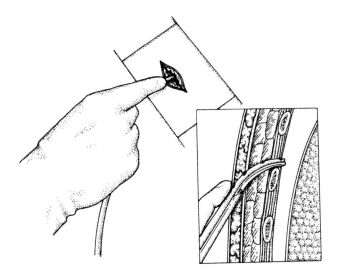

Figure 18-11 The tip of the thoracostomy tube is grasped with a Kelly clamp and directed into the pleural space posteriorly and superiorly

space posteriorly and superiorly (Fig. 18-11). Care should be taken not to introduce the catheter along the subcutaneous tissue outside the chest wall. Place the tube deeply enough so that the last hole in the catheter is well inside the pleural space and not in the subcutaneous tissue, thereby avoiding the development of subcutaneous emphysema.

The catheter is connected to a standard collection–suction apparatus that has a high volume flow, adjustable amount of suction, and an underwater seal with a compartment for accurately measuring liquid that drains from the chest tube. The suture material should be nonabsorbable, such as O silk, and used to secure the chest tube to the skin. The wound is dressed with Vaseline gauze, 4 × 4 dressing sponges, and elastoplast. All connection sites are taped together (Fig. 18-12 and 18-13). Obtain a chest radiograph immediately to evaluate tube placement and function. Never clamp the chest tube during transportation because a fatal tension pneumothorax may develop. Two chest tubes may be needed if a massive air leak is present or residual intrathoracic fluid is present with a single chest tube. Air leaks can be visualized at the base of the suction apparatus (Fig. 18-14). A gauge measures the volume of air leaking out in a semiquantitative way. There are various channels for bubbles to exit, corresponding to different rates.

Pneumothorax

The presence of a pneumothorax is the most common indication for chest tube placement.[13] Spontaneous pneumothoraces are most commonly seen in men with tall slender builds.[14] Traumatic pneumothoraces, both penetrating and nonpenetrating, are usually associated with some degree of hemothorax.[15,16] Pneumothoraces caused by blunt trauma are almost always associated with rib fractures.[15]

Minimal respiratory embarrassment may be present in patients with spontaneous or traumatic pneumothorax, but the diagnosis is rarely made incidently. The history of a spontaneous pneumothorax may include sudden onset of pleuritic chest pain. The usual

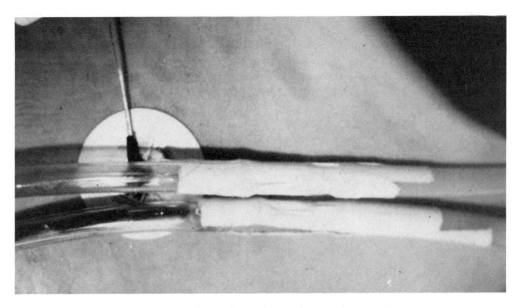

Figure 18-12 The attachment of the chest tube to the suction device usually incorporates a connector. When patients are turned in the bed or moved from bed to chair or stretcher, tension is often placed on those connections. A longitudinally placed strip of tape from chest tube across the connector to the suction tube should be reinforced with circumferential pieces of tape on each of the three components (tube, connector, rubber suction tubing).

clinical signs include diminished breath sounds, hyper-resonance to percussion (most diagnostic), tracheal deviation, and tachypnea.[15] A chest radiograph is required to rule out a minor pneumothorax, usually best seen on a view taken during expiration;[15,17] however, the chest radiograph does not take priority over deteriorating clinical signs, and tube thoracostomy should be performed without radiographic confirmation if a pneumothorax is suspected in the patient with worsening respiratory distress. A minimal pneumothorax, defined as <25% total collapse (<4-cm apical collapse), or <1-cm lateral collapse, may be observed without treatment providing the patient will not require positive pressure ventilation. Reabsorption of air occurs at the rate of about 1.25% of the lung volume per day.[18] Unfortunately estimates of the size of a pneumothorax are neither accurate nor reproducible.[19,20] Consideration of tube thoracostomy is then dependent on increase in the size of the pneumothorax and respiratory embarrassment of the patient.

A tension pneumothorax results when the communication between the lung parenchyma and the pleural cavity acts as a one-way valve, allowing air to enter the cavity during expiration but not to exit during inspiration. Air builds up in the pleural space under pressure, the diaphragm flattens, and the mediastinum shifts to the opposite side.[21] The trachea is shifted to the side opposite the tension, and little or no movement is present on the affected side. Jugular venous distension and arterial hypotension develop. As the contralateral lung and great vessels become compressed, ventilation and venous return are compromised,

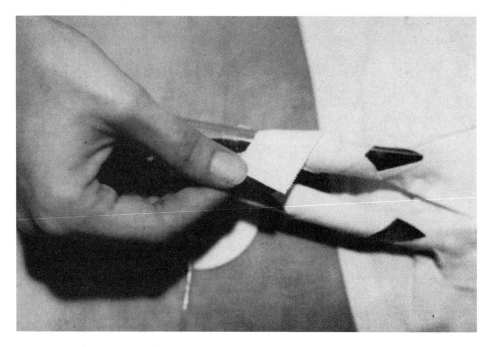

Figure 18-13 Another view of the chest tube–connector–suction tube assembly. Tape may also be split longitudinally and the halves wrapped around the connector and suction tubing in opposite directions.

leading to hypoxia and circulatory collapse.[15,22] Conscious patients may become extremely dyspneic and cyanotic.[22] The diagnosis is usually grossly apparent in advanced cases of tension pneumothorax and represents a life-threatening emergency for which immediate treatment is required. A large bore needle-catheter assembly may be placed in the second intercostal space anteriorly to decompress the pleural space while preparing to perform a tube thoracostomy.[15]

Iatrogenic causes of pneumothorax have increased with the advent of mechanical ventilation and central venous catheterization. The incidence of pneumothorax in patients who are mechanically ventilated is 3% to 4% and approaches 23% in those treated with mechanical ventilation and end-expiratory pressure.[23,24] Tension pneumothorax is present in 50% of ventilator-associated pneumothoraces.[23,24] Subclavian vein catheterization has a 3% to 6% incidence of pneumothorax.[25,26] Many other procedures have been noted to cause pneumothoraces, including thoracentesis, pleural biopsy, pulmonary artery catheterization,[27] invasive cardiac electrophysiologic procedures,[28] cardiopulmonary resuscitation, unusual gastroduodenal feeding tube placement,[29] esophageal obturator airways,[30] nerve conduction studies,[26] colonoscopy,[31] esophagoscopy,[32] acupuncture,[33] and aspiration of breast cysts.[34]

Pneumothorax has also been noted in patients who suffer from IV drug abuse[35] and generally results from central vein injection. Pneumothorax secondary to "free-base" cocaine use[36,37] requiring deep inspiration and Valsava maneuver has also been reported.

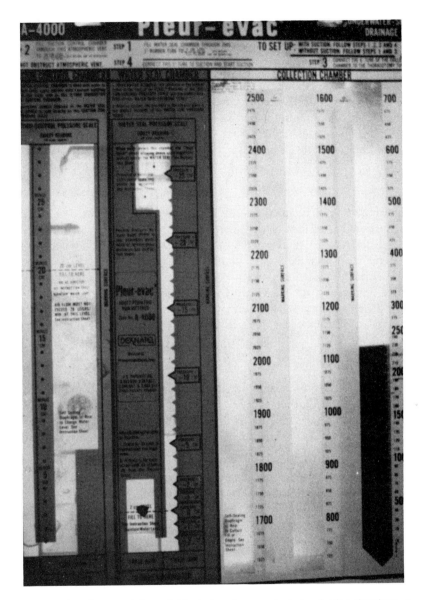

Figure 18-14 Commercially available devices have graduated collection chambers, a water seal device, and a suction chamber. This simplifies assembly and ensures that the components are connected in proper sequence.

Hemothorax

Most cases of traumatic hemothorax can be managed with tube thoracostomy alone. A large-caliber chest tube is needed (32–40 French) along with 20 cm H_2O of suction. Most intra-thoracic bleeding will stop spontaneously with simple re-expansion of the lung owing to the low pressure pulmonary vascular system.[38,39] The hemothorax must be completely drained; failure to do so can result in fibrothorax and significant impairment of respiratory function. Recommendations for a clotted hemothorax include a limited thoracotomy for evacuation.[40] Persistent bleeding is an indication for open thoracotomy, although guidelines vary regarding specific volumes of blood loss. The amount of the initial blood loss with insertion of tube thoracostomy and evidence of continued bleeding are included in most formulas. Siemens recommends open thoracotomy for an initial blood loss of >800 ml or for hypotension upon presentation (systolic blood pressure less than 90 mm Hg).[41] Others use an initial blood loss of 1000 to 1500 ml and continued loss of at least 150 to 200 ml/h for >4 hours as an indication for thoracotomy.[16,42–46]

Chylothorax

Chylothorax is the accumulation of lymphatic fluid in the pleural space. The problem is uncommon and usually related to trauma or malignant disease.[22,47] Filariasis, tuberculosis, and subclavian vein obstruction are also associated with chylothorax.[48] Lymphosarcoma is the most common malignancy associated with chylothorax, followed by metastatic disease and bronchiogenic carcinoma.[48] Chylothorax does not usually resolve spontaneously, and its presence rarely requires emergency action. Treatment includes repeated thoracentesis or tube thoracostomy and dietary restriction with enteral replacement of medium-chain triglycerides.[49] Thoracotomy and ligation of the thoracic duct are indicated if more conservative measures fail.

CHEST TUBE CARE

A chest tube should not be advanced further into the pleural cavity after the procedure has been completed, yet the tube can be withdrawn with care taken not to expose the drainage holes. A new site is necessary if a new tube needs to be inserted. The tube should not be clamped during transportation, nor should the drainage system be placed higher than the thorax. Movement of the fluid column with respiration is evidence for chest tube function. If respiratory variation is not present, the tube should be removed or replaced.

SUGGESTIONS

In the absence of a formal pleural collection system, an emergency one-way valve can be constructed by tying a rubber glove over the external end of the chest tube and cutting a small hole in the end of a glove finger. This will function as a one-way exit valve, providing temporary control of a simple or tension pneumothorax.

Similarly, the Heimlich valve, a one-way flutter valve placed at the distal end of the chest tube, was first developed in 1968 and used successfully in Vietnam and Israel.[50] Although developed for emergency use, the valve is currently used in selected patients for the outpatient management of spontaneous penumothorax.[51,52] The major drawback of this technology is the inability of the valve to keep the lung expanded in the face of a persistent air leak. Even in carefully selected patients, outpatient management fails in 25% of cases.[51] The Heimlich valve is rarely, if ever, indicated in the ICU patient population.

COMPLICATIONS

Technical complications associated with insertion of chest tubes should be rare, and they approach 1% when performed by experienced physicians.[53] Bleeding as a result of chest tube insertion is generally caused by the inadvertent laceration of an intercostal vessel or internal mammary vessel.[53] This complication can be prevented if care is taken to guide the instruments along the superior edge of the rib, avoiding the intercostal vessels, and by placing the anterior chest tube no closer to the sternum than the midclavicular line. Laceration of the lung can be avoided by grasping the clamp used to puncture the pleura so that the distance from hand to tip is just greater than the chest wall thickness.[54] Finding the proper tract with finger exploration will prevent improper placement of the chest tube.[54] Chest tube occlusion can be prevented by stripping the tube hourly and ensuring that a large sized tube is used for either a hemothorax or viscous pleural effusion.[54]

Persistent pneumothorax can be caused by a large bronchopleural fistula and may require thoracotomy for surgical closure. In general, a continued massive air leak (diagnosed as inadequate lung re-expansion on chest radiograph) despite two adequately functioning chest tubes on suction is an indication for early thoracotomy. Continued air leak after 1 week of treatment with a chest tube may also be an indication for thoracotomy, although patients with severe COPD may require a longer trial with tube thoracostomy.

The incidence of intrapleural infection is reported to be 1% to 16%;[55–57] however, most series report an incidence of less than 3%.[54] In general, prophylactic antibiotic therapy is not recommended for thoracostomy, whether placed for spontaneous pneumothorax or trauma.[58,59]

Chest tube removal may result in recurrent pneumothorax, but the incidence is uncommon (2.4%).[60] The most common abnormality seen after removal of a chest tube is the presence of pleural thickening or pleural fluid. Occasional atelectasis may be seen on follow-up chest radiograph. Fibrothorax may result from the inadequate drainage of a hemothorax.

CHEST TUBE BOTTLES

Although the three-bottle drainage system generally has been replaced by plastic portable units, the physical principles remain the same. The functioning chest drainage setup requires that the drainage tube from the chest be inserted beneath the level of water in a container. As the tubing is progressively submerged within the bottle, greater intrapleural pressure is needed to allow evacuation of the pleural contents. The usual distance is 1 to 2 cm under the surface (Fig. 18-15).[61] If the pressure in the chest rises above 1 to 2 cm H_2O, fluid or air will be evacuated. If the pressure within the chest falls below atmospheric pressure, fluid will be drawn up into the tube by an equivalent amount. The usual configuration of chest tube drainage systems is illustrated in Figure 18-16.

PARACENTESIS

Diagnostic paracentesis is often used in patients with ascites. Particular attention is directed toward the patient with unexplained fever or leukocytosis and suspicion of spontaneous bacterial peritonitis.[62] Also paracentesis is recommended in patients with a rapid increase in ascitic fluid, which was previously well controlled with medical therapy (diuretics and salt restriction).[62] Therapeutic paracentesis may be performed on patients with respiratory compromise caused by massive ascites.

Usual precautions in the performance of paracentesis include choosing an avascular site on the abdominal wall (preferably in the lower abdomen just lateral to the rectus

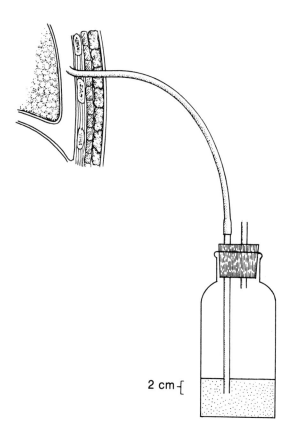

Figure 18-15 Underwater-seal drainage.

2 cm

abdominis muscle); correcting any underlying coagulopathy; and ensuring that the urinary bladder is well drained before the procedure. Avoid tapping a rare mesenteric cyst.

PROCEDURE

Place the patient in the supine position. Confirm the presence of ascitic fluid at the site intended for paracentesis by physical examination (*i.e.*, percussion). Ultrasound guidance also may be used (Fig. 18-17). Prepare the skin with povodine–iodine and create a sterile field with drapes. Using a 25-gauge needle, inject 1% lidocaine with epinephrine, first creating a skin wheal. Stretch the skin about 1 cm inferior to the point of the wheal (the z-track technique), which will make the needle track discontinuous and lessen the chance of an ascitic leak. Inject the lidocaine with a 21-gauge needle, first through the wheal then through the fascia and peritoneum (a "pop" may be felt). Aspirate as the needle is advanced, stopping when ascitic fluid is returned. Remove the needle. Next advance a 20-gauge Angiocath (needle through catheter) attached to a 10-ml syringe through the anesthetized area. Aspirate continuously. When ascitic fluid is returned, advance the catheter over the needle. Remove the needle and connect a 50-ml syringe to the catheter. The catheter should not be pulled back over the needle because this may shear the tip of the catheter within the

Figure 18-16 Removal of the second and third bottles leaves a simple water-seal drainage system. The effective suction pressure is equal to the difference in levels of bottles 1 and 2. The third bottle serves as a trap.

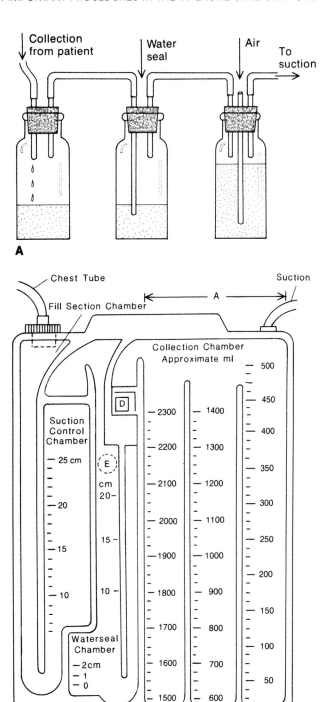

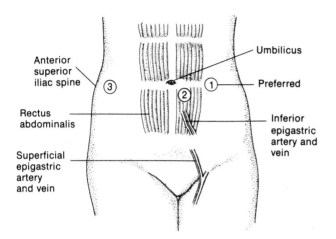

Figure 18-17 The preferred site for paracentesis is in the lower abdomen just lateral to the rectus abdominis muscle.

Anterior superior iliac spine

Rectus abdominalis

Superficial epigastric artery and vein

Umbilicus

Preferred

Inferior epigastric artery and vein

peritoneal cavity. Withdraw 50 ml of fluid (diagnostic tap) or the desired amount (therapeutic). Withdraw the catheter and cover with a sterile dressing.

The ascitic fluid should be sent for specific gravity, protein, cell count, cytology, cell block, Gram stain and culture, stain and culture for acid-fact bacilli, and amylase (Table 18-1).

Unless the patient has glycosuria or proteinuria, ascitic fluid will test positive and urine will test negative for protein and glucose, confirming that the bladder has not been inadvertently tapped.

COMPLICATIONS

Complications include bleeding, infection, bowel or bladder perforation, and persistent ascitic leak.[61] Hypotension may occur after therapeutic paracentesis if an excessive volume of fluid is withdrawn.[61]

DIAGNOSTIC PERITONEAL LAVAGE

The need for accurate detection of intra-abdominal injury in the trauma patient was first emphasized by Williams and Zollinger in 1959.[63] In 200 patients with blunt abdominal trauma, 80% of deaths were noted to be secondary to intra-abdominal hemorrhage, and one half of these were associated with a delay in diagnosis and treatment. Four quadrant taps (paracentesis) were known to have a high false-negative rate, failing to produce a representative sample of peritoneal fluid. Giacobine and Siler[64] showed a linear relationship in dogs between the amount of blood in the peritoneal space and a positive tap rate. An equivalent of 50 ml of defibrinated intraperitoneal blood yielded no true positives with paracentesis, and a 500-ml equivalent yielded a positive tap rate of only 78%. Root and colleagues demonstrated a 100% accuracy in detecting intraperitoneal blood with 1 liter of lavage fluid,[65] thus introducing peritoneal lavage as an efficacious method of evaluating intra-abdominal hemorrhage in the trauma patient.

Peritoneal lavage is routinely used to evaluate patients with blunt abdominal trauma and altered sensorium, as a result of an associated head injury or from other factors, including

TABLE 18-1 ASCITIC FLUID CHARACTERISTICS IN VARIOUS DISEASE-STATES

Condition	Gross Appearance	Specific Gravity	Protein (g/dl)	Cell Count		Other Tests
				Red Blood Cells (>10,000/mm³)	White Blood Cells (per mm³)	
Cirrhosis	Straw-colored or bile-stained	<1.016 (95%)*	<2.5 (95%)	1%	<250 (90%):* predominantly endothelial	
Neoplasm	Straw-colored, hemorrhagic, mucinous, or chylous	Variable, >1.016 (45%)	>2.5 (75%)	20%	>1000 (50%): variable cell types	Cytology, cell block, peritoneal biopsy
Tuberculous peritonitis	Clear, turbid, hemorrhagic, chylous	Variable, >1.016 (50%)	>2.5 (50%)	7%	>1000 (70%): usually >70% lymphocytes	Peritoneal biopsy, stain and culture for acid-fast bacilli
Pyogenic peritonitis	Turbid or purulent	If purulent, >1.016	If purulent, >2.5	Unusual	Predominantly polymorphonuclear leukocytes	+ Gram's stain, culture
Congestive heart failure	Straw-colored	Variable, <1.016 (60%)	Variable, 1.5–5.3	10%	<1000 (90%): usually mesothelial, mononuclear	
Nephrosis	Straw-colored or chylous	<1.016	<2.5 (100%)	Unusual	<250: mesothelial, mononuclear	If chylous, ether extraction, Sudan staining
Pancreatic ascites (pancreatitis, pseudocyst)	Turbid, hemorrhagic, or chylous	Variable, often >1.016	Variable, often >2.5	Variable, may be blood-stained	Variable	Increased amylase in ascitic fluid and serum

*Because the conditions of examining fluid and selecting patients were not identical in each series, the percentage figures (in the parentheses) should be taken as an indication of the order of magnitude rather than as the precise incidence of any abnormal finding.

drug or alcohol ingestion. In addition, peritoneal lavage is used to diagnose intra-abdominal trauma in patients with multiple injuries who require anesthesia for extra-abdominal procedures. More recently diagnostic lavage has been used in penetrating abdominal and thoracic trauma and perhaps may be helpful in the intensive care setting to evaluate nontraumatic intra-abdominal processes.

The only true contraindication to diagnostic peritoneal lavage is when laparotomy is already predetermined. Relative contraindications include a gravid uterus, lower midline abdominal scar (find another entry site), and abdominal wall hematomas (false-positive).

OPEN TECHNIQUE

If possible, take an upright chest radiograph before starting the procedure. Generally, the presence of free air under the diaphragm, suggestive of a perforated viscus, would mitigate against performing peritoneal lavage.

Place the patient in the supine position. Insert a Foley catheter to prevent inadvertent puncture of the bladder. In children, a nasogastric tube is inserted to prevent gastric perforation.

Prepare the skin with povodine–iodine solution and apply sterile drapes. For local anesthesia, administer 1% lidocaine with epinephrine (to minimize skin bleeding at the incision site which may contribute to a false-positive result) using a 25-gauge needle.

A 3- to 4-cm midline infraumbilical skin incision is created, which can be incorporated into a standard midline incision if laparotomy is necessary (Fig. 18-18). Select a different site if a surgical scar is present in the lower midline or if the abdomen is enlarged because of pregnancy. A midline incision above the umbilicus is an acceptable alternative, but do not extend too far cephalad (to avoid encountering the falciform ligament). Continue the incision through the subcutaneous tissue and through the linea alba.

Grasp the fascial edge on each side firmly with towel clips and elevate it to lift the abdominal wall away from the intra-abdominal structures (Fig. 18-19). Isolate the underlying peritoneum and open it under direct vision (Fig. 18-20).

Introduce a gloved finger into the peritoneal cavity to assure that adhesion is not present and to ensure a safe pathway for the lavage catheter. Insert the catheter without the trochar through the small peritoneal rent and carefully advance it into the pelvis (Fig. 18-22). Place a pursestring suture through the peritoneum, around the catheter with a 3-0 chromic suture (Fig. 18-23). Attach a 10-ml syringe to the dialysis catheter for aspiration. If gross blood is aspirated, no further procedure is necessary and laporatomy is indicated. If not, connect an IV infusion set to the catheter and infuse 1 liter of normal saline (15 ml/kg in children[66]). Leave a small amount of the lavage fluid in the container to establish a siphon effect when the container is placed on the floor. Lower the nearly empty saline bottle to the floor for return of the lavage fluid by gravity siphonage (Fig. 18-24). Draw a 50-ml sample of fluid from the connecting tubing during lavage return and submit it to the laboratory for analysis. After removing the catheter, tie the pursestring suture, approximate the linea alba with 2-0 suture material, and close the skin.

CLOSED TECHNIQUE

Although we prefer the open technique to avoid technical complications as a result of direct visualization of the peritoneum, the closed technique is also an accepted alternative. Two

Figure 18-18 A 3- to 4-cm midline infraumbilical skin incision is created, which can be incorporated into a standard midline incision if laparatomy is necessary. A different site is selected if a surgical scar is present in the lower midline.

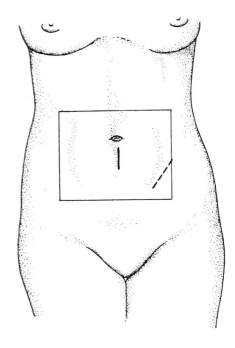

Figure 18-19 The fascial edge is grasped with towel clips and elevated to lift the abdominal wall away from the intra-abdominal structures.

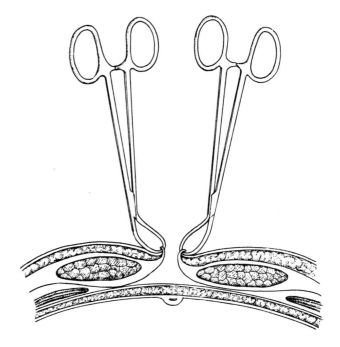

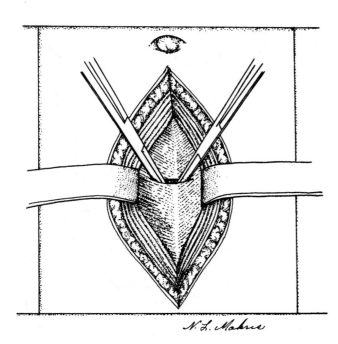

Figure 18-20 The underlying peritoneum is isolated and opened under direct vision.

N. L. Makris

methods are available: a prepackaged kit (Arrow) and a dialysis catheter kit with a trochar (Trocath-McCaw).

The skin preparation, draping, and local anesthesia are the same as for the open technique, as is the decompression of the bladder and stomach.

Dialysis Catheter and Trochar Method

Use a #11 scalpel to incise the skin 2 to 3 cm inferior to the umbilicus in the midline. Continue the incision to the linea alba. Administer more local anesthesia below the linea alba. Insert the trochar/catheter at a 45° angle toward the pelvis. Give a controlled thrust with both hands and stop all pressure when the "pop" through the peritoneum is felt (Fig. 18-24). Advance the catheter over the trochar into the peritoneal cavity and remove the trochar (Fig. 18-25). Connect the catheter to the infusion set and carry out the procedure identically to that of the open method.

Prepackaged Kit

Make a 3-mm skin incision with a #11 blade. Introduce the 18-gauge needle into the peritoneal cavity and angle it toward the center of the pelvis (Fig. 18-26). Then introduce a 15-cm guidewire through the needle (Fig. 18-27). If the wire does not advance easily, remove it and advance the needle. Remove the needle when half of the wire has been introduced. Place the catheter over the guidewire and thread it with a twisting motion to go past the fascia. Remove the guidewire when the catheter is within the abdomen. Proceed with the remainder of the procedure as with the open method.

Figure 18-21 The catheter without the trochar is inserted through the small peritoneal rent and directed into the pelvis.

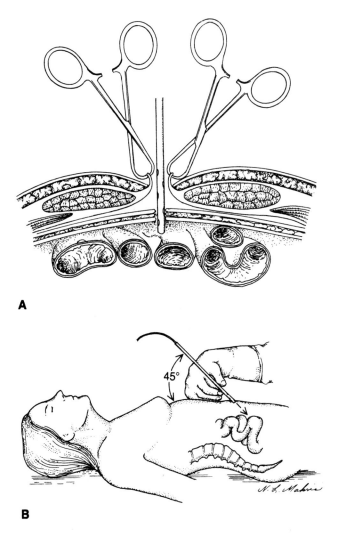

A

B

COMPLICATIONS

Technical complications occur at a rate of 1% to 3%[66] and include wound bleeding, misplacement of the catheter into the preperitoneal space, and perforation of intra-abdominal structures. Introduction of free air into the peritoneal cavity and loss of an accurate abdominal examination have been noted with the midline incision technique. When complications such as wound dehiscence and failure to return lavage fluid are considered, some studies report a complication rate of 9%.[67,68]

RESULTS

Interpretation of the lavage fluid has undergone considerable refinement since first introduced. Initially, positive results were determined by the presence of intra-abdominal hemorrhage alone and used only in blunt trauma. Many studies showed that 20 ml of freely

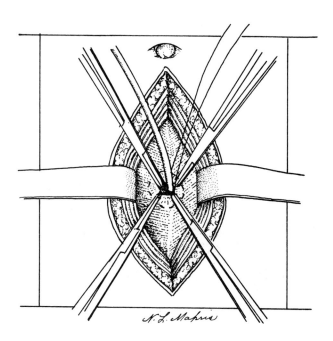

Figure 18-22 A purse-string suture is placed through the peritoneum, around the catheter with a 3-0 chromic suture.

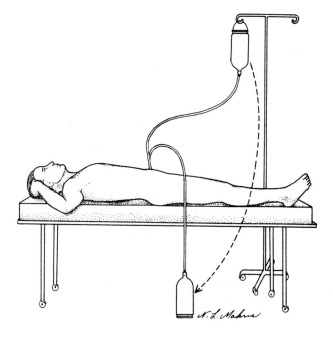

Figure 18-23 The saline bottle is lowered to the floor for return of the lavage fluid by gravity siphonage.

Figure 18-24 The catheter is inserted with a controlled thrust at a 45° angle toward the pelvis.

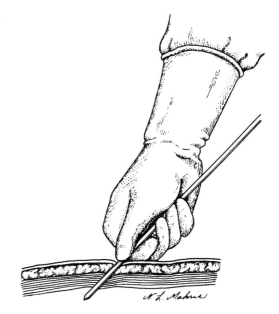

Figure 18-25 The catheter is advanced over the trochar into the peritoneal cavity, and the trochar is removed.

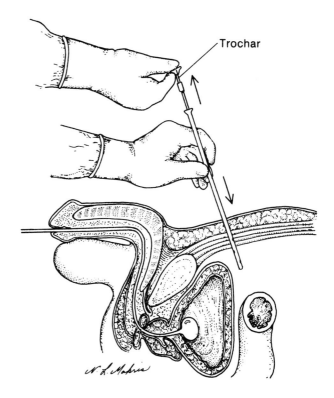

Trochar

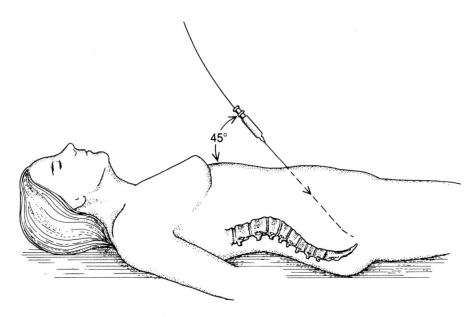

45°

Figure 18-26 The 18-gauge needle is introduced into the peritoneal cavity and angled toward the center of the pelvis.

aspirated gross intraperitoneal blood had a 100% correlation with intraperitoneal injury.[69–71] Peritoneal lavage for blunt trauma has an accuracy rate of 96%.[72] The organ-systems most commonly involved in false-negative studies include ruptured diaphragm, ruptured spleen, lacerated liver, and intraperitoneal bladder rupture.[68,73] When history and physical examination alone are used, the error rate is 25% to 45%.[74–77]

The red blood cell (RBC) count should be measured rather than estimated, and counted on a hemocytometer rather than by Coulter counter, since the latter may falsely increase the count by including macrophages and debris.[78] Other recommendations have included attempting to read newspaper through IV tubing and spinning a hematocrit of the lavage fluid. Cell counts remain the most accurate method of determining a positive lavage (Table 18-2).[69]

Studies in animals have shown that, after injury resulting from a perforated viscus, it may take 3 hours for the white blood cell (WBC) count to become elevated enough to produce a positive result.[79] Most diagnostic peritoneal lavage procedures are performed within several hours of injury, raising concern as to the potential for false-negative studies. However, Engrav and colleagues demonstrated an 83% correlation of significant intraperitoneal injury with an elevated lavage WBC count (>500 cells/mm^3) in early peritoneal lavage, although an unspecified number also had significant hemoperitoneum.[80]

Currently, lavage fluid is routinely sent for RBC and WBC counts and amylase and analyzed for the presence of bile, food particles, and bacteria. All patients with a positive lavage are prepared for exploratory laparotomy. The management of indeterminate lavage results remains controversial, and some have suggested repeated lavage in several hours.[81,82]

Several studies have evaluated the efficacy of diagnostic peritoneal lavage in penetrating trauma. Most institutions consider gunshot wounds to the anterior abdomen as an absolute indication for exploratory laparotomy. Thal and associates performed diagnostic

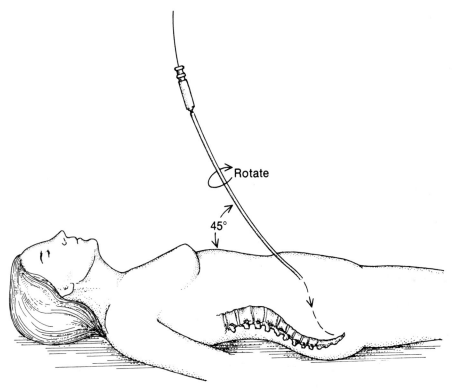

Figure 18-27 A 15-cm guidewire is introduced through the needle. The needle is removed when half of the wire has been introduced. The catheter is placed over the guidewire and threaded with a twisting motion to go past the fascia.

peritoneal lavage in patients with gunshot wounds to the lower chest and anterior abdomen before exploratory laporatomy and found a false-negative rate of 25%, using a lavage fluid RBC count greater than 100,000 as criteria for a positive result.[83] Merlotti and coworkers performed diagnostic peritoneal lavage on patients with penetrating trauma between the nipples and subcostal margins, with flank and back trauma, and with tangential gunshot wounds to the anterior abdominal wall.[84] In this study, an RBC count of greater than 10,000 was considered positive. There was a 13.6% false-positive and 1% false-negative rate, with

TABLE 18-2 INTERPRETATION OF PERITONEAL LAVAGE

Positive
  Aspiration of >10 ml of blood
  Lavage fluid exits by means of Foley catheter
    or chest tube
  Grossly bloody lavage return
  RBC >100,000/mm^3
  WBC >500/mm^3
  Amylase >175 U/dl
  Presence of bile, bacteria, or particulate matter

Negative (nonpenetrating trauma)
  RBC <50,000/mm^3
  WBC <100/mm^3
  Amylase <75 U/dl

Indeterminant
  Dialysis catheter fills with blood
  RBC >50,000–<100,000/mm^3
  WBC >100–<500/mm^3
  Amylase >75–<175 U/dl

an overall accuracy rate of 96.6%. If one had used 100,000 RBC/mm^3 as being diagnostic of a positive lavage, then there would have been no false-positives but a prohibitively high false-negative rate of 11.1%. Similarly, Thal evaluated patients with stab wounds below the fifth intercostal space between anterior axillary lines or if local exploration of an anterior abdominal stab wound showed penetration of the posterior fascia.[85] With greater than 100,000 RBC considered as a positive lavage, the false-positive rate was 2.4%. However, the false-negative rate of 4.9% included patients with serious visceral injuries that could have caused serious morbidity if missed.

Diagnostic peritoneal lavage has recently been noted to be useful for evaluating suspected nontraumatic peritonitis in elderly patients or in those with altered sensorium and an uninterpretable abdominal examination.[86,87] In general, surgery was performed if there was an elevated WBC count (>500 mm^3) in the lavage fluid.

Overall a diagnostic peritoneal lavage is believed to be reliable, safe, and efficacious in rapidly detecting intra-abdominal injury and leads to an organized plan of care in the trauma patient.

VENOUS CUTDOWN

The need to perform venous cutdowns has diminished as a result of the improved techniques and technology for cannulating the central venous space. On occasion the venous cutdown may be helpful in caring for the markedly hypovolemic patient who requires urgent IV therapy when the veins are collapsed and a large caliber conduit is needed for fluid and blood administration or in the rare instance when percutaneous central or peripheral venous cannulation is unsuccessful (Table 18-3). Multiple access sites are available, and anatomic knowledge and attention to technique are essential for successful cannulation.

PROCEDURE

Prepare the skin with 10% povodine-iodine solution and apply sterile drapes. Administer lidocaine 1% without epinephrine as local anesthesia by means of a 25-gauge needle (Fig. 18-28). Make a 2- to 3-cm transverse incision over the vein (Fig. 18-29). Mobilize a 2-cm segment of the vein with blunt dissection (Fig. 18-30). Pass two silk ligatures beneath the vein and place the distal suture on tension by attaching to the drapes with a Kelly clamp (Fig. 18-31). Insert the catheter percutaneously through the skin distal to the cutdown incision. Place tension on the distal ligature and insert the cannula into the vein with the bevel facing the back wall (Fig. 18-32). Relax the proximal ligature and advance the plastic cannula. Remove the inner needle. Assure good backflow of blood to confirm the position

TABLE 18-3 SALINE FLOW RATES THROUGH VARIOUS CATHETERS

Catheter Type	Diameter	Length (in)	Flow Rate (Gravity) (ml/sec)	Flow Rate (Pressure) (ml/sec)
Deseret Intracath	16 g	8	1.6	2.5
Vicra Quik-Cath	14 g	2	2.9	4.8
McGaw Extension Set	3 mm	12	3.6	6.5

Figure 18-28 Lidocaine 1% is used as local anesthesia.

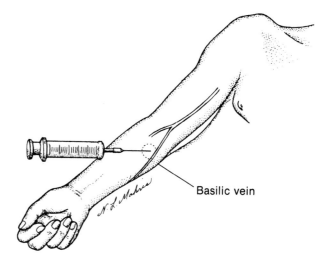

Basilic vein

of the catheter in the lumen of the vein. Connect the IV tubing and suture the skin with 3–0 nylon. Secure the cannula to the skin at the exit point.

Alternatively, use a catheter with the cannula within the needle. Pass the 14-gauge needle through the skin, from inside out (Fig. 18-33), then pass the cannula through the needle, from outside in. Remove the needle (Fig. 18-34). Incise the vein with a #11 blade, first by hemisecting the vein in the horizontal plane and then by turning the blade 90° upward. This will create a flap that will extend through the radius of the vein and allow easy access for the venous cannula (Fig. 18-35). Insert the cannula into the vein. A mosquito clamp may be needed to dilate the vein and guide the catheter (Fig. 18-36). Close the skin and secure as described above.

Preferred sites of veins include the median basilic, basilic, and cephalic veins. The proximal saphenous vein can be used when other sites are not available or when intravenous tubing is inserted in the vein directly to achieve high infusion rates ("Vietnam" lines).

Ankle

The saphenous vein begins at the junction of the medial end of the dorsal venous arch of the foot and the medial dorsal vein of the great toe. The vein ascends anterior to the medial

Figure 18-29 Make a 2- to 3-cm transverse incision over the vein.

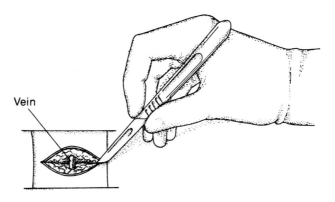

Vein

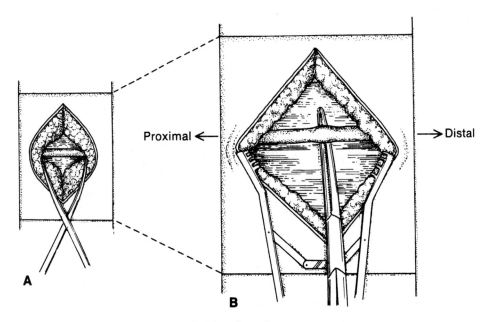

Figure 18-30 The vein is mobilized with blunt dissection.

Figure 18-31 Pass two silk ligatures beneath the vein and place the distal suture on tension by attaching to the drape with a Kelly clamp.

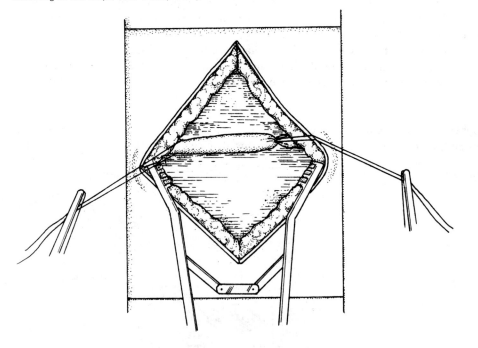

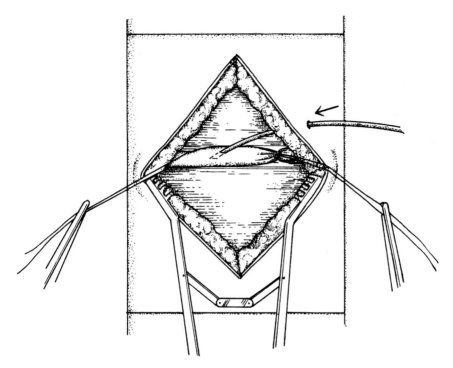

Figure 18-32 Insert the catheter percutaneously through the skin distal to the cutdown incision. Place tension on the distal ligature and insert the cannula into the vein with the bevel facing the back wall.

malleolus, where it lies on tough periosteum (Fig. 18-37). The only associated structure at this point is the terminal segment of the saphenous nerve.[88]

The advantage of using this vein is that it can be cannulated during an arrest situation when most of the clinical activity is centered around the upper torso. Access using this vein should be converted to another site when clinically feasible. Potential disadvantages include thrombophlebitis and loss of a vein valuable for arterial bypass. This site should not be used if there is suspicion that the inferior vena cava and femoral or iliac veins are disrupted.[89]

Groin

The proximal saphenous vein is 4 to 5 mm in diameter and joins the femoral vein 3 in inferior to the inguinal ligament, along the anteromedial aspect of the thigh. The proximal saphenous vein may be confused with the anterior lateral femoral vein, which is smaller (2–3 mm) and more anterior.[88]

Rotate the thigh externally and make a transverse incision in the anterior medial thigh 5 cm distal to the femoral pulse. The saphenous vein is medial to the femoral artery (Fig. 18-38).

If no pulse is palpable, make the incision 5 cm below the junction of the medial and middle thirds of the inguinal ligament. The incision should be 5 to 7 cm long. Bluntly dissect the subcutaneous tissue (Fig. 18-39).

Intracath
needle

Intracath
cannula

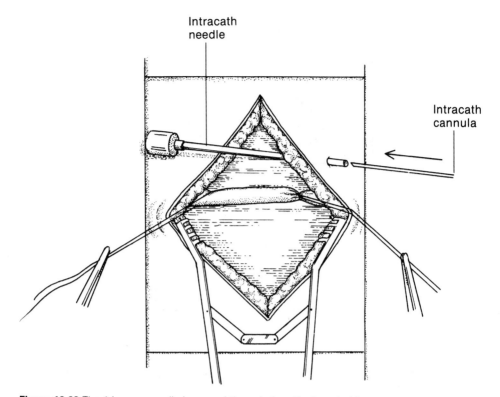

Figure 18-33 The 14-gauge needle is passed through the skin, from inside out.

The "Vietnam" catheter uses a beveled IV extension tubing inserted 8 to 12 cm into the vein. This is used when maximal fluid and blood infusion rates are needed.[90]

The disadvantages of this method include anatomic variability and loss of a potential vein for coronary artery bypass, arterial reconstruction, and dialysis.[89]

Antecubital Fossa

The basilic vein is a continuation of the ulnar end of the dorsal venous arch of the hand. The vein ascends along the ulnar border of the forearm into the antecubital fossa anterior to the medial epicondyle. After the vein is joined by the median antecubital vein it ascends in the bicipital groove, accompanied by the medial cutaneous nerve (see Fig. 18-40).[88]

Make the incision 1 to 2 cm lateral and superior to the medial epicondyle of the humerus. Alternatively, extend the skin incision from the brachial artery pulse at the proximal flexor crease of the antecubital fossa toward the medial epicondyle.

The advantages of the approach are the consistently large diameter of the vein, the superficial location, and the capability to place a long line for central venous pressure measurement.[89]

Damage to the medial cutaneous nerve results in loss of sensation over the medial aspect of the forearm. Deeper dissection presents a risk to the brachial artery and median nerve.

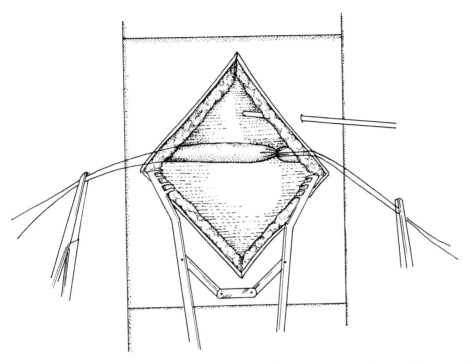

Figure 18-34 The cannula is passed through the needle, from outside in, and the needle is removed.

Figure 18-35 Incise the vein by hemisecting the vein in the horizontal plane and turning the blade 90° upward.

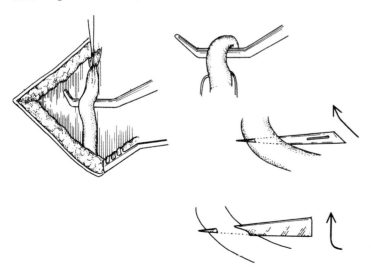

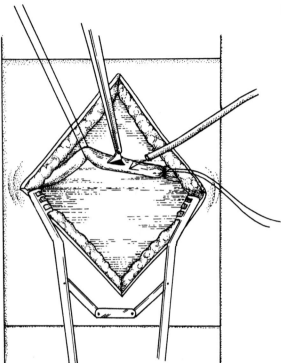

Figure 18-36 Insert the cannula into the vein.

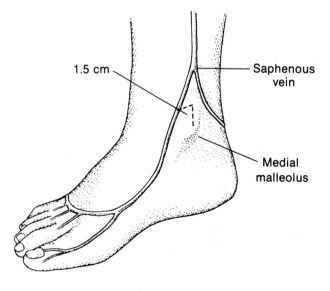

Figure 18-37 The saphenous vein.

1.5 cm

Saphenous vein

Medial malleolus

Figure 18-38 The proximal saphenous vein.

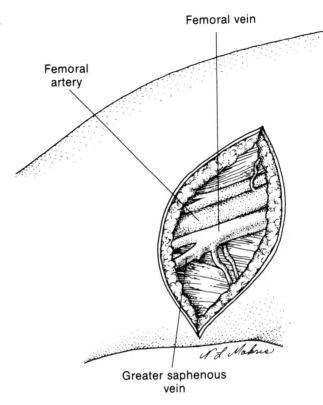

Femoral vein

Femoral artery

Greater saphenous vein

Figure 18-39 Femoral artery runs directly across midpoint of line drawn between anterior superior iliac spine and symphysis pubis.

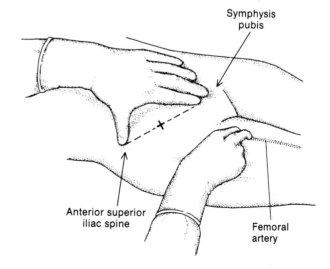

Symphysis pubis

Anterior superior iliac spine

Femoral artery

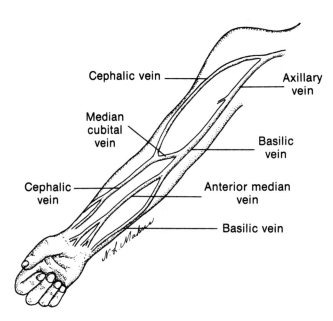

Figure 18-40 The basilic and cephalic veins.

Cephalic vein

Axillary vein

Median cubital vein

Basilic vein

Cephalic vein

Anterior median vein

Basilic vein

The cephalic vein is a radial continuation of the dorsal venous arch of the hand and ascends parallel to the brachioradialis muscle into the antecubital fossa. At the point where it connects with the basilic vein by the obliquely ascending median cubital vein, the diameter may be greatly reduced in size. The vein ascends in the lateral bicipital groove to the deltopectoral groove and empties into the axillary vein (see Fig. 18-40).[88] Make the incision at the distal flexor crease of the antecubital fossa lateral to the midline.

The disadvantage of this approach is the variability in size of the vein. In addition, this method cannot be easily used for central venous access because the vein traverses the clavipectoral fascia at right angles, making passage into the central venous system difficult.[89]

COMPLICATIONS

Local complications of venous cutdown include thrombophlebitis. Because most cutdowns are placed during initial fluid resuscitation of hemorrhagic shock, sterile technique is often compromised, leading to an increased incidence of phlebitis. Therefore emergency cutdowns should be removed within 24 hours.[89]

Generalized sepsis is a more serious complication of venous cutdowns. In addition to early removal of contaminated or infected catheters, precautionary measures to prevent contamination include secure fixation of the cannula to avoid the to-and-fro movement, keeping the puncture site dry and sterile, and avoiding antibiotic ointment, which encourages fungal growth.[91]

DEFIBRILLATION

Ventricular fibrillation is the most disorganized of all dysrhythmias and is thought to be maintained by a "critical mass" of fibrillating myocardium.[92] The only practical treatment for ventricular fibrillation is electrical defibrillation, which is dependent upon depolarizing a sufficient portion of the fibrillating ventricle.

Defibrillation was first described in 1899 by Prevost and Batelli.[93] The first successful human defibrillation was 1947 with an open chest technique.[94] Initially AC defibrillators were used but have since been replaced by DC monophasic defibrillators, which are more effective, portable, and less dangerous.[95,96] The strength of energy delivery is expressed in joules (J) or watt-seconds (Wsec; product of power and duration) and produces several thousand volts during a 4- to 12-msec monophasic energy delivery.[97]

The indication for defibrillation is ventricular fibrillation that does not revert with a precordial thump.[98] The patient is defibrillated initially with 200 to 300 J and the paddles left in place. If ventricular fibrillation continues, the patient is defibrillated again immediately while the transthoracic resistance is reduced.[99] Basic life support is continued if ventricular fibrillation persists, epinephrine is given IV, and defibrillation is attempted again.

PROCEDURE

Turn the cardioverter on and the synchronizer switch off. Select the energy level (usually 200–300 watt-seconds). Apply electrode jelly to the paddles. (Do not use alcohol pads.) Apply one paddle below the right clavicle just lateral to the upper sternum and one just lateral to the left nipple in the anterior axillary line (Fig. 18-41). Assure that there is no patient or bed

Figure 18-41 Apply the paddles—one below the right clavicle just lateral to the upper sternum and one just lateral to the left nipple in the anterior axillary line.

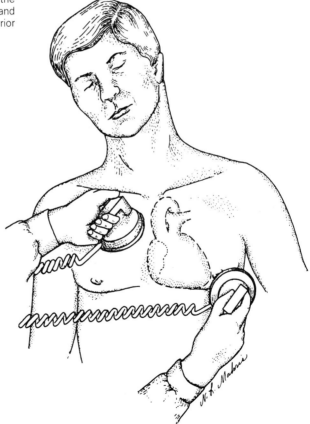

contact by the operator or assistants. Administer the shock. Check the pulse, EKG, and airway. If unsuccessful, continue CPR and repeat at 300 and 360 J.

COMPLICATIONS

Complications include asystole, unsuccessful defibrillation, and skin burns from inadequate electrode contact to skin (caused either by arcing or inadequate amount of electrode jelly).[100]

Pacemaker failure has been noted infrequently after defibrillation. Diodes were incorporated into the pacer circuitry in the early 1960s, giving them a degree of safety from shocks of less than 400 Wsec.[101] Recommendations for defibrillation in pacemaker patients include use of low energy, placement of the paddles in the anterior–posterior position at least 10 cm from electrodes and pulse generator, reconfirmation of pacemaker function after shock, and availability of a standby temporary pacemaker.[101–107]

The success of defibrillation depends on many factors. The longer the duration of ventricular fibrillation, the less likely it is that electrical defibrillation will be successful.[98] The environment and the condition of the myocardium are extremely important, and poor outcome is associated with hypoxemia, acidosis, hypothermia, electrolyte imbalance, and drug toxicity.[108] A larger heart size is associated with a larger critical fibrillating mass and thought to require more energy delivery for defibrillation.[109] A relation between body weight and energy requirements has been shown in animal studies, although this association has not been proved in humans.[110,111] Previous countershocks delivered tend to diminish transthoracic resistance, thereby decreasing energy requirements.[112] The ideal paddle size for defibrillators in adults has not yet been established, but current recommendations suggest a 10- to 13-cm diameter.[113,114] The paddle–skin interface is best with a low impedance medium.[115,116] Alcohol may ignite and should not be used. Firm pressure with the paddles can improve energy delivery, and paddle contact pressure of about 10 kg (25 lb) can decrease the transthoracic resistance by 25%.[114]

CARDIOVERSION

Cardioversion is used to treat ventricular and supraventricular tachydysrhythmias in clinical settings that mandate rapid dysrhythmia termination to prevent further clinical deterioration (*i.e.*, severe hypotension, chest pain).

Figure 18-42 Atrial tachycardia. Initially, normal sinus rhythm is present. This is interrupted by PAC (*arrow*) which initiates episode of atrial tachycardia with rate of 185/min. The proposed reentry mechanism at AV node level is illustrated ladder diagram. Abbreviations: *A*, atrium; *AVN*, AV node; *V*, ventricle.

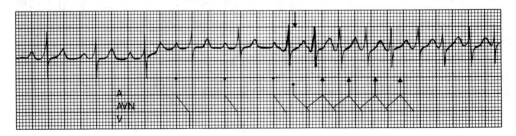

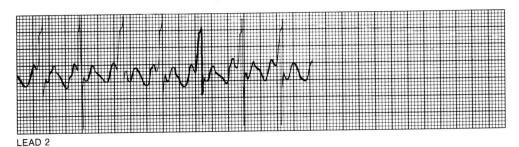

LEAD 2

Figure 18-43 Atrial flutter. Atrial rate is 250/min and rhythm is regular. Every other F wave is conducted to ventricles (2:1 block) resulting in regular ventricular rhythm at rate of 125/min.

Paroxysmal atrial tachycardia (PAT) is characterized by the sudden onset of repeated episodes of atrial tachycardia (Fig. 18-42).[117,118] The episodes last several minutes to hours and usually end abruptly. The dysrhythmia is thought to be due to a re-entrant phenomenon and the EKG findings include 1:1 AV conduction or 2:1 conduction when the atrial rate exceeds 200.

Atrial flutter is due to re-entry at the atrial level and seldom occurs without organic heart disease (Fig. 18-43).[98] Atrial flutter is usually the intermediate rhythm between normal sinus rhythm and atrial fibrillation. Characteristic EKG findings include flutter (F) waves at a regular rate of about 300. The ventricular rate is regular with constant conduction, usually at a ratio of 2:1.

Atrial fibrillation results from multiple ectopic foci, each depolarizing only a small islet of atrial myocardium (Fig. 18-44).[98] Impulses are randomly transmitted through the AV node, causing an irregular ventricular rhythm of 160 to 180. No P waves are visible on EKG.

Ventricular tachycardia is defined as three or more consecutive beats of ventricular origin (Fig. 18-45).[119] The dysrhythmia may be well tolerated or may be life-threatening, which usually depends on the presence or absence of underlying myocardial dysfunction. Cardioversion is not indicated for dysrhythmias possibly related to digitalis toxicity.

A synchronizing circuit allows the delivery of a countershock to be "programmed" to occur during a specific part of the QRS complex. This has been shown to reduce energy requirements and secondary complicating dysrhythmias.

Figure 18-44 Atrial fibrillation with controlled ventricular response. Note irregular undulations of baseline representing atrial electrical activity (f waves). The f waves vary in size and shape and are irregular in rhythm. Conduction through AV node occurs at random, hence ventricular rhythm is irregular.

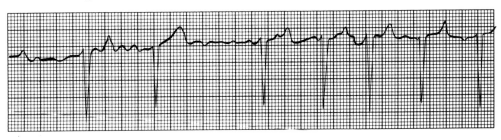

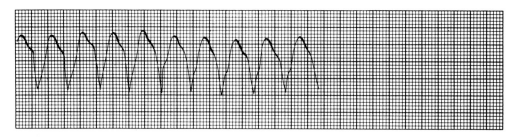

Figure 18-45 Ventricular tachycardia. The rhythm is regular at rate of 158/min. The QRS is wide. No evidence of atrial depolarization is seen.

PROCEDURE

Attach the patient's electrodes to the cardioverter for sensing. Turn the cardioverter and the synchronizer switch on. Use the lead with an upright QRS complex and maximum R-wave height, since the inverted QRS may not trigger the synchronizing circuit or may cause discharge on the T wave.

Select the appropriate energy level: ventricular tachycardia, 200 Wsec; atrial arrhythmias, begin at 10 Wsec if patient is on digitalis and increase sequentially to 50, 100, 200, 300, or 400 Wsec if needed. Ninety-five percent with atrial flutter have their rhythm corrected with less than 50 Wsec, whereas 95% of patients with atrial fibrillation revert with less than 200 Wsec.[100]

If the patient is awake, give an amnesic drug, such as diazepam (Valium), 5mg initially with 2.5 mg IV additionally every 2 minutes until sedation and amnesia are obtained, or methohexital (Brevital), 1 mg/kg IV, while monitoring blood pressure and respiratory rate. Apply electrode jelly to the paddles. Assure that the operator has no patient or bed contact. Administer the shock, holding the firing buttons down until the patient receives the current. Check the pulse, EKG, and airway. If the rhythm does not revert, increase the energy level and repeat the cardioversion. If ventricular fibrillation develops, turn off the synchronizer circuit, charge to 200 to 300 J, and defibrillate.

COMPLICATIONS

Complications include additional cardiac dysrhythmias, most being transient and innocuous.[120] Serious dysrhythmias are related to high electrical discharge, overdigitalization, severity of the heart disease, and electrolyte abnormalities. Animal studies have demonstrated a 2000-fold increase in sensitivity to electrical discharge with ouabain toxicity, manifested by ventricular tachycardia.[121] Electric shock releases cardiac potassium, which is accentuated in digitalized patients.[122] Ventricular fibrillation after cardioversion is usually related to improper synchronization and begins immediately after the shock.[120] Late onset of ventricular fibrillation suggests digitalis or quinidine toxicity.[123–125]

Transient elevations of CPK and LDH enzymes have been noted with repeated high-energy shocks,[126,127] but cardioversion rarely obscures the diagnosis of myocardial infarction and rarely are both enzymes elevated from cardioversion alone.

Pulmonary edema may occur immediately or up to several hours after cardioversion.[128] The cause is not known but postulated to be related to delayed return of left atrial function.

Systemic embolization after cardioversion in patients with atrial fibrillation occurs in

1.2% to 1.5% of those reverted to sinus rhythm.[129,130] Anticoagulation is recommended for 3 weeks before and 4 weeks after cardioversion if the atrial fibrillation has been present for more than a week.[99,120]

PRECORDIAL THUMP

The precordial thump is effective in evoking ventricular depolarization. The precordial thump is used only in two monitored situations: The first indication is the monitored, witnessed onset of ventricular tachycardia or ventricular fibrillation; the second situation is during ventricular asystole caused by complete heart block when rhythmic thumps produce a QRS complex and associated myocardial contraction (pulse) until a pacemaker is inserted. The precordial thump is not recommended in the pediatric population.[98]

PERICARDIOCENTESIS

Pericardiocentesis is indicated for the relief of cardiac tamponade or when a fluid sample would be helpful for the etiologic diagnosis of a pericardial effusion.

PROCEDURE

Place the pateint in the supine position or with the upper torso elevated 20° to 30°. Atropine may be used as a premedication to prevent vagal reactions associated with pericardial puncture. Lidocaine without epinephrine should be used as the local anesthetic. The paraxiphoid subcostal approach is most common and avoids both the pleura and the coronary vessels. The left parasternal approach through the fourth intercostal space may also be used (Fig. 18-46).

Attach a long (12–18 cm) large bore (16–18 gauge) cardiac needle with a short bevel (to minimize the risk of cardiac laceration) to a 50-ml syringe. Connect the metal needle to the V lead of the EKG with a sterile alligator clip and place a 10-ml syringe on the needle

Figure 18-46 The paraxiphoid approach is most common and avoids both the pleura and coronary vessels.

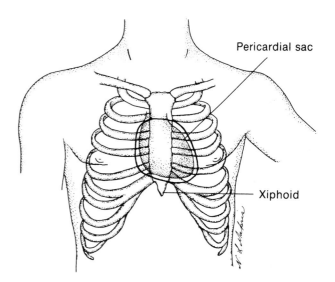

Pericardial sac

Xiphoid

(Fig. 18-47). For the paraxiphoid approach, enter the skin just below the costal margin adjacent to the xiphoid and advance the needle slowly at a 45° horizontal angle under the ribs toward the midpoint of the left clavicle. Apply gentle suction to the syringe.

For the left parasternal approach, advance the needle slowly through the fourth intercostal space just at the sternal border and perpendicular to the chest wall. Insert the needle in the anesthetized tract. When the needle tip is deep to the costal arch, depress the hub and advance the needle toward the left shoulder, aspirating during advancement. Monitor for injury current. ST elevation is present with ventricular epicardial contact (Fig. 18-49), and PR segment elevation is present with atrial epicardial contact. With epicardial contact, withdraw the needle slightly or reposition. If fluid is not obtained, redirect the needle toward the head or right shoulder. A characteristic resistance of the pericardium may often be felt at the needle tip. A "popping" sensation may be noted as the pericardium is penetrated.

When fluid is returned, the needle is stabilized by attaching a hemostat at the skin surface, preventing inadvertent overpenetration and also providing depth reference for future aspiration attempts. Removal of as little as 25 to 50 ml of blood may result in immediate

Figure 18-47 Connect the metal needle to the V lead of the EKG with a sterile alligator clip and place a 10-ml syringe on the needle.

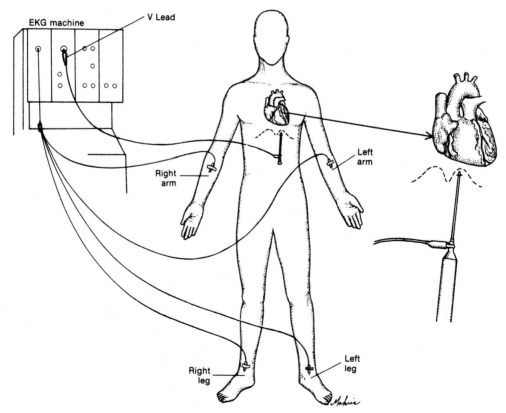

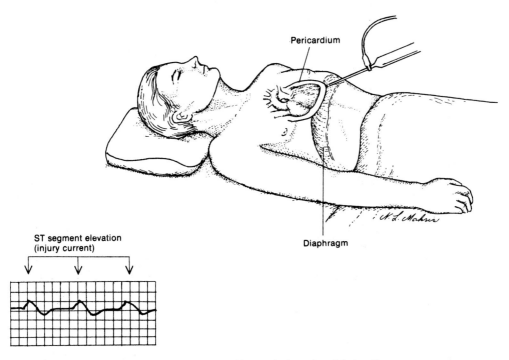

Figure 18-48 ST segment elevation is present with ventricular epicardial elevation.

improvement in the patient's condition, with a decrease in venous pressure and rise in systolic pressure.

The beating heart usually defibrinates blood that has been in the pericardial space. Clotting suggests that a cardiac chamber has been entered inadvertently.

If no improvement in the patient's condition occurs after aspiration for suspected acute traumatic tamponade, immediate thoracotomy is mandatory. Pericardiocentesis to remove bloody fluid following trauma should be considered a temporary measure to be followed in most cases by thoracotomy. If V-lead monitoring from the pericardiocentesis needle is not feasible, an alternate approach is to use a 20-gauge spinal needle as an exploring needle over which a 14-gauge needle has been placed. Once the pericardial space has been entered with the spinal needle, the large-bore needle is advanced over the spinal needle into the pericardial space and the spinal needle is removed.

The pericardial sac normally contains up to 50 ml of fluid, which has the same composition as serum.[131]. Pericardial tamponade results from the accumulation of fluid within the pericardial sac, which restricts ventricular diastolic filling and reduces stroke volume, cardiac output, and arterial blood pressure.[132–135] The fluid emanates from trauma, infection, or neoplastic diseases.[136] As intrapericardial pressure rises, systemic arterial pressure cannot be maintained, and Beck's triad of hypotension, increased venous pressure, and a small quiet heart is often fulfilled.[132,137] Volume infusion to increase ventricular filling pressure will likely help to maintain adequate systemic pressure while the clinician prepares for pericardiocentesis.[138]

The earliest response to increased intrapericardial pressure is a compensatory increase in central venous pressure; thus an elevated central venous pressure is seen in nearly all cases of cardiac tamponade.[132–137,139] The Y descent in the venous pulse and early filling dip in the ventricles are diminished with inhibition of early ventricular filling with increased intrapericardial pressure during diastole. Equalization of intracardiac pressures (CVP, RA, LA, PCWP, LV, RV) is noted during diastole when measured by pulmonary artery catheterization. In the face of left ventricular dysfunction, left-sided filling pressures will exceed the RA and RV, but right-sided filling pressures will still be elevated and equal to pericardial pressures.[132–137,139]

Pulsus paradoxus (greater than 10 mm Hg decline in systolic arterial pressure with normal inspiration), usually present in pericardial tamponade, is due to a leftward shift of the septum as the ventricles compete for space within the distended pericardial sac. This leads to selective impairment of ventricular filling.[132–137,139] Reduced ventricular filling also results from increased pulmonary venous capacitance owing to the discrepancy in intrapericardial pressure and pulmonary venous pressure.[132–137,139] Pulsus paradoxus may be difficult to detect in the presence of severe hypotension, cardiac dysrhythmias, or erratic respiratory patterns. Direct arterial tracings may be more sensitive in detecting respiratory variation than is cuff measurement. Pulsus paradoxus may occur in other disease-states such as obstructive airway disease, restrictive cardiomyopathy, constrictive pericarditis, hypovolemia, or mechanical ventilation.[139]

Narrowing of the pulse pressure occurs with rising systemic vascular resistance and decreased stroke volume. Hypotension is a late finding in pericardial tamponade.[132–137,139]

The chest radiograph may show evidence of a pericardial effusion with an enlarged cardiac silhouette, although it is rarely helpful in acute pericardial tamponade. Although bulging sac-like and globular heart shapes are characteristic for pericardial effusion, no size or shape is obligatory.[140] Patients with acute tamponade can die with as little as 200 ml of pericardial fluid, yet 300 ml or more may be present without a detectable increase in cardiac silhouette. Subtle clues may be noted acutely, such as a central venous catheter lodged against the right atrial wall but more than 5 mm from the cardiac silhouette, indicating an effusion.[140]

The echocardiogram may show evidence of pericardial effusion or right ventricular compression indicative of tamponade.[141–144] The right ventricular compression resolves after pericardiocentesis.

The EKG may show low voltage and nonspecific ST-T wave changes. Electrical alternans may be present, showing beat-to-beat changes in the axis as the heart swings within the pericardial effusion.[145] Electromechanical dissociation may be a manifestation of pericardial tamponade.[132–137,139]

Needle pericardiocentesis is indicated for cardiac tamponade when it is immediately life-threatening or when it is progressive and produces increasingly severe hemodynamic impairment. Pericardiocentesis should be performed for any patient with acute tamponade in whom systolic blood pressure has fallen >30 mm Hg from the baseline level.[131,146]

COMPLICATIONS

A complication of pericardiocentesis includes ventricular puncture, which usually has no sequelae. The patient should be observed for tamponade.[147] Cardiac dysrhythmias and laceration of the cardiac chambers or coronary arteries are potential complications, as are hydrothorax and pneumothorax.[136,146,147]

TRANSTRACHEAL ASPIRATION

Transtracheal aspiration was first described by Pecora and Brook in 1959 after the discovery that sputum specimens did not accurately reflect the bacteriology of the lower respiratory tract because of contamination with mouth organisms.[148] More recently, studies have shown that transtracheal aspiration is efficacious in documenting anaerobic pulmonary infections.[149] Currently transtracheal aspiration is used to obtain a sputum specimen in the nonintubated patient who cannot raise sputum or who is likely to be infected with an unusual organism.

PROCEDURE

Place the patient in the supine position with a pillow or roll under the shoulders to extend the neck. Locate the cricothyroid space (Fig. 18-49). Inject the local anesthetic, first raising a skin wheal, then infiltrating down to the membrane. Avoid injecting the lidocaine into the trachea—it is bacteriostatic. Puncture the cricothyroid membrane with a 14-gauge Intracath needle, with the bevel up on a syringe. Aim caudally and 45° to the skin. Thrust the needle through the membrane. Aspirate to confirm intratracheal position. Remove the syringe. Quickly thread the catheter down into the trachea. Remove the stylette and slide the needle from the trachea over the cannula (Fig. 18-51). Aspirate the specimen during cough only. If the specimen is inadequate, inject 2 to 3 ml of sterile, nonbacteriostatic saline

Figure 18-49 Locate the cricothyroid space.

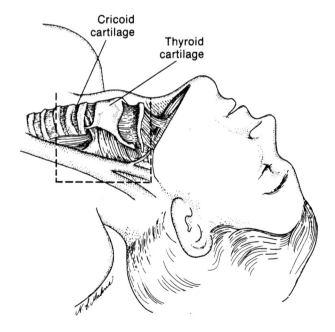

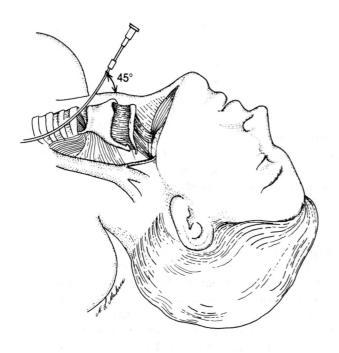

Figure 18-50 Thread the catheter down into the trachea. Remove the stylette, and slide the needle out of the trachea over the cannula.

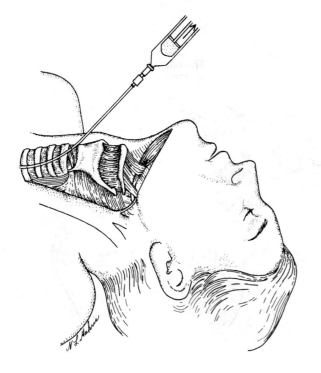

Figure 18-51 Aspirate the specimen during cough only.

and aspirate again (Fig. 18-51). Remove the syringe and inoculate the media immediately. Withdraw the catheter and needle as a single unit and apply a dressing.

COMPLICATIONS

Because complications include bleeding into the trachea, evaluation for bleeding diathesis should be performed before the study. Cardiac arrest may be caused by vagal stimulation in a hypoxemic patient. Infection is rare. Subcutaneous emphysema has been reported to be more prominent in patients with persistent coughing after the procedure, and the incidence was less if the patient was placed at bedrest for 8 to 12 hours.[150,151]

REFERENCES

1. Langston HT: The thorax, pleura and lungs. In Davis L (ed): *Christopher's Textbook of Surgery.* Philadelphia, WB Saunders, 1968
2. Gott PH: A simplified method for thoracentesis and pleural fluid drainage. *Am Rev Respir Dis* 1965; 92:295
3. Hoffman L: A modified thoracentesis technique. *Am Rev Respir Dis* 1964; 89:106
4. Light RW, Girard WM, Jenkinson SG, et al: Parapneumonic effusions. *Am J Med* 1980; 69:507
5. Light RW: Parapneumonic effusions and empyema. *Clin Chest Med* 1985; 6:55
6. Light RW, MacGregor MI, Luchsinger PC, et al: Pleural effusions: The diagnostic separation of transudates and exudates. *Ann Intern Med* 1972; 77:507
7. Light RW, Ball WC Jr: Glucose and amylase in pleural effusions. *JAMA* 1973; 225:257
8. Light RW, MacGregor MI, Ball WC Jr, et al: Diagnostic significance of pleural fluid pH and PCO_2. *Chest* 1973; 64:591
9. Potts DE, Levin DC, Sahn SA: Pleural pH in parapneumonic effusions. *Chest* 1976; 70:328
10. Light RW: Management of parapneumonic effusions. *Chest* 1976; 70:325
11. Hewett FC: Thoracentesis: The plan of continuous aspiration. *Br Med J* 1876; 1:317
12. Betts RH, Less WM: Military thoracic surgery in forward area. *J Thorac Surg* 1946; 15:44
13. Kovarik JL, Brown RK: Tube and trochar thoracostomy. *Surg Clin North Am* 1969; 49:1455
14. Melton LJ III, Hepper WG, Offord KP: Influence of height on the risk of spontaneous pneumothorax. *Mayo Clin Proc* 1981; 56:678
15. Rutherford RB: Thoracic injuries. In Ballinger (ed): *The Management of Trauma,* 2nd ed. Philadelphia, WB Saunders, 1973
16. Cordice JWV, Cabezon J: Chest trauma with pneumothorax and hemothorax. Review of experience with 502 cases. *J Cardiovasc Thorac Surg* 1965; 50:316
17. Kattan KR: Trauma of the bony thorax. *Semin Roentgenol* 1978; 13:69
18. Kircher LT Jr, Swartzel RL: Spontaneous pneumothorax and its treatment. *JAMA* 1954; 155:24
19. Greene R, McCloud TC, Stark P: Pneumothorax. *Semin Roentgenol* 1977; 12:313
20. Rhea JT, Deluca SA, Greene RE: Determining the size of pneumothorax in the upright patient. *Radiology* 1982; 144:733
21. Sabiston DC, Spencer FC: *Gibbon's Surgery of the Chest,* 3rd ed. Philadelphia, WB Saunders, 1976
22. Vukich DJ: Pneumothorax, hemothorax, and other abnormalities of the pleural space. *Emerg Med Clin North Am* 1983; 1:431
23. Zimmerman JE, Dunbar RS, Klingenmaier CH: Management of subcutaneous emphysema, pneumomediastinum and pneumothorax during respirator therapy. *Crit Care Med* 1975; 3:69
24. Zwillich DW, Pierson DJ, Creagh CE, et al: Complications of assisted ventilation. A prospective study of 354 consecutive cases. *Am J Med* 1974; 57:161
25. Bernard RW, Stahl WM: Subclavian vein catheterizations: A prospective study. I. Noninfecting complications. *Ann Surg* 1971; 173:184
26. Christenson KH: Complications of percutaneous catheterization of the subclavian vein in 129 cases. *Acta Chir Scand* 1967; 113:615
27. Farber DL, Rose DM, Bassell GM, et al: Hemoptysis and pneumothorax after removal of a persistently wedged pulmonary artery catheter. *Crit Care Med* 1981; 9:494
28. Dimarco JP, Hasan G, Ruskin JN, et al: Complications of patients undergoing cardiac electrophysiologic procedures. *Ann Intern Med* 1982; 97:490
29. Culpepper JA, Veremakis C, Guntapalli KK, et al: Malpositioned nasogastric tube causing pneumothorax and bronchopleural fistula (lett). *Chest* 1982; 81:389

30. Sarr MG: Bilateral pneumothoraces after resuscitation with esophageal airway (lett). *JAMA* 1980; 243:2154
31. Thomas JH, Perce GE, MacArthur RI: Bilateral pneumothoraces secondary to colonic endoscopy. *J Natl Med Assoc* 1979; 71:701
32. McDonald HF: Right pneumothorax following fiberoptic oesophageal dilation. *Endoscopy* 1978; 10:130
33. Ritter HG, Tarala R: Pneumothorax after acupuncture. *Br Med J* 1978; 2:602
34. Orr KB, Magarey CJ: Pneumothorax after aspiration of breast cysts (lett). *Med J Aust* 1978; 1:101
35. Lewis JW, Elliott JF Jr, Obeid FN: Complications of attempted central venous injections by drug abusers. *Chest* 1980; 78:613
36. Cohen S: Coca past and freebase: New fashion in cocaine use. *Drug Abuse Alcholism Newslett* 1980; 9:April
37. Shesser R, David C, Edelstein S: Pneumomediastinum and pneumothorax after inhaling alkaloidal cocaine. *Ann Emerg Med* 1981; 10:213
38. Graham JM, Mattox KL, Beall AC: Penetrating trauma to the lung. *J Trauma* 1979; 19:665
39. Griffith GL, Todd EF, McMillin RD, et al: Acute traumatic hemothorax. *Ann Thorac Surg* 1978; 26:204
40. Coselli JS, Mattox KL, Beall AC Jr: Reevaluation of early evacuation of clotted hemothorax. *Am J Surg* 1984; 148:786
41. Siemens R, Polk HC, Gray LA, et al: Indications for thoracotomy following penetrating thoracic injury. *J Trauma* 1977; 17:493
42. NcNamara JJ, Messersmith JK, Dunn RA, et al: Thoracic injuries in combat casualties in Vietnam. *Ann Thorac Surg* 1970; 10:389
43. Sandrasagra FA: Management of penetrating stab wounds of the chest: An assessment of the indication for early operation. *Thorax* 1978; 33:474
44. Webb WR: Thoracic trauma. *Surg Clin North Am* 1974; 54:1179
45. Oparah SS, Mandal AK: Penetrating stab wound of the chest: Experience with 200 consecutive cases. *J Trauma* 1976; 16:868
46. Oparah SS, Mandal AK: Penetrating gunshot wounds of the chest in civilian practice: Experience with 250 consecutive cases. *Br J Surg* 1978; 65:45
47. Schulman P, Cheng E, Cvitkovic E, et al: Spontaneous pneumothorax as a result of cytotoxic chemotherapy. *Chest* 1979; 75:194
48. McFarlane JR, Cranston WH: Chylothorax. *Am Rev Respir Dis* 1972; 105:207
49. Bessone LN, Ferguson TB, Burford TH: Chylothorax. *Ann Thorac Surg* 1971; 12:527
50. Heimlich HJ: Valve drainage of the pleural cavity. *Dis Chest* 1968; 53:282
51. Mercier C, Page A, Verdant A, et al: Outpatient management of intercostal tube drainage in spontaneous pneumothorax. *Ann Thorac Surg* 1976; 22:163
52. Page A, Cossette R, Dontigny L, et al: Spontaneous pneumothorax: Outpatient management with intercostal tube drainage. *Can Med Assoc J* 1975; 112:707
53. Millikan JS, Moore EE, Steiner E, et al: Complications of tube thoracostomy for acute trauma. *Am J Surg* 1980; 140:739
54. VanderSalm TJ: Chest tube insertion (closed thoracostomy). In VanderSalm TJ (ed): *Atlas of Bedside Procedures.* Boston, Little, Brown, 1979
55. Beall AC Jr, Crawford HW, DeBakey M: Considerations in the management of acute traumatic hemothorax. 1966; 52:351
56. Beall AC Jr, Bricker DL, Crawford WH, et al: Considerations in the management of penetrating thoracic trauma. *J Trauma* 1968; 8:408
57. Grover FL, Richardson JD, Fewel JG, et al: Prophylactic antibiotics in the treatment of penetrating chest wounds. *J Thorac Cardiovasc Surg* 1977; 74:528
58. Neugebauer MK, Fosburg RG, Trummer MJ: Routine antibiotic therapy following pleural space intubation; A reappraisal. *J Thorac Cardiovasc Surg* 1971; 61:882
59. LeBlanc KA, Tucker WY: Prophylactic antibiotics and closed tube thoracostomy. *Surg Gynecol Obstet* 1985; 160:259
60. Daly RC, Mucha P, Pairolero PC, et al: The risk of percutaneous chest tube thoracostomy for blunt thoracic trauma. *Ann Emerg Med* 1985; 14:865
61. Nealon TF Jr: Diagnostic procedures. In Nealon TF Jr (ed): *Fundamental Skills in Surgery,* 3rd ed. Philadelphia, WB Saunders, 1979
62. Glickman RM, Isselbacker KJ: Abdominal swelling and ascites. In Petersdorf RG, Adams RD, Braunwald E, et al (eds): *Harrison's Principles of Internal Medicine,* 10th ed. New York, McGraw–Hill, 1983
63. Williams RD, Zollinger RM: Diagnostic and prognostic factors in abdominal trauma. *Am J Surg* 1959; 97:575
64. Giacobine JW, Siler VE: Evaluation of diagnostic abdominal paracentesis with experimental and clinical studies. *Surg Gynecol Obstet* 1960; 110:676
65. Root HD, Keizer PJ, Perry JF: The clinical and experimental aspects of peritoneal response to injury. *Arch Surg* 1967; 95:531
66. Drew T, Perry JF Jr, Fischer RP: The expediency of peritoneal lavage for blunt trauma in children. *Surg Gynecol Obstet* 1977; 145:885

67. Cochran W, Sobat WS: Open versus closed diagnostic peritoneal lavage. *Ann Surg* 1984; 200:24
68. Fischer RP, Beverlin BC, Engrav LH, et al: Diagnostic peritoneal lavage: Fourteen years and 2586 patients later. *Am J Surg* 1978; 136:701
69. Engrav LH, Benjamin CI, Strate RG, et al: Diagnostic peritoneal lavage in blunt abdominal trauma. *J Trauma* 1975; 15:854
70. Olsen WR, Redman HC, Hildreth DH: Quantitative peritoneal lavage in blunt abdominal trauma. *Arch Surg* 1972; 104:536
71. Thal ER, Shires GT: Peritoneal lavage in blunt abdominal trauma. *Am J Surg* 1973; 125:64
72. Perry JF, DeMueles JE, Root HD: Diagnostic peritoneal lavage in blunt abdominal trauma. *Surg Gynecol Obstet* 1970; 131:742
73. Fischer RP, Freeman T: The inadequacy of peritoneal lavage in diagnosing acute diaphragmatic rupture. *J Trauma* 1976; 16:538
74. Parvin S, Smith D, Asher M, et al: Effectiveness of peritoneal lavage in blunt abdominal trauma. *Ann Surg* 1975; 181:255
75. Bivins BA, Jona JZ, Belin RP: Diagnostic peritoneal lavage in pediatric trauma. *J Trauma* 1976; 16:739
76. Olsen WR, Hildreth DM: Abdominal paracentesis and peritoneal lavage in blunt abdominal trauma. *J Trauma* 1971; 11:824
77. Pacey J, Forward AD, Preto AD: Peritoneal tap and lavage in patients with abdominal trauma. *Can Med Assoc J* 1971; 105:365
78. Jergens ME: Peritoneal lavage. *Am J Surg* 1977; 133:365
79. Marx JA, Moore EE, Bar-Or D: Peritoneal lavage in penetrating injuries of the small bowel and colon: Value of enzyme determinations. *Ann Emerg Med* 1983; 12:13
80. Engrav LH, Benjamin CI, Strate RG, et al: Diagnostic peritoneal lavage in blunt abdominal trauma. *J Trauma* 1975; 15:854
81. Hornyak SW, Shaftan GW: Value of "inconclusive lavage" in abdominal trauma management. *J Trauma* 1979; 19:329
82. Alyono DA, Perry JF: Significance of repeating diagnostic peritoneal lavage. *Surgery* 1982; 91:656
83. Thal ER, May RA, Beesinger D: Peritoneal lavage; its unreliability in gunshot wounds of the lower chest and abdomen. *Arch Surg* 1980; 115:430
84. Merlotti GJ, Marcet E, Sheaff CM, et al: Use of peritoneal lavage to evaluate abdominal penetration. *J Trauma* 1985; 25:228
85. Thal ER: Evaluation of peritoneal lavage and local exploration in lower chest and abdominal stab wounds. *J Trauma* 1977; 17:642
86. Lobbato V, Cioroiu M, LaRaja RD, et al: Peritoneal lavage as an aid to diagnosis of peritonitis in debilitated and elderly patients. *Am Surg* 1985; 51:508
87. Richardson JD, Flint LM, Polk HC: Peritoneal lavage: A useful diagnostic adjunct for peritonitis. *Surgery* 1983; 94:826
88. Woodburn RT: *Essentials of Human Anatomy,* 5th ed. New York, Oxford University Press, 1973
89. Moore FA: Venous access. In Moore EE, Eisman B, Van Way CW III (eds): *Critical Decisions in Trauma.* St. Louis, CV Mosby, 1984
90. Dronen SC, Yee AS, Tamlonovich MC: Proximal saphenous vein cutdown. *Ann Emerg Med* 1981; 10:238
91. Ellis BW, Dudley HA: Intravenous therapy and blood transfusion. In Dudley HA (ed): *Hamilton Bailey's Emergency Surgery,* 10th ed. Chicago, Year Book Medical Publishers, 1977
92. Zipes DP, Fischer J, King RM, et al: Termination of ventricular fibrillation in dogs by depolarizing a critical amount of myocardium. *Am J Cardiol* 1975; 36:37
93. Prevost JL, Batelli F: Sur quelques effets des decharges electriques sur le coeur des mammiferers. *CR Acad Sci (Paris)* 1899; 129:1267
94. Beck CS, Pritchard WH, Feil H: Ventricular fibrillation of long duration abolished by electrical shock. *JAMA* 1947; 135:985
95. Lown B, Neuman J, Amarasingham R, et al: Comparison of alternating current with direct current electroshock across the closed chest. *Am J Cardiol* 1962; 10:223
96. Nachias MM, Box HH, Mower MM, et al: Observations on defibrillators, defibrillation and synchronized countershock. *Prog Cardiovasc Dis* 1966; 9:64
97. *American National Standard for Cardiac Defibrillator Devices.* Arlington, Virginia, American Association for the Advancement of Medical Instrumentation, 1981
98. Creed JD, Packard JM, Lambrew CT, et al: Defibrillation and synchronized cardioversion. In (McIntyre KM, Lewis AJ (eds): *Textbook of Advanced Cardiac Life Support.* Dallas, American Heart Association (publisher) 1983
99. Dahl CF, Ewy GA, Ewy MD, et al: Transthoracic impedance to direct current discharge: Effect of repeated countershocks. *Med Instrum* 1976; 10:151
100. DeSilva RA, Graboys TB, Podrid PJ, et al: Cardioversion and defibrillation. *Am Heart J* 1980; 100:881
101. Lau Fy: Protection of implanted pacemakers from excessive electrical energy of DC shock. *Am J Cardiol* 1969; 23:244

102. Cordis Corporation: *Cordis Gemini Pulse Generator Technical Manual.* Miami, Cordis Corporation, 1983
103. Cordis Corporation: *Cordis Sequicor Pulse Generator Technical Manual.* Miami, Cordis Corporation, 1982
104. Gould L, Patel S, Gomes GI: Pacemaker failure following external defibrillation. *PACE* 1981; 4:575
105. Medtronic, Inc: *Medtronic Mirel VL 5988/5989 Pulse Generator Technical Manual.* Minneapolis, Medtronic, 1978
106. Medtronic, Inc: *Medtronic Spectrax SXT Pulse Generator Technical Manual.* Minneapolis, Medtronic, 1981
107. Springrose S: CPI *Technical Issues, Technical Memorandum and Recommendations for Defibrillator Procedures for Pacemaker Patients.* St. Paul, Cardiac Pacemakers, 1979
108. Lown B, Amarasingham R, Neuman J: New methods for terminating cardiac arrhythmias: Use of synchronized capacitor discharge. *JAMA* 1962; 182:548
109. Zipes DP: Electrophysiological mechanisms involved in ventricular fibrillation. *Circulation* 1975; 52(suppl13):120
110. Geddes LA, Tacker WA, Rosborough JP, et al: Electrical dose for ventricular defibrillation of large and small animals using precordial electrodes. *J Clin Invest* 1974; 53:310
111. Lown B, Crampton RS, DeSilva RA, et al: The energy for ventricular defibrillation—too little or too much? *N Engl J Med* 1978; 298:1252
112. Geddes LA, Tacker WA, Cablar P, et al: The decrease in transthoracic impedance during successive ventricular defibrillation trials. *Med Instrum* 1975; 9:179
113. Thomas ED, Ewy GA, Dahl CF, et al: Effectiveness of direct current defibrillation: Role of paddle electrode size. *Am Heart J* 1977; 93:463
114. Kerber RE, Grayzel J, Hoyt R, et al: Transthoracic resistance in human defibrillation: Effects of body weight, chest size, serial same-energy shocks, paddle size, and paddle contact pressure, abstracted. *Med Instrum* 1980; 14:56
115. Patton JN, Pantridge JF: Current required from ventricular defibrillation. *Br Med J* 1979; 1:513
116. Ewy GA, Taren D: Impedance to transthoracic direct current discharge: A model for testing interface material. *Med Instrum* 1978; 12:47
117. Marriott HJ, Myerburg RJ: Recognition and treatment of cardiac arrhythmias and conduction disturbances. In Hurst JW, Logue RB, Schlant TC (eds): *The Heart: Arteries and Veins,* 4th ed. New York, McGraw-Hill, 1978
118. Goldreyer BN, Bigger JT Jr: Site of reentry in paroxysmal supraventricular tachycardia in man. *Circulation* 1971; 43:15
119. Wellens HF, Bar FW, Lie KI: The value of the electrocardiogram in the differential diagnosis of a tachycardia with a widened QRS complex. *Am J Med* 1978; 64:27
120. Lown B, DeSilva RA: The technique of cardioversion. In Hurst JW (ed): *The Heart.* New York, McGraw-Hill, 1986
121. Lown B, Cannon RL III, Rossi MA: Electrical stimulation and digitalis drugs: Repetitive response in diastole. *Proc Soc Exp Biol Med* 1967; 126:698
122. Regan TJ, Markov A, Oldewurtel HA, et al: Myocardial K loss after countershock and the relation to ventricular arrhythmias after nontoxic doses of acetyl strophanthidin. *Am Heart J* 1969; 77:367
123. Rabbino, MD, Likoff W, Dreifus LS: Complications and limitations of direct current countershock. *JAMA* 1964; 190:147
124. Ross EM: Cardioversion causing ventricular fibrillation. *Arch Intern Med* 1964; 114:811
125. Castellanos A, Lamberg L, Gilmore H, et al: Countershock exposed quinidine syncope. *Am J Med Sci* 1965; 260:254
126. Ehsani A, Ewy GA, Sobe BE: Effects of electrical countershock on serum creatinine phosphokinase (CPK) isoenzyme activity. *Am J Cardiol* 1976; 37:12
127. Reiffel JA, McCarthy DM, Leakey EB: Does DC cardioversion affect isoenzyme recognition of myocardial infarction? *Am Heart J* 1974; 97:810
128. Resnekov L, McDonald L: Complications in 220 patients with cardiac dysrhythmias treated by phased direct current shock and indications for electroversion. *Br Heart H* 1967; 29:926
129. Lown B: Electrical reversion of cardiac arrhythmias. *Br Heart J* 1967; 29:469
130. Goldman MJ: The management of chronic atrial fibrillation: Indications for and method of conversion to sinus rhythm. *Prog Cardiovasc Dis* 1960; 2:465
131. Roberts WC, Spray TL: Pericardial heart disease: A study of its causes, consequences, and morphologic features. In Spodick D (ed): *Pericardial Diseases. Cardiovascular Clinics,* vol 7, no 3. Philadelphia, FA Davis, 1976
132. Fowler NO: Physiology of cardiac tamponade and pulses paradoxus: II. Physiological, circulatory, and pharmacological responses in cardiac tamponade. *Mod Concepts Cardiovasc Dis* 1978; 47:115
133. Shabetai R: The pathophysiology of cardiac tamponade and constriction. In Spodick D (ed): *Pericardial Diseases. Cardiovascular Clinics,* vol 7, no 3. Philadelphia, FA Davis, 1976
134. Shabetai R, Fowler NO, Guntheroth WG: The hemodynamics of cardiac tamponade and constrictive pericarditis. *Am J Cardiol* 1970; 26:480
135. Fowler NO: Physiology of cardiac tamponade and pulsus paradoxus in cardiac tamponade. *Mod Concepts Cardiovasc Dis* 1978; 47:109

136. Fowler NO: The recognition and management of pericardial disease and its complications. In Hurst JW, Logue RB, Schlant RC, et al (eds): *The Heart: Arteries and Veins.* New York, McGraw-Hill, 1978
137. Beck CS: Two cardiac compression triads. *JAMA* 1935; 104:714
138. Cooper FW Jr, Stead EA Jr, Warren JV: Beneficial effect of intravenous infusions in acute pericardial tamponade. *Ann Surg* 1944; 120:822
139. Hancock EW: Management of pericardial disease. *Mod Concepts Cardiovasc Dis* 1979; 48:1
140. Spodick DH: Acute cardiac tamponade pathologic physiology, diagnosis and management. *Prog Cardiovasc Dis* 1967; 10:64
141. D'Cruz IA, Cohen HC, Prabhu R, et al: Diagnosis of cardiac tamponade by echocardiography. Changes in mitral valve motion and ventricular dimensions, with special reference to paradoxical pulse. *Circulation* 1975; 52:460
142. Settle HP, Adolph RJ, Fowler NO, et al: Echocardiographic study of cardiac tamponade. *Circulation* 1977; 56:951
143. Schiller NB, Botvinick EH: Right ventricular compression as a sign of cardiac tamponade. An analysis of echocardiographic ventricular dimensions and their clinical implications. *Circulation* 1977; 56:774
144. Vignola PA, Phohst GM, Curfman GD, et al: Correlation of echocardiographic and clinical findings in patients with pericardial effusion. *Am J Cardiol* 1976; 37:701
145. Usher BW, Popp RL: Electrical alternans: Mechanism in pericardial effusion. *Am Heart J* 1972; 83:459
146. Kilpatrick ZM, Chapman CB: On pericardiocentesis. *Am J Cardiol* 1965; 16:722
147. Pories WJ, Guadiani VA: Cardiac tamponade. *Surg Clin North Am* 1975; 55:573
148. Pecora DV, Brook R: A method of securing uncontaminated tracheal secretions for bacterial examination. *J Thorac Surg* 1959; 37:653
149. Bartlett JG, Rosenblatt JE, Finegold SM: Percutaneous transtracheal aspiration in the diagnosis of anaerobic pulmonary infection. *Ann Intern Med* 1973; 79:535
150. Kalinske RW, Parker RH, Brandt D, et al: Diagnostic usefulness and safety of transtracheal aspiration. *N Engl J Med* 1967; 276:604
151. Spencer CD, Beaty HN: Complications of transtracheal aspiration. *N Engl J Med* 1972; 286:304

CHAPTER NINETEEN

FIBEROPTIC BRONCHOSCOPY IN CRITICAL CARE

John J. Marini
Arthur P. Wheeler

Fiberoptic bronchoscopy (FOB) has gained great popularity since its introduction in 1968. It is a welcome advance over rigid bronchoscopy because it offers extensive visualization of the bronchi[1] while decreasing cost, risk, and patient discomfort. Flexible instruments (Fig. 19-1) allow inspection, sampling, and therapy in the airways of many patients who cannot be examined by rigid techniques. Further, whereas rigid bronchoscopy is limited to the operating suite, FOB can be done at the bedside, is easily mastered, and therefore is well suited for use in the ICU.

The uses of FOB range from the investigation of lung masses and hemoptysis to localization of bronchopleural fistula and bronchography (Table 19-1). Even in experienced hands, however, FOB carries a small but real risk of morbidity, especially when used in the critical care setting.[2]

Many physicians have little or no experience with FOB. They may encounter some difficulty until they familiarize themselves with the instrument. The depth of the vocal cords is exaggerated. The visual field constricts as the fiberscope aproaches each structure. Secretions and blood easily obstruct the view. With practice, however, these problems are easily overcome. The basic technique is summarized in Table 19-2. Typical views obtained during FOB are shown in Figures 19-2 and 19-3.

Care must be taken to maintain the fiberscope in the midline to avoid entering the pyriform sinuses, which resemble the glottic entrance. An oral airway intubator allows insertion of the bronchoscope into the mouth in the midline, protecting it from the teeth and directing it near the larynx. In general, FOB is not indicated for apneic, cyanotic patients because it is time consuming. However, it is of unmatched value during difficult but non-emergency situations.

Certain problems must be kept in mind. An adult FOB with an outside diameter of 5.2 mm requires lubrication and a minimum 7.5-mm inside diameter (ID) endotracheal or tracheostomy tube in intubated patients. If manual or mechanical ventilatory support is used, the minimum ID is 8.0 mm. Increased outflow resistance to exhaled gas may lead to unwanted positive end-expiratory pressure (PEEP) and the potential for pulmonary barotrauma. This untoward effect can be minimized by using the largest possible endotracheal

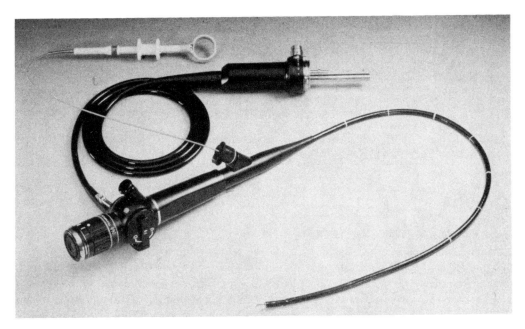

Figure 19-1 Olympus BF 20D bronchoscope with distal suction port. (Courtesy of Olympus Corporation, Lake Success, New York)

tube and 100% oxygen, discontinuing externally applied PEEP, and limiting the duration of suctioning.

Inadequate gas exchange must be considered as a possible cause of patient uncooperativeness and should be ruled out before administering sedative or narcotic drugs. Local anesthetic toxicity can occur because of the very rapid uptake of agent from the airway mucosa.

TABLE 19-1   INDICATIONS FOR BRONCHOSCOPY (PARTIAL LISTING)

Diagnostic Indications	Therapeutic Indications
Cough	Difficult intubation
Hemoptysis	Foreign body extraction
Wheezing	Accumulated secretions
Atelectasis	Atelectasis
Unresolved pneumonia	Aspiration
Positive sputum cytology	Lung abscess
Abnormal chest radiographic findings	
Diffuse lung disease	**Preoperative Evaluation**
Hoarseness	R/O multiple primary tumors
Diaphragmatic paralysis	Metastases
Selective bronchography	Bronchiectasis (with bronchography)
Acute inhalation injury	
Verification of endotracheal tube position	
Pneumonia	
Upper airway obstruction	
Pleural effusion	
Suspicion of bronchial rupture	

TABLE 19-2 TECHNIQUE OF FIBEROPTIC BRONCHOSCOPY

1. Sedation and anticholinergic drug administration before endoscopy (as necessary)
2. Check light source, objective, and ocular lenses
3. Adjust eyepiece with diopter adjuster ring
4. Lubricate insertion tube (not objective lens)
5. Hold instrument in right hand with deflection knob between thumb and index finger
6. Use left hand to insert and to advance fiberscope (keep in midline to avoid pyriform sinuses)

INDICATIONS

INTUBATION AND AIRWAY CONTROL

Fiberoptic bronchoscopy has diagnostic and therapeutic value in airway control, playing a key role in identifying acute airway obstruction in high-risk patients. It permits diagnosis of numerous conditions that produce acute airway obstruction, including supraglottitis, vocal cord dysfunction or paralysis, laryngeal edema, tracheal stenosis, tumors, and airway hemorrhage.[2] Smoke inhalation and heat injury also can be diagnosed quickly and reliably. Findings of severe inflammation and edema of the larynx are predictive of impending airway obstruction and the need for tracheal intubation or tracheostomy.[3] If supraglottic edema is

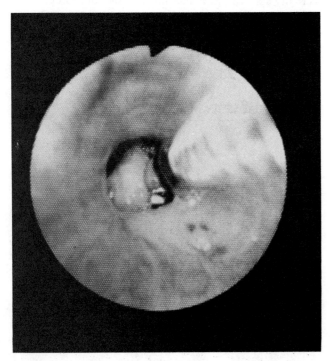

Figure 19-2 Polypoid tumor invading bronchiolar lumen. (Courtesy of Olympus Corporation, Lake Success, New York)

Figure 19-3 Small cell carcinoma producing stenosis and hyperemia (Courtesy of Olympus Corporation, Lake Success, New York)

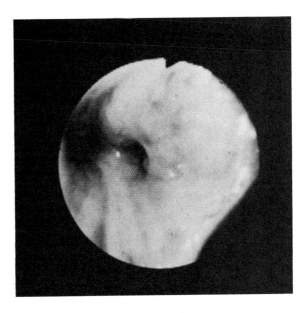

found, intubation can be carried out with an endotracheal tube placed over the bronchoscope. Serial examinations define the course of upper airway abnormalities and help to predict the timing of safe extubation. Supraglottic mucosal edema usually resolves within 4 to 6 days of onset, whereas vocal cord abnormalities may persist for 3 to 4 weeks. Although bronchoscopy can predict airway obstruction, when used alone it provides no reliable information about the risk of developing adult respiratory distress syndrome (ARDS) in smoke inhalation.[3]

The difficulty and complications of intubation increase dramatically in emergency settings. Fiberoptic bronchoscopy is helpful in the placement of endotracheal tubes in patients with cervical spine trauma, massive obesity, oropharyngeal tumors, rheumatoid arthritis, ankylosing spondylitis, and other conditions limiting access to the trachea (Table 19-3). Patients with abnormalities that prevent mouth opening, such as temporomandibular joint disorders and status epilepticus, can be intubated using transnasal FOB. The replacement of endotracheal tubes with leaking cuffs and the accurate positioning of double lumen endotracheal tubes are facilitated by FOB (Fig. 19-4). Fiberoptic bronchoscopes are even used in placing nasogastric tubes when insertion proves difficult in the critically ill. However, the nasotracheal route should not be used for any type of intubation in patients with bleeding or clotting disorders because of the potential for serious hemorrhage.

MECHANICAL VENTILATION

After tracheal intubation, bronchoscopy maintains a role in the treatment of the mechanically ventilated patient. Main-stem bronchus intubation and endotracheal tube obstruction by secretions, malposition, or cuff herniation can be promptly diagnosed and corrected.[4] Bronchial trauma from endotracheal tubes or suction catheters is easily diagnosed. Such data may prove useful when tracheostomy is considered after extended intubation.

**TABLE 19-3 CONDITIONS PREDISPOSING TO DIFFICULT
TRACHEAL INTUBATION**

Obesity
"Bull neck"
Oropharyngeal tumors
Cellulitis
Maxillofacial deformities
Ankylosing spondylitis
Cervical rheumatoid arthritis
Cervical fracture
Trismus
Prior history of
  difficult intubation
Airway edema

Because airway resistance increases rapidly when a bronchoscope is introduced into an endotracheal tube, the size of endotracheal tube that will safely allow passage of the instrument is limited. This problem is accentuated when the bronchoscope diameter is large in comparison to the endotracheal tube lumen (Fig. 19-5). Obstruction produces significant increases in expiratory time and a (PEEP) effect, especially at higher rates of ventilation. Increases in airway resistance limit examination with standard bronchoscopes to endotracheal tubes of $\geq$ 8-mm internal diameter. Smaller bronchoscopes have been developed to avoid excessive increases in airway pressure. Extraluminal bronchoscopy, performed by passing the bronchoscope alongside the endotracheal tube after temporarily deflating the cuff, is another useful option.

If inflation volume is lost as a result of pressure limitation of the ventilator, reduction in flow rate settings may reduce peak airway pressures to acceptable levels. For safe completion of the procedure, it may be necessary to withdraw the bronchoscope to the Y connector of the ventilator circuit at 15-second to 30-second intervals to allow unimpeded, intermittent ventilation. High-frequency ventilation may reduce peak airway pressures during bronchoscopy, permitting use of the procedure in patients with smaller endotracheal tubes than would be possible with conventional ventilation. Helium–oxygen gas mixtures can also be used to enable FOB to be performed through small endotracheal tubes without generating limiting increases in airway pressure.[5] Time- or volume-cycled ventilators are preferable to deliver adequate tidal volumes without pressure limitation. Many adaptors allow adequate movement of the bronchoscope while maintaining a sealed airway; nonetheless, some air leak is inevitable. Loss of inflation volume owing to excessive suctioning may also produce inadequate alveolar ventilation. Therefore, constant monitoring of exhaled lung volume or end-tidal carbon dioxide is needed to guarantee adequate alveolar ventilation.

ATELECTASIS

Lobar atelectasis is frequently encountered in critically ill patients, particularly in the setting of upper abdominal and thoracic surgery. This process must be reversed because unresolved atelectasis leads to poor gas exchange, infection, and eventual fibrosis. Collapse occurs

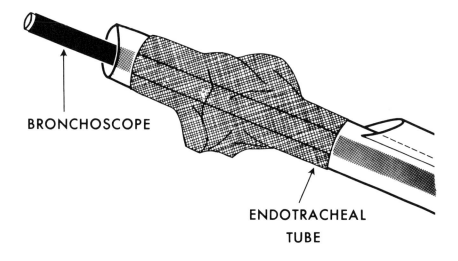

BRONCHOSCOPE

ENDOTRACHEAL
TUBE

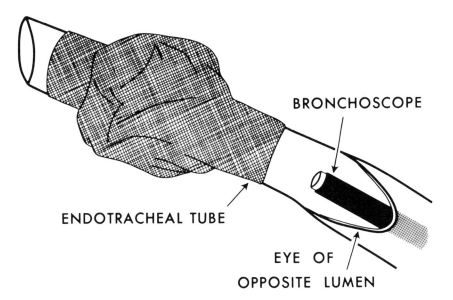

BRONCHOSCOPE

ENDOTRACHEAL TUBE

EYE OF
OPPOSITE LUMEN

Figure 19-4 Placement of a double-lumen endobronchial tube using FOB. **A.** A pediatric bronchoscope is inserted through the bronchial lumen to ensure appropriate positioning. **B.** The bronchoscope is in the tracheal lumen from which the position of the endobronchial cuff and the orientation of the tracheal lumen orifice can be ascertained. (Dellinger RP: Fiberoptic bronchoscopy in acute respiratory failure. In Kirby RR, Taylor RW (eds): *Respiratory Failure.* Chicago, Year Book Medical Publishers, 1986, pp. 434–447)

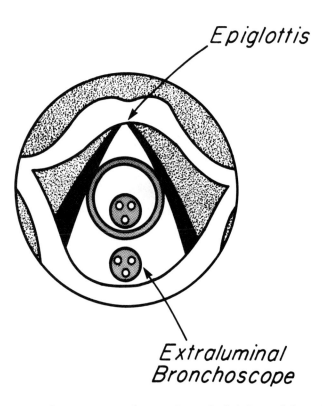

Epiglottis

Extraluminal Bronchoscope

Figure 19-5 Two routes for passage of the fiber-optic bronchoscope in an intubated patient. Intra-luminal placement occludes a substantial percentage of the airway, an effect greatly accentuated at small lumen diameters. Ineffective ventilation and sustained positive alveolar pressure may result. In such cases reintubation with a larger tube, use of a smaller bronchoscope, or passage of the instrument alongside the main airway lumen may be required.

almost twice as frequently in the left lower lobe as in the right lower lobe. This region may be disproportionately affected because of its long, narrow, angulated airway and the associated difficulty in providing effective suctioning. Cannulation of the left main bronchus with a suction catheter is achieved in fewer than 60% of cases when it is attempted through an endotracheal or tracheostomy tube.[6] Although acute atelectasis frequently results from impaired regional mechanics and failure of the cough mechanism to clear retained secretions, other causes in the critically ill include tumors, endotracheal tube malposition, bronchial disruption, and foreign bodies.

The literature abounds with reports of successful treatment of lobar atelectasis by bronchoscopy. Radiographic improvement is reported in the great majority of cases. Air bronchograms branching distally into areas of collapse suggest that atelectasis without plugging of central airways is present and that bronchial suctioning alone is not likely to cause re-expansion (Fig. 19-6).[7] The most likely mechanisms by which FOB improves atelectasis include removal of secretions, stimulation of coughing, and, in the intubated patient, a PEEP effect produced by partial airway occlusion and increased airway pressure. Selective application of positive pressure with the bronchoscope has been used for refractory atelectasis but carries the risks of air embolization and barotrauma.[8] Aggressive respiratory therapy, when applied early, is as effective as FOB for acute atelectasis.[7] Further, patients who can be treated by vigorous respiratory care techniques do not experience the frequent recurrence of atelectasis seen in patients treated by bronchoscopy.[7]

In summary, FOB is a useful adjunct to respiratory therapy and suctioning for atelectasis that is refractory to standard measures. In patients with flail chest or spinal or cranial

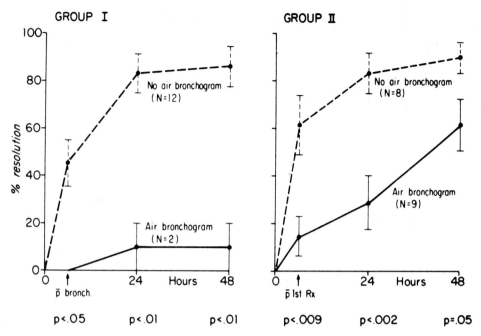

Figure 19-6 Effect of bronchoscopy and air bronchograms on percentage resolution of atelectasis over a 2-day period. Patients with acute lobar atelectasis in group I received bronchoscopy followed by 48 hours of vigorous respiratory therapy. Patients in group II received respiratory therapy alone. Note that bronchoscopy did not accelerate the pace of resolution and that an air bronchogram branching into the area of collapse predicted a delayed response to treatment. (Lundgren R, Haggmarks S, Reiz S: Hemodynamic effects of flexible fiberoptic bronchoscopy performed under topical anesthesia. *Chest* 1982; 82:295)

injuries who cannot undergo vigorous coughing and manipulation, FOB may be the procedure of choice when nasotracheal suctioning fails. Because of cost, risk to the patient, and the effectiveness of less invasive procedures, FOB should be reserved for cases with specific indications.

HEMOPTYSIS

The primary danger of massive hemoptysis is asphyxiation. Potential sources of hemoptysis are numerous, with bronchitis and bronchiectasis being the leading causes in most series (Table 19-4). To avoid high mortality rates, massive hemoptysis requires rapid localization and definitive correction by surgery, endobronchial tamponade, or bronchial artery embolization. Chest radiographic abnormalities alone are inadequate for guiding resection of the bleeding area.[9]

Rigid bronchoscopy remains the diagnostic procedure of choice for massive hemoptysis because of improved visualization. It also allows tamponade of bleeding and suctioning of large volumes of blood from the airways. However, massive hemoptysis has been diagnosed and managed successfully by FOB.

Minor hemoptysis is best evaluated with FOB. In the intubated patient, a frequent source of minor hemoptysis is mucosal trauma induced by catheter suctioning. Many pul-

TABLE 19-4   SOME CONDITIONS IN WHICH HEMOPTYSIS MAY OCCUR

Bacterial Infections
Pulmonary tuberculosis
Lung abscess
Bronchitis
Bronchiectasis
Pseudomonas pneumonias
Staphylococcus pneumonias
Klebsiella pneumonias

Vascular Conditions
Mitral stenosis
Pulmonary embolism and infarction
Flushing of wedged Swan Ganz catheters
Aortic aneurysm
Arteriovenous fistula
Venous obstructive condition
Anomalous vessel
Primary pulmonary hypertension

Fungal Infections
Aspergillosis
Coccidioidomycosis
Actinomycosis
Mucormycosis
Candidiasis

Neoplastic Conditions
Bronchogenic carcinoma
Bronchial adenoma
Choriocarcinoma
Endometriosis
Metastatic neoplasms

Parasitic Diseases
Paragonimiasis
Strongyloidiasis
Ancylostomiasis
Echinococcosis

Miscellaneous
Cystic fibrosis
Idiopathic hemosiderosis
Occult pulmonary hemorrhage
Goodpasture's syndrome
Broncholithiasis
Cysts and bullae
Vicarious menstruation
Malingering
Wegeners granulomatosis
Foreign bodies
Polyarteritis nodosa
SLE
Bronchial endometriosis
Suction catheter trauma

monologists advocate bronchoscopy of essentially *all* patients with an initial episode of bleeding. By contrast, Weaver and colleagues propose specific criteria to gauge the need for bronchoscopy in the patient with minor hemoptysis.[10] In their studies, the factors most commonly associated with a productive bronchoscopic procedure included an abnormal chest radiograph, age greater than 40 years, and prolonged hemoptysis (>1 week).

Success in identifying the source and nature of the bleeding site varies with timing, technique, and etiology. Extensive visualization of distal bronchi, particularly in the upper lobes, is possible with FOB, which consequently yields a higher diagnostic rate than does rigid bronchoscopy. Therefore, FOB is the technique of choice, except in some cases of massive hemoptysis where airway control and operating potential are important considerations.

The optimal timing of bronchoscopy in hemoptysis is controversial. Although early reports favored delaying evaluation of hemoptysis until bleeding had stopped or stabilized, subsequent studies showed the safety and effectiveness of bronchoscopy in active hemoptysis.[9] When used during active hemorrhage, FOB identifies up to 90% of bleeding sites. Localization is three times more likely in patients undergoing FOB within 48 hours of the cessation of hemoptysis than in patients who receive a more delayed evaluation.

Diffuse pulmonary infiltrates in patients with abnormal hemostasis occasionally result from pulmonary hemorrhage. This condition is often overlooked and rarely diagnosed in living patients. Intrapulmonary hemorrhage should be suspected when large numbers of hemosiderin-laden alveolar macrophages are recovered from bronchial lavage fluid.

As many as 75% of patients presenting with hemoptysis have a normal chest radiograph, The site of bleeding is identified in a minority of these patients, with a firm diagnosis established in only 40%. A normal chest radiograph with nondiagnostic bronchoscopy is seen in 5% to 15% of patients with hemoptysis.[11] Long-term follow-up of this group demonstrates that in the majority bleeding stops within 6 months and occult carcinoma or tuberculosis is unlikely.[11] In general, hemoptysis is a late symptom of lung cancer, and carcinoma is rare in patients with hemoptysis and a normal chest radiograph.

Techniques for controlling endobronchial bleeding include epinephrine instillation, bronchoscopic tamponade, Fogarty balloon tamponade, intravenous vasopressin infusion, and selective bronchial intubation. Balloon tamponade is effective primary therapy in patients unable to undergo definitive pulmonary resection and is a temporizing maneuver for patients awaiting surgery. Balloon tamponade is also advised as a diagnostic tool to isolate bleeding lung segments.

INFECTION

Diagnosis of infection in the critically ill by FOB is difficult because of the problems of colonization and oropharyngeal contamination.[12] Even when the bronchoscope is passed through a freshly placed endotracheal tube, specimens are frequently contaminated by bacteria of the mouth and upper airways. Several approaches have been used in attempts to overcome such problems, including combining Gram staining with culture, quantitative culturing, and the use of transbronchoscopic protected brushes. Many of these specialized techniques reduce the frequency of bacterial contamination, but none eliminates it entirely.

Transtracheal aspiration consistently yields lower colony counts of contaminating bacteria than either bronchoscopy or sputum examination but still does not produce 100% specificity. Although accurate bacteriologic diagnosis by bronchoscopic washings has been suggested, debate continues because culture results of bronchoscopic washings often disagree with those of other methods. Bronchoscopic washings do not accurately reflect bronchial flora when collected in the customary manner. Contamination by upper airway bacteria is minimized if less then 3 ml of lidocaine is used and bronchial brushings are collected *before* aspirating through the suction channel.[13] Gram stains of bronchoscopic washings can be useful when correlated with culture results at a later time. Organisms present in large numbers on Gram stain are likely to be the pathogens later demonstrated in culture.

Quantitative culture is another technique that potentially can help to distinguish true infection from contamination. Although controversy remains, such cultures are probably of little value in practice, largely because processing delays alter the relative proportions of bacteria in the sample. Bronchoscopic washings that yield a single pathogen at a concentration of $>10^5$ colonies per milliliter probably indicate infection. True infections usually evoke a host response that coats bacteria with antibody. Fluorescent antibody coating, based on this principle, is a technique that seeks evidence of infection rather than colonization. Overall, such methods are reported to have nearly 75% sensitivity and 100% specificity. Fluorescent antibody coating may be used to diagnose infection when empiric antibiotic therapy has been started or when the use of lidocaine may suppress culture results.

Although catheters wedged in a peripheral airway have been used to help address questions of infection versus colonization, the distinction is still difficult. The "protected" or telescoping brush catheter was designed to improve sensitivity and specificity in diagnosing infection. Plugged catheters appear to have fewer problems with contamination than do unplugged catheters, but, when compared to percutaneous transthoracic needle aspiration or transtracheal aspiration, the plugged catheter produces disturbingly high rates of false-positive and false-negative results. Protected brush specimens have yielded up to 30% false negatives and 10% false positives in studies of animals with bacterial pneumonia.

Fiberoptic bronchoscopy is superior to rigid bronchoscopy in the diagnosis of pulmonary fungal infections. Diagnostic bronchoscopy is indicated in most cases of lung abscess to exclude endobronchial blockage by a malignancy or foreign body. Although FOB is advocated as an effective means of draining a lung abscess, the procedure is potentially dangerous and presents a substantial risk of intrapleural drainage and massive postprocedural aspiration of purulent material. Even diagnostic FOB is performed most safely when delayed until the abscess cavity no longer contains a large collection of fluid. Lung abscess may form after transbronchial biopsy of a tumor mass.

The Normal Host

The efficacy of bronchoscopy for diagnosis of diffuse pulmonary infiltrates in the normal host is controversial, with diagnostic rates ranging from 60% to 85%.[14] The diagnostic yield appears to be largely independent of the number of biopsy specimens taken. In evaluating vasculitis, FOB yields little information and is prone to sampling errors. Many investigators believe transbronchial biopsy to be so markedly inferior to open lung biopsy for the diagnosis of diffuse infiltrative lung disease that open lung biopsy is chosen as the initial diagnostic procedure.[15]

Although this approach is defensible when the etiology is totally uncertain or there is a high index of suspicion for a noninfectious process, transbronchial biopsy is often successful in common diffuse lung disease. Diagnostic rates of 80% for sarcoidosis, 77% for diffuse malignancy, and 57% for diffuse interstitial lung disease have been reported. Nonetheless, one third to one half of all transbronchial biopsies in immune-competent hosts yield nonspecific results.[16] In the great majority of such patients, a specific diagnosis may be made at open lung biopsy. Diagnoses suggested by transbronchial biopsy are confirmed approximately 70% of the time by material obtained from open lung biopsy.

The Compromised Host

Pulmonary infection is frequent in the immunocompromised host and carries a high mortality when the lung involvement is diffuse. Even an aggressive approach to diagnosis fails to yield an infectious cause in a sizeable percentage of cases. Controversy regarding the value of invasive procedures in the compromised host continues. Open lung biopsy if performed early holds the greatest prospect of accurate diagnosis. However, therapy is frequently unaffected by the biopsy results, and there is little evidence that outcome is consistently improved when a specific diagnosis is made. Diagnosis is further complicated by the fact that as many as one third of infected patients have more than one pathogen present. Further, many noninfectious problems, including alveolar hemorrhage, pulmonary edema, drug toxicity, leukostasis, and oxygen toxicity, mimic or accompany infection. Unfortunately, chest radiographs are seldom helpful in predicting a specific pathogen in these patients.

The reported diagnostic accuracy of FOB in this patient population varies widely. The consensus is that FOB provides a specific diagnosis in approximately 50% of patients with diffuse infiltrates,[14] a rate comparable to that of open lung biopsy. The success rate is cut by about half in patients with localized infiltrates. The nature and frequency of complications are highly dependent on the patient population. In well-selected candidates, the incidence of major problems averages 10% to 15%.

Bronchoalveolar lavage (BAL) is an effective adjunct for the diagnosis of diffuse infiltrates in the compromised host. Diagnostic rates vary widely, but most investigators agree that BAL's success in defining opportunistic pathogens exceeds that in establishing diagnoses of malignant or drug-induced lung disease.[17] The technique adds to the diagnostic rate of bronchoscopic brushing, washing, and transbronchial biopsy, but it must still be considered a research tool in the diagnosis of noninfectious processes.

Pneumocystis carinii, a common infection in the immunocompromised host, can be diagnosed by FOB in up to 80% of cases. Brushing and forceps biopsy are particularly useful for diagnosing *P. carinii* in distinction to other pathogens. If infection by *P. carinii* is suspected, silver-stained touch preparations of transbronchial biopsies are frequently diagnostic. When the patient cannot undergo biopsy procedures because of the presence of coagulopathy or the need for mechanical ventilation, BAL is sometimes useful.

Aspergillus infections are also encountered frequently in immunocompromised patients. Fiberoptic bronchoscopy identifies approximately 50% of all cases of *aspergillus* infections in patients with acute leukemia; bronchial washings are the diagnostic component of the procedure in most proven cases.

Transbronchial biopsy in the compromised host can also reliably establish the diagnosis of pneumonia caused by fungi and protozoa. Compiled data from numerous series indicate that transbronchial biopsy alone provides a specific diagnosis in approximately 40% of cases (range, 26% to 68%). Brushing is less effective, producing a diagnosis only about 25% of the time (range, 8% to 63%). However, brushing does add to the yield of transbronchial biopsy alone.

Transbronchial biopsy reveals nonspecific inflammation in nearly half of all immunocompromised patients with diffuse infiltrates. This finding often generates controversy regarding the need for further invasive procedures, particularly open lung biopsy. Nishio and Lynch found a specific diagnosis by open lung biopsy in nearly 45% of patients with a nonspecific transbronchial biopsy.[18] However, at least four other groups of investigators reported sensitivity greater than 80% and specificity approaching 100% for transbronchial biopsy in the setting of diffuse infiltrates. It appears that open biopsy improves the chances of making a specific diagnosis after an unrevealing bronchoscopy, but only a minority of patients benefit.

In summary, FOB provides a specific diagnosis in about half of immunocompromised patients with diffuse infiltrates and in the majority of those in whom a diagnosis is eventually made. Therefore, when formulating a strategy for approaching such patients, we consider FOB to be the initial procedure of choice, provided that a nondiagnostic bronchoscopy does not unduly delay further diagnostic procedures.

Acquired Immune Deficiency Syndrome. Pulmonary infections are common in acquired immune deficiency syndrome (AIDS) and behave differently than they do in other immunocompromising diseases. Initially, open lung biopsy was the preferred method for diagnosis. However, it soon became evident that transbronchial biopsy was unusually effective in these patients.[19] Fluoroscopy was used to guide biopsies until evidence surfaced that a "blind" technique was both safe and effective, owing to the unusually widespread, diffuse, and proliferative nature of the infectious process.

Subsequently, BAL was discovered to be effective in diagnosing the most common infection associated with AIDS, *Pneumocystis carinii*. The profusion of intra-alveolar organisms may account for the unusual success in diagnosing atypical mycobacteriosis and cytomegalovirus, as well as *P. carinii* pneumonia. The reported diagnostic success of BAL in this illness approaches 90%.[20] Further study demonstrated that BAL could be performed safely and effectively using disposable fiberoptic catheters, without the need for FOB. More recently, induced sputum was found to be an effective diagnostic method in as many as 50% of cases.[21] Rapid-staining techniques for *P. carinii* assist in the prompt diagnosis of this pathogen. Nonetheless, FOB is undoubtedly superior to the examination of induced sputum, recovering *P. carinii* at a higher rate (90% versus 50%) and providing the opportunity to recover coexisting pathogens. Because almost any bacterium, fungus, virus, or protozoan may cause pulmonary infection in the patient with AIDS, FOB provides a valuable diagnostic tool.

Tuberculosis. Tuberculosis is a deceptive and potentially fatal disease that often pursues a fulminant course. All too often, it remains undiagnosed until autopsy. Currently, a low level of suspicion of the disease is maintained because of its declining prevalence. Many ICU patients are at risk for recrudescence of tuberculosis by virtue of the immune system compromise that attends malnutrition and multi-organ-system failure. Cutaneous anergy and abnormal chest radiographs further obscure the diagnosis. Half of all chest radiographic abnormalities in patients with undiagnosed tuberculosis are interpreted as secondary to underlying disease.[22]

When tuberculosis is considered in the differential diagnosis, FOB plays an important role. Perhaps the primary value of bronchoscopy is its ability to establish the diagnosis before culture results are available, allowing the early institution of therapy. The early diagnosis of tuberculosis can be accomplished by demonstration of acid-fast bacilli (AFB) in bronchial washings or brushings or in postbronchoscopy sputum and has been reported in 34% to 61% of culture-positive cases.

In patients with proven tuberculosis who are initially sputum-smear-negative, sputum cultures eventually grow AFB in 59% to 75% of cases.[23] The bronchial washings of patients whose sputum is smear-negative contain visible AFB in 12% to 42% of cases. Positive cultures of bronchial washings are seen in 66% to 95% of these patients. Bronchial brushings add to the diagnostic yield of washing and sputum examination, although widely divergent rates of positive brushings are reported. Transbronchial biopsy is diagnostic in 16% to 54% of cases of pulmonary tuberculosis, and provides the sole positive bronchoscopic specimen on smear or culture in up to 50% of successful procedures. Postbronchoscopy sputum is reported to be culture-positive in 3.3% to 58% of cases.

In summary, FOB has a high success rate in the diagnosis of tuberculosis.[23] The likelihood of making a bronchoscopic diagnosis of tuberculosis exceeds that associated with sputum smear and culture. Brushing, transbronchial biopsy, and postbronchoscopic sputum collection add to the diagnostic yield of bronchial washing and suctioning. A small but definite percentage of patients will be diagnosed only by transbronchial biopsy or by post-bronchoscopy sputum studies. Therefore, unless contraindicated, these procedures should be performed whenever FOB is undertaken.

New techniques of mycobacterial isolation and culture may improve the sensitivity of FOB and speed the growth of *Mycobacterium tuberculosis* but often isolate nonpathogenic atypical mycobacterial species. However, it can be argued that nonspecificity is a secondary consideration in the critically ill patient. Transmission of mycobacterial infections by FOB has been described in cases where iodophor solutions were used for decontamination. Therefore, sterilization procedures following a case in which *M. tuberculosis* is suspected should include application of glutaraldehyde or ethylene oxide for a sufficient time to achieve total microbial kill.

Local Anesthetics and Culture Results

Bronchoscopy without anesthesia is difficult in patients who are awake. Unfortunately, most local anesthetics, including those commonly used for bronchoscopic examinations, are potent inhibitors of numerous microorganisms.[24] For example, lidocaine in 2% concentrations inhibits growth of 80% of all bacterial isolates. All species of gram-negative organisms except *Pseudomonas aeruginosa* are sensitive to this concentration of lidocaine. Grampositive bacteria are less sensitive. *Cryptococcus neoformans* is uniformly inhibited by 1% lidocaine, but all species of *Candida* are resistant to its effects. Topical anesthetics clearly impede the growth of mycobacterial pathogens.[24]

Wimberly and associates strongly suggest that the concentrations of lidocaine in clinical use should not prevent the bronchoscopic diagnosis of pneumonia, although definite reductions in bacterial counts occur.[25] Nonetheless, the suppressive effect of local anesthetics increases the importance of performing transbronchial biopsy and minimizing the use of lidocaine during bronchoscopy, especially when culture results are critical. Topical anesthesia may be circumvented by bilateral injection of the superior laryngeal nerve in the awake patient or by paralysis and sedation in the intubated patient.

FOREIGN MATERIALS

Children below 3 years of age and adults with disordered swallowing, altered consciousness, or trauma are the most frequent victims of foreign body aspiration. Coughing, wheezing, and reduced air flow constitute the diagnostic triad signaling the presence of a foreign body. Rigid bronchoscopy has been used for the removal of foreign bodies because of the reported advantages of better visualization, improved airway control, operating potential, and ability to control hemorrhage. With the wide range of hardware available, 90% to 95% of all foreign bodies can be removed successfully using the rigid instrument.

In recent years, FOB also has gained popularity for foreign body retrieval. Specific advantages include its use at the bedside and in patients with conditions that preclude rigid bronchoscopy. A further advantage is that FOB can be used to retrieve objects lodged in the upper lobes (admittedly an unusual circumstance) and in areas beyond the range of rigid instruments. In many instances, foreign bodies can be retrieved by FOB with less morbidity than is associated with rigid techniques.

The sensitivity of FOB in detecting acid aspiration is claimed to exceed 90%, and on occasion food may be visualized in the airway.[26] Certain organic objects (*e.g.*, peanuts) are notorious for inciting a necrotizing endobronchial reaction, with resultant airway stenosis, atelectasis, and other long-term adverse consequences unless they are promptly removed.

Broncholiths (calcified lymph nodes eroding into airways) are a special subgroup of foreign bodies presenting with symptoms similar to those of foreign body aspiration. They are usually located in the segmental bronchi of the right lung and often produce coughing or hemoptysis. Broncholiths are identified by FOB much more frequently than by rigid bronchoscopy. However, whereas up to 90% of rigid bronchoscopies are successful in stone removal, FOB is frequently unsuccessful.[27] At least one episode of massive hemoptysis complicating the attempted removal of the broncholith with FOB has been reported.

Fiberoptic bronchoscopy appears to be an appropriate first approach to establishing a diagnosis and removing objects that are not lodged too firmly within the airway. Specialized forceps for object retrieval are available for this purpose. Rigid bronchoscopy remains the treatment of choice for extracting foreign bodies refractory to these attempts.

BRONCHIAL DISRUPTION OR TRAUMA

Bronchial or tracheal disruption is an unusual and serious outcome of severe closed or penetrating chest trauma. Pulmonary vessels are rarely injured in closed chest trauma. However, the relatively fixed position of the trachea and bronchi put these structures at risk from rapid deceleration injury or from chest compression against a closed glottis.

Patients with bronchial rupture may present with acute respiratory failure, pneumothorax, pneumomediastinum, atelectasis, and, perhaps most commonly, minimal respiratory symptoms. Pneumothorax that persists despite tube thoracostomy should arouse suspicion of bronchial disruption. Tracheobronchial disruption should be suspected in any patient sustaining closed chest trauma who presents with an unexplained hemothorax, subcutaneous emphysema, pneumothorax, pneumomediastinum, hemoptysis, and lobar atelectasis. More than 80% of bronchial injuries occur within 2.5 cm of the carina, with a slight predominance of injuries to the right main bronchus. An isolated pneumothorax occurs if the right or distal left main bronchus is disrupted, whereas deep cervical and mediastinal emphysema results from a rupture of the proximal left mainstem bronchus. Two thirds of bronchial injuries are missed until infection or atelectasis supervenes.

In all cases of suspected bronchial rupture, FOB should be performed through an endotracheal tube as soon as possible. The bronchoscope facilitates placement of the endotracheal tube cuff distal to the disruption. Morbidity and mortality are increased when bronchial disruption goes unrecognized, with the consequences dependent on whether disruption is complete or partial. Partial bronchial rupture leads to chronic fibrous stricture, frequently accompanied by atelectasis, infection, and subsequent bronchiectasis. Complete bronchial transection leads to sterile atelectasis in most cases and is usually associated with a better outcome than partial disruption. Symptoms of airway compromise or infection usually are not apparent for 7 to 10 days, and atelectasis produced by bronchial granulation tissue is often mistakenly attributed to retained secretions. Immediate repair of the bronchus is the preferred treatment approach, although bronchial repair undertaken as long as 15 years after the initial injury has been successful.

COMPLICATIONS

Flexible fiberoptic bronchoscopy is a generally safe and effective procedure, with an overall complication rate of less than 11%[14] and a major complication rate of less than 1%.[25] These figures are deceptive, however, because retrospective reviews underestimate complication rates when compared to prospective studies. Clearly, FOB should not be considered innocuous in the critical care setting. Complications of bronchoscopy include those related to premedication and anesthesia (hypotension and allergic reactions), those induced by the procedure itself (bronchospasm, dysrhythmias, and hypoxia), and those related to tissue sampling (pneumothorax and hemorrhage). While overall complication rates are low, many unusual complications have been reported, especially in the critically ill (Table 19-5).

DRUG TOXICITY

Nearly one third of the major complications of FOB relate to toxicity of topical anesthetic agents or premedications.[27] Adverse occurrences from topical anesthesia are not unexpected, considering that for the most commonly used mucosal anesthetics, serum levels approach those obtained with intravenous use. Respiratory arrest, seizures, laryngospasm, cardiovascular collapse, and methemoglobinemia have been described.

Tetracaine is the drug most frequently implicated in toxic side-effects, because of its narrow therapeutic range in relation to the volume necessary to anesthetize the bronchi. Total dose of this drug should be limited to 80 mg. Topical cocaine is also rapidly absorbed through the mucosa and is sufficiently toxic that its use should be restricted to a total dose of 200 mg or less.

Lidocaine is a safer alternative to tetracaine or cocaine for anesthesia during endoscopy, and its toxic effects are more predictable. Low-grade central nervous system signs (drowsiness and confusion) usually occur prior to cardiovascular deterioration. During an average bronchoscopic procedure, patients receive significant doses of lidocaine, usually in the range of 200 to 400 mg. Corresponding serum concentrations usually remain below 3 mg/dl. Because the majority of the dose is administered during the first 5 minutes, serum levels tend to peak from 5 to 30 minutes after beginning the procedure. The drug is rapidly metabolized on the first pass through the liver in patients free of cardiac or hepatic failure, and toxicity is rare in such individuals. Lidocaine is associated with sinus arrest and atrioventricular block, particularly in patients with underlying heart disease. In these patients, total doses for a procedure of average duration should be limited to 200 to 300 mg.

Premedications also are implicated in the morbidity and mortality that attend bronchoscopy. Many practitioners administer atropine and a narcotic analgesic or sedative, although these drugs are deemed unnecessary by most patients. Respiratory depression and hypotension appear to be the most common problems. When premedication is given well in advance of the procedure, perhaps the greatest risk is unobserved respiratory arrest. Intravenous sedation with small aliquots of diazepam, midazolam, or an opiate may be a preferable alternative. Because deep sedation can supervene as the stimulation of bronchoscopy wanes, the patient must be observed closely after the procedure. In our opinion, patients with borderline cardiac or respiratory failure should not receive narcotic or sedative premedications without formal assessment and specific indications.

TABLE 19-5 COMPLICATIONS OF FOB

Premedication	Procedural
Respiratory depression	Laryngospasm/bronchospasm
Hypertension	Hypoventilation/hypoxemia
Excitement	Hyper/hypotension
	Dysrhythmias
Anesthesia	Bacteremia/pneumonia
Laryngospasm/bronchospasm	
Hypoventilation/hypoxemia	**Tissue sampling**
Dysrhythmias	Pneumothorax
Cardiac arrest	Hemorrhage

While concerns have been raised about atropine as a premedication, there is little evidence of adverse effects with modest intramuscular doses (0.4 to 1.2 mg). Conversely, considerable data support the salutary effects of atropine in maintaining cardiac rhythm and preventing bronchospasm.

BRONCHOSPASM/LARYNGOSPASM

Bronchospasm may be encountered in any patient undergoing FOB;[28] those with asthma appear to be at particular risk.[14] In rare cases, bronchospasm results from an allergic reaction to a topical anesthetic. Mechanical or chemical stimulation of irritant receptors in the larynx and central airways may also produce bronchoconstriction by a vagal mechanism. Airway obstruction is usually transient following bronchoscopy, with pulmonary function tests reverting to baseline values within 24 hours.[28] Life-threatening laryngospasm is rare, while mild laryngospasm is perhaps the most frequent of all airway complications. It generally resolves without intervention, but in very severe cases tracheal intubation may be necessary. A laryngoscope, endotracheal tube, and paralytic agent must be readily available during all bronchoscopic procedures.

Risk factors for bronchospasm appear to consist of inadequate topical anesthesia, reactive airway disease, carinal stimulation, and hypoxemia. Bronchospasm induced by the histamine-releasing effect of opiate drugs is a theoretical risk but seldom occurs at the usual therapeutic doses. Isoproterenol and atropine alleviate the bronchoconstrictive response to FOB.[28] Addition of a β-adrenergic agonist to local anesthetics is advocated to avert bronchospasm in asthmatic subjects. The benefits of atropine in preventing bradycardia and reducing bronchial secretion volume were noted previously. Pretreatment with aminophylline or corticosteroids in addition to atropine may also be beneficial in minimizing bronchospasm.

HYPOXEMIA

Hypoxemia is an almost universal finding during FOB in both normal volunteers and patients. Arterial oxygen tension declines by an average of 20 to 30 mm Hg in response to bronchoscopy.[29] However, wide fluctuations are reported. Fortunately, FOB-induced hypoxemia is usually short-lived, lasting only 1 to 4 hours after an uncomplicated procedure. Bronchial lavage exacerbates hypoxemia. The duration of the procedure and length of suctioning are independent contributing factors. Hypoxemia during suctioning results from excessive removal of intrathoracic gas (decreasing lung volume below functional residual capacity) or from replacing oxygen mixtures with ambient air. Persistent suctioning of intrathoracic gas can reduce the effective tidal volume and, in conjunction with anesthesia, can elevate Pa_{CO_2}. Loss of tidal volume can be compensated if exhaled lung volumes are monitored during the procedure.

Radionuclide lung scanning demonstrates mismatching of ventilation perfusion ($\dot{V}/\dot{Q}$) induced by bronchoalveolar lavage, which may require a prolonged time for resolution. Arterial blood gas abnormalities tend to resolve before resolution of $\dot{V}/\dot{Q}$ defects. In subjects with delayed resolution of hypoxemia, perfusion defects resolve first.

Fiberoptic bronchoscopy may actually improve oxygenation in patients with excessive secretions or atelectasis. Pierson and associates demonstrated a mean increase in Pa_{O_2} of 14 mm Hg in 10 critically ill intubated patients following bronchoscopy.[30] Slight elevations in Pa_{CO_2}, indicative of reduced alveolar ventilation, were also seen. Some mechanically ventilated patients experience a slow rise in Pa_{CO_2} during bronchoscopy, an effect not consistently seen in spontaneously breathing patients. Improved oxygenation and increased Pa_{CO_2} may reflect the air-trapping (PEEP) effect produced when the bronchoscope partially obstructs the endotracheal tube lumen. Continuous earlobe and pulse oximetry are safe, noninvasive methods to monitor oxygen saturation during bronchoscopy and can be helpful in preventing hypoxemia and attendant dysrhythmias.

CARDIAC DYSRHYTHMIAS

Although deaths from FOB are rare, the serious complications and fatalities that do occur often result from cardiac dysrhythmias. Large retrospective surveys report a low risk of serious dysrhythmias during bronchoscopy. Credle and coworkers found only 8 minor dysrhythmias, 2 major dysrhythmias, and one cardiac death among 22,521 bronchoscopies.[31] Pereira and associates reported a 0.9% incidence of arrhythmias.[32]

All studies demonstrate sinus tachycardia. Dysrhythmias and electrocardiographic evidence of myocardial ischemia are unusually prevalent during translaryngeal passage of the bronchoscope and during suctioning.[33] Prospective studies of dysrhythmias during bronchoscopy document hypoxemia, defined by Pa_{O_2} <60 mm Hg, as a major risk factor. Katz and associates found that 40% of all patients experienced dysrhythmias, half of which were ventricular in origin.[34] The incidence correlated well with the nadir in oxygen saturation.

HYPOTENSION

Vasovagal reactions to drugs or airway manipulation are common, especially when atropine is not administered as a premedication. Intrathoracic pressure can build to high levels in intubated, mechanically ventilated patients when bronchoscopic occlusion produces air trapping. Impeded venous return and barotrauma sometimes follow.

HEMORRHAGE

Hemorrhage during bronchoscopy is rare unless transbronchial biopsy is performed. Early published reports emphasized that biopsy was a low-risk procedure associated with a small incidence of minor bleeding. Credle and colleagues found only 2 episodes of serious bleeding in more than 25,000 bronchoscopies.[31] The first report of fatal hemorrhage following transbronchial biopsy did not appear until 1975.[35] Some form of clinically significant hemoptysis occurs following this procedure in up to 20% of patients. The overall incidence of serious hemorrhage is almost 10%. When "high risk" patients are removed from consideration, the incidence declines to less than 5%.[36] For immunocompromised patients, however, the risk of hemorrhage is nearly 30%. Except for anticoagulated patients, the patients at highest risk are those with uremia, who experience significant hemorrhage in approximately 45% of biopsy attempts.[36] Despite the frequency of bleeding complications, death is rare.

These complications are minimized by restricting transbronchial biopsy to patients with more than 50,000 platelets/cu mm and normal prothrombin and partial thromboplastin times. In cases where platelet function may be impaired, it is useful to obtain bleeding times before bronchoscopy. Performance of transbronchial biopsy through an endotracheal tube under fluoroscopic guidance is recommended to minimize bleeding.[36]

Therapy of biopsy-related bleeding must be directed first toward maintenance of a clear airway and then toward control of the bleeding site. Techniques for control include placing the bleeding lung in a dependent position to prevent endobronchial spread of blood; instilling epinephrine locally as a vasoconstrictor; and performing endobronchial tamponade with the bronchoscope or with a Fogarty catheter.[36] "Wedging" the bronchoscope in a segmental bronchus prior to biopsy is also advocated. Proper patient selection, prophylaxis by transfusion of platelets, and replacement of deficient clotting factors may minimize the hazard. Patients with uremia remain at high risk for bronchoscopic bleeding and do not respond readily to blood component supplementation. Investigations into the use of vasopressin analogs to correct uremia-induced bleeding hold future promise.

PNEUMOTHORAX

Pneumothorax is a well-recognized complication of transbronchial biopsy but is virtually unreported in the absence of a biopsy procedure. Large retrospective reviews indicate that pneumothorax occurs in less than 5% to 6% of cases in which a biopsy is performed.[31,32] The incidence in prospective studies ranges from 1% to 19%[12] and compares favorably with rigid bronchoscopy and percutaneous cutting or aspiration needle biopsy. In the immunocompromised patient, the risk of pneumothorax approaches 20%. Positive-pressure ventilation and PEEP (intentional or inadvertent) are risk factors. The size or number of biopsies and operator experience do not appear to affect risk. One study favors fluoroscopic guidance to lower the risk of biopsy-induced pneumothorax, and, in the absence of extensive data, most physicians concur.[16] Chest tube drainage is required in more than 50% of cases.

BACTEREMIA, PNEUMONIA, AND FEVER

Bacteremia occurs in up to 15% of patients following rigid bronchoscopy and in a small fraction of patients after tracheal intubation. Antibiotic prophylaxis is recommended for patients with valvular heart disease undergoing FOB. Major concern regarding bacteremia is probably unwarranted, although there have been isolated reports of bacteremia following bronchoscopy and even of failure of prophylactic antibiotics. However, two prospective studies failed to document a single episode of bacteremia in a total of 143 patients who underwent bronchoscopy.[37,38]

Fever and pneumonia are more common infectious complications of this procedure. In a prospective study, Pereira and colleagues serially examined the temperature curves and chest radiographs of 100 patients after bronchoscopy.[37] Fever developed in 16% of these patients and pneumonia in 6%. No patient became bacteremic. Neither the type of bacteria isolated from bronchoscopic washings nor the performance of biopsy procedures was related to fever. Advanced age (>60 years), endobronchial abnormalities, and bronchoscopic brushing emerged as major risk factors for fever. Isolated fever following bronchoscopy in most other studies appears to occur at a lower rate, about 4%.

Tuberculosis and other pathogenic gram-negative rods have been transmitted by the fiberoptic bronchoscope on rare occasions. Saprophytic fungi and atypical mycobacteria contaminating bronchoscopy equipment have led to "pseudoepidemics."

REFERENCES

1. Kovnat DM, Rath GS, Anderson WM, et al: Maximal extent of visualization of the bronchial tree by flexible fiberoptic bronchoscopy. *Am Rev Respir Dis* 1974; 110:88
2. Giudice JC, Komansky H, Gordon R, et al: Acute upper airway obstruction—Fiberoptic bronchoscopy in diagnosis and therapy. *Crit Care Med* 1981; 9:878
3. Wanner A, Cutchavaree A: Early recognition of upper airway obstruction following smoke inhalation. *Am Rev Respir Dis* 1973; 108:1421
4. Barrett CR, Vecchione JJ, Bell AL: Flexible fiberoptic bronchoscopy for airway management during acute respiratory failure. *Am Rev Respir Dis* 1974; 109:429

5. Pingleton SK, Bone RC, Ruth WC: Helium-oxygen mixtures during bronchoscopy. *Crit Care Med* 1980; 8:50
6. Anthony JS, Sieniewicz DJ: Suctioning the left bronchial tree in critically ill patients. *Crit Care Med* 1977; 5:161
7. Marini JJ, Pierson DJ, Hudson LD: Acute lobar atelectasis: A prospective comparison of fiberoptic bronchoscopy and respiratory therapy. *Am Rev Respir Dis* 1979; 119:971
8. Harada K, Mutsuda T, Sadyama N, et al: Re-expansion of refractory atelectasis using a bronchofiberscope with a balloon cuff. *Chest* 1983; 84:725
9. Selecky PA: Evaluation of hemoptysis through the bronchoscope. *Chest* 1978; 73:741
10. Weaver LT, Solliday N, Cugell DW: Selection of patients with hemoptysis for fiberoptic bronchoscopy. *Chest* 1979; 76:7
11. Adelman M, Haponik EF, Bleeker ER, et al: Cryptogenic hemoptysis: Clinical features, bronchoscopic findings, and natural history in 67 patients. *Ann Intern Med* 1985; 102:829
12. Guckian JC, Christensen WD: Quantitative culture and Gram stain of sputum in pneumonia. *Am Rev Respir Dis* 1978; 118:997
13. Teague RB, Wallace RJ, Awe RJ: The use of quantitative sterile brush culture and Gram stain in the diagnosis of lower respiratory tract infection. *Chest* 1981; 79:157
14. Dreisin RB, Albert RK, Talley PA: Flexible fiberoptic bronchoscopy in a teaching hospital: Yield and complications. *Chest* 1978; 74:144
15. Wall CP, Gaensler EA, Carrington CB, et al: Comparison of transbronchial and open lung biopsy in chronic infiltrative lung disease. *Am Rev Respir Dis* 1981; 123:280
16. Ellis JH: Transbronchial biopsy via the fiberoptic bronchoscope: Experience with 107 consecutive cases and comparison with bronchial brushing. *Chest* 1975; 68:524
17. Stover DE, Zaman MB, Hajdu SI, et al: Bronchoalveolar lavage in the diagnosis of diffuse pulmonary infiltrates in the immunosuppressed host. *Ann Intern Med* 1984; 101:1
18. Nishio, JN, Lynch JP: Fiberoptic bronchoscopy in the immunocompromised host: The significance of a "nonspecific" transbronchial biopsy. *Am Rev Respir Dis* 1980; 121:307
19. Coleman DL, Dodek PM, Luce JM, et al: Diagnostic utility of fiberoptic bronchoscopy in patients with *Pneumocystis carinii* pneumonia and the acquired immunodeficiency syndrome. *Am Rev Respir Dis* 1983; 128:795
20. Stover DE, White DA, Romano PA, et al: Diagnosis of pulmonary disease in acquired immunodeficiency syndrome (AIDS): Role of bronchoscopy and bronchoalveolar lavage. *Am Rev Respir Dis* 1984; 130:659
21. Pitchenik AE, Ganjei P, Torres A, et al: Sputum examination for the diagnosis of *Pneumocystis carinii* pneumonia in the acquired immunodeficiency syndrome. *Am Rev Respir Dis* 1986; 133:226
22. Katz I, Rosenthal T, Michaeli D: Undiagnosed tuberculosis in hospital patients. *Chest* 1985; 87:770
23. Danek JJ, Bower JS: Diagnosis of pulmonary tuberculosis by fiberoptic bronchoscopy. *Am Rev Respir Dis* 1979; 119:677
24. Schmidt RM, Rosenkranz HS: Antimicrobial activity of local anesthetics: Lidocaine and procaine. *J Infect Dis* 1970; 121:597
25. Wimberly N, Willey S, Sullivan N, et al: Antibacterial properties of lidocaine. *Chest* 1979; 76:37
26. Ristagno RL, Kornstein MJ, Hasen-Flasch JH: Diagnosis of occult meat aspiration by fiberoptic bronchoscopy. *Am J Med* 1986; 80:154
27. Dixon GF, Donnerberg RL, Schonfeld SA, et al: Advances in the diagnosis and treatment of broncholithiasis. *Am Rev Respir Dis* 1984; 129:1028
28. Neuhaus A, Markowitz D, Rotman HH, et al: The effects of fiberoptic bronchoscopy with and without atropine premedication on pulmonary function in humans. *Ann Thorac Surg* 1978; 25:393
29. Albertini RE, Harrell JH, Kurihara N: Arterial hypoxemia induced by fiberoptic bronchoscopy. *JAMA* 1974; 230:1666
30. Pierson DJ, Iseman MD, Sutton FD, et al: Arterial blood gas changes in fiberoptic bronchoscopy during mechanical ventilation. *Chest* 1974; 66:495
31. Credle WF, Smiddy JF, Elliott RC: Complications of fiberoptic bronchoscopy. *Am Rev Respir Dis* 1974; 109:67
32. Pereira W, Kovnat DM, Snider GL: A prospective cooperative study of complications following flexible fiberoptic bronchoscopy. *Chest* 1978; 73:813
33. Lundgren R, Haggmarks S, Reiz S: Hemodynamic effects of flexible fiberoptic bronchoscopy performed under topical anesthesia. *Chest* 1982; 82:295
34. Katz AS, Michelson EL, Stanicki J: Cardiac arrhythmias: Frequency during fiberoptic bronchoscopy and correlation with hypoxemia. *Arch Intern Med* 1981; 141:603
35. Flick MR, Wasson K, Dunn LJ, et al: Fatal pulmonary hemorrhage after transbronchial lung biopsy through the fiberoptic bronchoscope. *Am Rev Respir Dis* 1975; 111:853
36. Zavala DC: Pulmonary hemorrhage in fiberoptic transbronchial biopsy. *Chest* 1976; 70:584
37. Pereira W, Kovnat DM, Khan MA, et al: Fever and pneumonia after flexible fiberoptic bronchoscopy. *Am Rev Respir Dis* 1975; 112:59
38. Kane RC, Cohen MH, Fossieck BE, et al: Absence of bacteremia after fiberoptic bronchoscopy. *Am Rev Respir Dis* 1975; 111:102

CHAPTER TWENTY

TEMPORARY CARDIAC PACEMAKERS

James R. Higgins

INDICATIONS FOR TEMPORARY PACING

GENERAL

Symptoms of organ hypoperfusion secondary to bradyarrhythmias (*i.e.*, sinus bradycardia or high-degree AV block) form the primary indications for temporary cardiac pacing (Table 20-1). Although pharmacologic therapy is usually needed acutely, it is unreliable for long-term use (hours to days) as the improvement in rate may not be sustained or conduction and other intolerable side-effects may occur. Occasionally, certain patients may develop angina or congestive heart failure because bradycardia results in a low cardiac output state, and symptoms may improve with pacing. Prophylactic temporary cardiac pacing is occasionally warranted, as in patients with Mobitz type II second-degree AV block or right bundle branch block and left axis deviation in the setting of acute myocardial infarction. Temporary pacing may also be used to prevent or terminate a variety of tachyarrhythmias.

BRADYARRHYTHMIAS

Deciding when temporary pacing is indicated in the setting of symptomatic bradycardia is usually not difficult (Fig. 20-1). Dysfunction of the sinoatrial node (sick sinus syndrome) in the form of severe sinus bradycardia or bradycardia-tachycardia syndrome is a common indication for temporary pacing. Temporary pacing is obviously effective for high-degree AV block and slow ventricular escape rhythms.

PROPHYLACTIC PACING

When symptomatic bradycardia is likely to occur, temporary pacing is indicated (Fig. 20-2). Because of an increased incidence of high-degree AV block, Mobitz II second-degree AV block should be managed with temporary pacing, even without symptoms. Mobitz type I second-degree AV block rarely progresses to high-grade block, and thus temporary pacing is infrequently needed. Other times when prophylactic pacing is used include [1] after cardiac surgery; [2] during right heart catheterization in patients with left bundle branch block; [3] during therapeutic administration of drugs that produce bradycardia; and [4] during acute myocardial infarction (see below).

TABLE 20-1 INDICATIONS FOR TEMPORARY CARDIAC PACING

1. Symptomatic bradyarrhythmias
   Sick sinus syndrome
   Bradycardia-tachycardia syndrome
   Complete heart block
   Carotid sinus hypersensitivity
   Other miscellaneous bradyarrhythmias
2. Prophylactic pacing
   Mobitz II second-degree AV block
   After cardiac surgery
   Right heart catheterization with left bundle
   branch block (LBBB)

3. During acute myocardial infarction
   Symptomatic bradycardia
   Type II second-degree AV block
   Third-degree AV block
   New bifascicular block
   New LBBB or RBBB with anterior myocar-
   dial infarction
4. Tachycardias
   Atrial flutter
   Torsades de Pointes ventricular tachycardia
   Other miscellaneous tachyarrhythmias

Figure 20-1 Symptomatic bradycardia. **A.** Rhythm strip taken from a patient presenting with severe fatigue, dizziness, and orthostatic syncope. Sinus bradycardia at 27 beats per minute and a first-degree AV block are demonstrated. A 12-lead electrocardiogram also verified left bundle branch block morphology. Although the first-degree AV block and left bundle branch block may suggest another cause for this patient's syncope, the primary indication for temporary pacing is the patient's significant symptomatic sinus bradycardia. **B.** A 5.2-second episode of sinus arrest in a patient presenting to the emergency room with three syncopal episodes in the past week. **C.** A 3.2-second pause following the self-terminating episode of atrial fibrillation with a rapid ventricular response. Symptoms secondary to the "tachycardia–bradycardia syndrome" are common indications for temporary and permanent cardiac pacing. **D.** Rhythm strip showing complete AV block with a sinus rate of 75 beats per minute and a ventricular escape rhythm of 36 beats per minute.

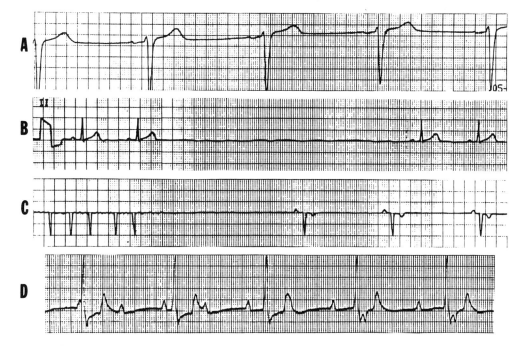

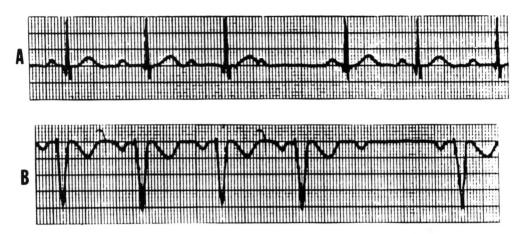

Figure 20-2 A. Mobitz type I second-degree AV block. This form of second-degree AV block rarely progresses to high-degree AV block, and thus temporary pacing is rarely indicated. **B.** Mobitz II second-degree AV block. This form of AV block is usually associated with a QRS morphology of greater than 120 msec, and indicates a need for prophylactic temporary pacing, especially in the setting of an acute myocardial infarction.

DURING ACUTE MYOCARDIAL INFARCTION

For certain types of AV conduction disturbances and bundle branch block occurring during an acute myocardial infarction (Figs. 20-3 and 20-4), temporary pacing may be indicated. However, because the risk-to-benefit ratio has not been well established, there are differing points of view. First-degree AV block that develops during an acute myocardial infarction as an isolated finding is not an indication for temporary pacing. In general, type I second-degree AV block (Wenckebach), associated with an acute inferior myocardial infarction, is not associated with symptoms, and thus does not require pacing. Type II second-degree AV block more commonly occurs during an acute anterior myocardial infarction and may progress to complete AV block. Thus, this type of second-degree AV block requires temporary pacing. Development of complete AV block requires temporary pacing.

Temporary pacing in the setting of an acute myocardial infarction is also indicated in patients who develop bifascicular block. Bifascicular block is defined as alternating right and left bundle branch block, right bundle branch block with left axis deviation, right bundle branch block with right axis deviation, and left bundle branch block with first-degree AV block. Although there is no consensus concerning prophylactic pacing in the setting of an acute anterior myocardial infarction with new right bundle branch block and normal axis or with a new left bundle branch block and a normal PR interval, I believe that these patients should undergo prophylactic pacing provided that the anticipated complication rate of inserting a temporary pacing catheter is low. In patients with a preexisting stable right bundle branch block or left bundle branch block with or without axis deviation, there is no indication for prophylactic pacing.

In summary, prophylactic temporary pacing in the setting of an acute myocardial infarction is appropriate with [1] symptomatic bradycardia of any type that responds poorly to drug therapy; [2] type II second-degree AV block; [3] third-degree AV block; [4] bifascicular block of recent onset; [5] new right bundle branch block; or [6] left bundle branch block with an anterior myocardial infarction.

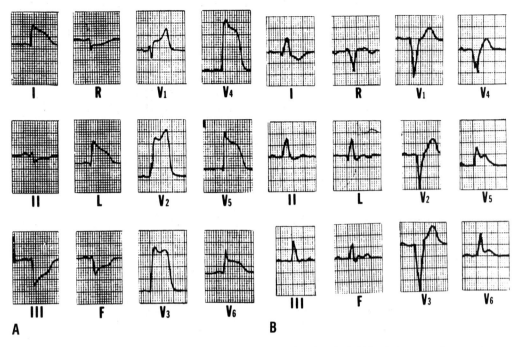

Figure 20-3 Prophylactic pacing during an acute myocardial infarction. **A.** A 12-lead electrocardiogram shows "massive" ST segment elevation in the anterior and lateral leads, pathognomonic for transmural, anterior, and lateral ischemia. **B.** This patient subsequently developed a left bundle branch block and first-degree AV block, a finding that prompted the insertion of a prophylactic temporary pacemaker.

TACHYCARDIAS

Temporary pacing can be used to *terminate* arrhythmias. Rapid atrial overdrive pacing has been used to terminate atrial flutter (Fig. 20-5). However, re-entrant arrhythmias involving the SA node, AV node, and accessory pathways as well as ventricular tachyarrhythmias have been terminated by various pacing modalities (Fig. 20-6). Termination is achieved when the pacing initiated depolarization penetrates the re-entrant tachycardia circuit, disrupting conduction or altering refractoriness within the circuit, or both, causing extinction of the re-entrant process.

Pacing can also be used to *prevent* several tachyarrhythmias. Pacing at rates faster than an automatic focus results in depolarization of the focus and "overdrives" the abnormal rhythm. This is especially useful when atrial pacing can be used to overdrive a ventricular arrhythmia. Clinically, ventricular arrhythmias of the Torsades-de-Pointes type, associated with a prolonged Q-T interval, can be suppressed with rapid atrial or ventricular pacing, or both (Fig. 20-7).

ELECTRODE CATHETERS AND EXTERNAL PACEMAKER UNITS

Catheter electrodes and external pacing "boxes" that produce electrical impulses are the basic essentials needed for temporary transvenous cardiac pacing. Transvenous electrode

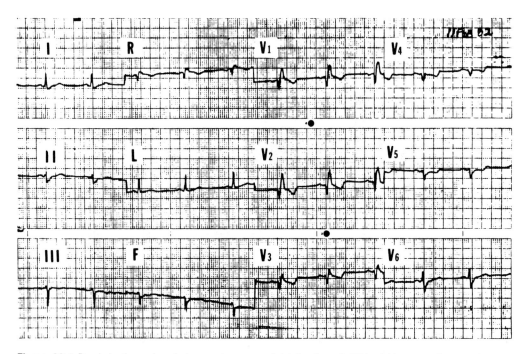

Figure 20-4 Prophylactic pacing during acute myocardial infarction. A 12-lead electrocardiogram demonstrates a right bundle branch block and left anterior fascicular block along with findings of an anterior myocardial infarction. Since this electrocardiogram was taken 1 day after one similar to that shown in Figure 20-3A, a temporary transvenous pacemaker was prophylactically inserted. This patient subsequently developed complete heart block, and permanent pacing was performed.

catheters are available in various circumferential sizes (most commonly 4 to 6 French) but, more important clinically, vary in flexibility (Fig. 20-8). Electrode catheters constructed of woven Dacron are relatively firm, whereas extruded plastic electrodes are soft and pliable. The placement of a balloon between the proximal and distal electrodes of an extruded plastic catheter allows "blood-flow assisted" catheter placement. When fluoroscopic equipment (including a radiolucent bed) is not available and urgent transvenous pacing is needed, the use of a balloon-tipped electrode is preferred. However, the electrodes of soft catheters are less stable. These catheters are also less maneuverable, which is especially important in patients with structural heart disease (*i.e.*, atrial or ventricular enlargement, tricuspid regurgitation, low cardiac output states). Thus, because of characteristics favoring manipulation and stability of position, woven Dacron firm catheters are preferable, although even with fluoroscopic guidance one must be careful not to perforate vessels or endocardium during insertion.

Most temporary electrode catheters are bipolar, that is, both the distal (cathodal) and proximal (anodal) electrodes are within the heart chamber being paced. Comparatively, unipolar catheters have only one distal electrode, used for cathodal stimulation, with the skin used as the anodal "electrode." Bipolar electrodes are preferred because they are less susceptible to external electrical interference but, if needed, can be converted to a functional unipolar electrode (Fig. 20-9).

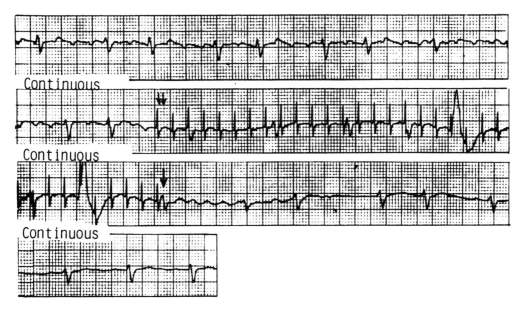

Figure 20-5 Temporary pacing to terminate tachyarrhythmias. The tracings shown are continuous and from day 1 after coronary artery bypass surgery. Atrial flutter with a varied ventricular response has developed. At the arrows, atrial pacing (through epicardial temporary leads) has begun at a rate slightly greater than 300 per minute. Upon termination of pacing *(larger arrow),* atrial fibrillation is present that rapidly and spontaneously converts to sinus rhythm.

Modified pacing catheters are now available that allow AV sequential pacing and intracardiac pressure measurements. Multielectrode catheters with electrodes positioned so that both atrial and ventricular endocardial contact occur allow temporary AV pacing with a single catheter (Fig. 20-10). Preformed electrode catheters have been designed to facilitate placement into the right atrial appendage or coronary sinus, and thus allow atrial pacing (Fig. 20-11). Electrode catheters incorporating a lumen are also available and allow fluid or drug administration as well as pressure determinations.

Figure 20-6 Temporary pacing to terminate tachyarrhythmias. A nine-beat run of ventricular tachycardia is terminated by six rapidly delivered ventricular pacing stimuli. The first pacing stimulus is delivered synchronous with the last beat of ventricular tachycardia and is not readily seen on this rhythm strip; however, the last five pacing stimuli change the QRS morphology, and, when pacing is stopped, normal sinus rhythm returns.

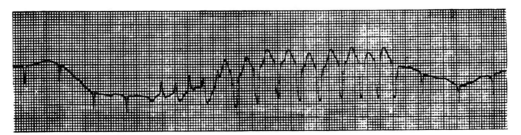

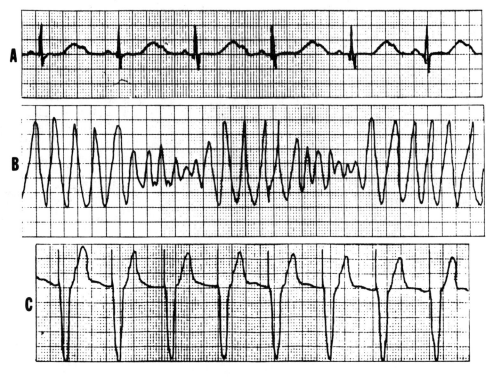

Figure 20-7 Pacing to prevent tachyarrhythmias. **A.** Sinus rhythm with a greatly prolonged QT (QT-U) interval. **B.** The patient subsequently developed "Torsades de Pointes" ventricular tachycardia. Note the characteristic varying QRS morphology with "turning of the points." **C.** When this arrhythmia is associated with a slow sinus rhythm (as in this case), temporary pacing can be effective in preventing arrhythmia recurrence by instituting pacing at a higher rate.

The external temporary pacemaker unit controls the stimulus output and frequency (Fig. 20-12). The range of output varies from 0 to 20 (ma) and the frequency from 30 to 180 pulses per minute (ppm). Easily readable and usable dials on the unit allow control of these variables as well as sensitivity. The latter variable adjusts the amplitude of intrinsic QRS voltage (millivolts) that must be sensed before the external pacemaker unit suppresses its output. Adjustment of this control can result in fully asynchronous pacing, where no sensing occurs and the pacemaker fires at the set rate regardless of the patient's own rhythm, or the most sensitive ("full demand") setting can result in oversensing of T waves or extrinsic electrical signals and can partially or fully suppress generator output. Thus, careful adjustment of this control is necessary for successful temporary pacing.

PROCEDURE FOR TEMPORARY PACEMAKER INSERTION

GENERAL

Temporary transvenous pacing electrode catheters can be inserted through several venous access sites, including brachial, femoral, subclavian, internal jugular, and external jugular veins. Virtually all temporary ventricular pacing electrodes are positioned in the right ven-

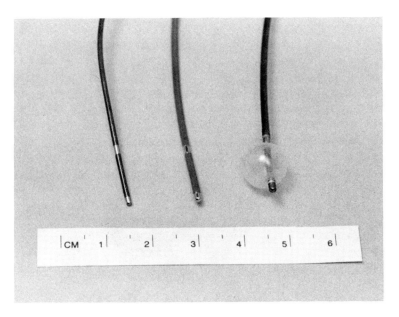

Figure 20-8 Electrode catheters. Transvenous electrode catheters are available in various sizes (commonly 4 French to 6 French). The left electrode catheter is constructed of woven Dacron and is a firm, relatively nonpliable catheter. The middle catheter is formed from extruded plastic and is soft and pliable. The electrode catheter on the right is formed from extruded plastic and has a balloon located between the distal and proximal electrodes to allow "blood-flow-assisted" catheter placement.

tricular apex, while atrial temporary pacing electrodes are positioned in the right atrial appendage. Percutaneous transthoracic cardiac electrode placement is rarely indicated, especially since external noninvasive temporary cardiac pacing became available.

PREPARATION

The placement of a temporary pacing electrode should not be undertaken without adequate technical support. Continuous electrocardiographic monitoring and a defibrillator at the bedside must be available. Ideally, fluoroscopy and a fluoroscopic bed should be available, but, if not, a balloon-tipped electrode catheter should be used. Standard sterile technique, including sterile gowns and gloves for the inserting physician and assistants, are necessary. Sterile drapes and sterile preparation of the insertion site are also mandatory. Subcutaneous and deep local anesthesia using standard anesthetics such as lidocaine or bupivacaine should be available.

PERCUTANEOUS SELDINGER TECHNIQUE

The percutaneous Seldinger technique has become a standard method of introducing various catheters into the cardiac chambers. A needle is inserted into the vein and free blood flow established. A flexible guidewire is inserted through the needle and passed gently into the venous lumen. The needle is removed. A small puncture wound is then made with a scalpel blade at the skin insertion site and blunt dissection used to create a pathway for the dilator

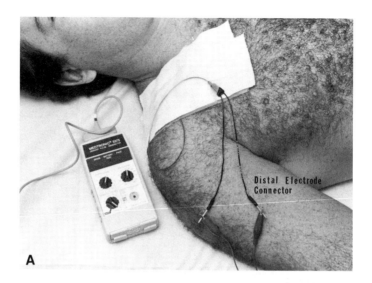

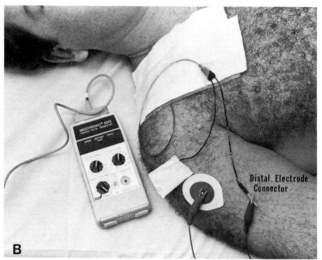

Figure 20-9 Converting a bipolar to a unipolar pacemaker. Conversion of a bipolar electrode to a unipolar electrode is sometimes useful if under-sensing of the bipolar electrogram occurs or if one electrode becomes electrically disrupted, thus preventing the electrical circuit from being completed. **A.** Typical bipolar connection. Attachment of the negative and positive poles of the generator to the respective distal and proximal catheter electrodes is shown using connecting cable and alligator clamps. **B.** Conversion to a unipolar pacemaker. The alligator connector to the distal electrode remains unchanged, whereas proximal electrode pin is covered with adhesive tape (or other insulator). The other alligator connector is attached to a skin electrode to complete of the circuit back to the generator.

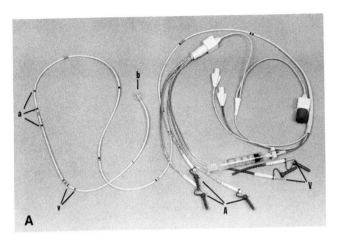

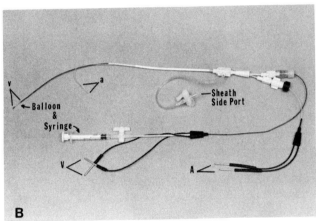

Figure 20-10 Multielectrode catheters. Electrode catheters have been designed with distal and proximal electrodes so that AV sequential pacing can be performed. **A.** A "pacing pulmonary artery" catheter, designed to provide atrial and ventricular sequential pacing while maintaining the ability for right atrial, pulmonary artery, or pulmonary wedge pressures as well as thermodilution cardiac output measurement. Three atrial electrodes (a) at approximately 30 cm and two ventricular electrodes at 20 cm from the balloon tip (b) with respective pin connectors (A, V) are additions to a standard thermodilution pulmonary artery catheter. **B.** The system shown has a ventricular balloon flotation electrode that is placed into the right ventricular apex. A small atrial "J" electrode can then be positioned through a catheter lumen in the right atrium.

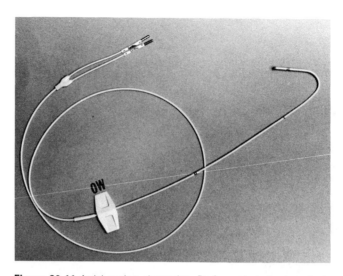

Figure 20-11 Atrial pacing electrodes. Preformed electrode catheters have been designed with a "permanent J" to facilitate placement into the right atrial appendage. The "orientation wing" *(OW)* provided with this electrode catheter allows relatively easy placement into the right atrial appendage, in experienced hands, even without fluoroscopic guidance. Because of stability, these preformed atrial J wires are a preferred form of atrial pacing.

and sheath. A tapered vessel dilator with a shorter surrounding sheath is then introduced over the guidewire and inserted into the vessel. The dilator and wire are removed, leaving the sheath in place. Venous access is thus established, allowing passage of the temporary electrode catheter into the vascular system. A number of sheath sets are available, several of which have infusion side-ports that allow the sheath to be used for intravenous fluid or drug administration.

A modification of the Seldinger technique allows the placement of two sheaths into the vein by a single percutaneous "stick." The technique is similar to that described previously with the following exceptions: Once the sheath, dilator, and guidewire are in the venous system, the dilator is removed, leaving the sheath and guidewire in place. A second guidewire is then placed through the sheath and into the venous system. The sheath is subsequently removed, leaving two guidewires in the vein. Finger pressure at the site of guidewire entrance into the venous system significantly reduces back-bleeding. Now that two guidewires are in the venous system, separate sheath and dilator systems are passed down each wire into the vein. The guidewires and dilators are then removed, leaving two sheaths in the venous system. This technique is very useful when AV sequential pacing is contemplated because it allows for the passage of separate atrial and ventricular leads.

BRACHIAL APPROACH

The medial superficial vein in the antecubital fossa drains into the basilic vein and provides a direct pathway to the central venous circulation. Using a tourniquet and the percutaneous Seldinger technique as described previously, a venous sheath can frequently be placed into the vein, allowing access to the circulation. The passage of the electrode catheter from the

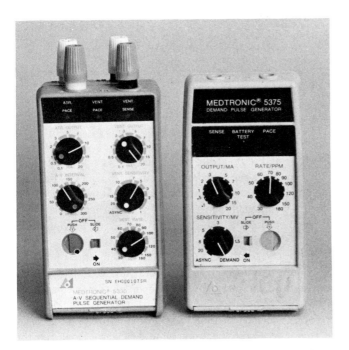

Figure 20-12 External temporary pacemaker generators. External pulse generators provide reliable output and pacing rates. Powered by a 9.0-v battery, they can provide 20 ma output and pacing rates of up to 800 pulses per minute (specially designed units—not shown here). Dual channel units (*left* in picture) are provided that allow AV synchronous pacing while controlling the AV interval (in milliseconds), ventricular sensitivity, and atrial/ventricular outputs.

arm to the subclavian vein may be difficult in some patients but can be facilitated by patient shoulder and head movements. Occasionally, the brachial vein can be cannulated percutaneously, but more commonly a cutdown is performed to isolate the vein. The cutdown technique minimizes the risk of damaging associated structures such as the brachial artery. The use of the brachial approach avoids disturbing the subclavian vein, which may be important if permanent pacemaker implantation is contemplated. However, arm movement can produce significant catheter movement, which in turn may lead to dislodgement or perforation.

FEMORAL APPROACH

The femoral vein lies just medial to the femoral artery and is generally easily cannulated by the percutaneous technique. Positioning of the electrode catheter into the right heart chambers by this technique is more difficult. Thus, maneuverability is very important, and a stiff, woven Dacron catheter and fluoroscopy should be used. The mobility of the patient is restricted once the catheter is in place because the patient cannot flex at the hip joint. There may be an increased risk of thromboembolic phenomena and an increased risk of infection with the catheter in the femoral position. At present I rarely use this approach unless the patient is undergoing cardiac catheterization utilizing the femoral approach (usually in the acute myocardial infarction setting when thrombolytic therapy is being administered) and a temporary pacemaker is necessary.

SUBCLAVIAN APPROACH

Either the right or left subclavian vein has become a favored site for venous access by many physicians. The heart chambers are readily accessible and catheter positioning relatively easy from either the right or left subclavian approach. Although supraclavicular approaches to the subclavian vein have been described, the infraclavicular approach is most commonly used. Because the subclavian vein arches over the first rib and beneath the clavicle, advancement of a needle just under the outer one half to one third of the clavicle and directed about 2 cm above the sternal notch will puncture the subclavian vein (see also Chapter 12, "Vascular Cannulation"). Using the previously described technique will allow either one or two venous sheaths to be placed in the subclavian vein. The electrode catheter position is stable because the catheter can be taped securely to the chest wall and little movement of the catheter occurs, unlike the brachial approach.

Complications include [1] hemothorax secondary to inadvertent puncture of the innominate or subclavian artery; [2] pneumothorax from inadvertent puncture of the apical pleura; [3] hydrothorax if infusion of fluid is started before proper placement has been ascertained; and [4] air embolism because of negative intrathoracic pressure "sucking" air in through the syringe. With operator experience, meticulous care to anatomic landmarks, and use of the Trendelenburg position, these complications should be rare. However, the subclavian approach for temporary pacemaker insertion may preclude the vein's later use for the insertion of a permanent pacemaker.

INTERNAL JUGULAR APPROACH

The internal jugular veins on the right and the left provide easy venous access to the right heart chambers. With proper taping and suturing of the catheter, catheter movement is minimal even with neck motion. Various approaches to the internal jugular vein have been proposed, based on the anatomic relationship of the vein to the sternocleidomastoid muscle. One approach involves skin access medial to the sternal head, a second between the sternal and clavicular head, and a third lateral to the clavicular head. Each method can be equally successful; however, with each approach it is important to avoid puncture of the carotid artery. Pneumothorax is less frequent with this approach than with the subclavian approach, a complication especially important to avoid in patients with compromised lung function. This port of venous access leaves both subclavian veins free for permanent pacemaker insertion, if necessary. Internal jugular cannulation has become my preferred approach to temporary cardiac pacing.

TRANSTHORACIC APPROACH

Although the transthoracic approach (Fig. 20-13) has been used successfully on many occasions, it is uncommon that temporary pacing is so acutely needed that the risk of this procedure is warranted. This seems especially true since the introduction of effective external noninvasive temporary cardiac pacing. I prefer a transthoracic entry site just to the left of the sternum in the fourth intercostal space with the needle and stylette directed perpendicular to the chest wall, rather than the subxiphoid approach. Connecting the stylette and needle to the V1 lead of a standard electrocardiograph provides an "injury current" upon

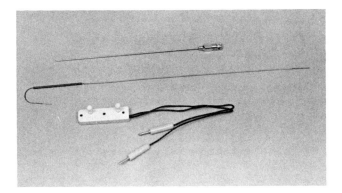

Figure 20-13 Transthoracic temporary pacing. Transthoracic pacing kits are provided, supplying a needle with stylette *(top)*, pacing electrode *(middle)*, and electrode connector *(bottom)*. The transthoracic approach now is rarely indicated, especially since the introduction of the external noninvasive pacing (see Fig. 20-14).

penetration of the right ventricular wall (providing that there is not complete ventricular asystole). Subsequent removal of the stylette and aspiration of blood allows the pacing electrode to be passed through the needle and into the right heart chamber. The needle is then removed and the electrodes are connected to a standard pacing box. This method of temporary pacing has several severe complications, including pneumothorax, coronary artery perforation, mediastinal bleeding, and cardiac tamponade. It thus should be considered an approach of "last resort."

EXTERNAL NONINVASIVE APPROACH

A modified external noninvasive temporary pacemaker monitor (Fig. 20-14) was introduced in 1981. Since that time there have been several published reports documenting good stimulation thresholds, patient comfort, and stimulation effectiveness. Although almost all patients complain of pectoral muscle stimulation, it is frequently tolerable and uncommonly prevents successful short-term external stimulation. Initial reports indicate that noninvasive pacing is technically ineffective in producing electrical ventricular responses in 22% of the patients in whom it is applied. Thus, although external noninvasive temporary cardiac pacing has been extremely useful in initiating rapid electrical stimulation, patient discomfort limits long-term use and is technically ineffective in greater than 20% of patients. However, it remains an important modality to consider when acute cardiac pacing is necessary and other means of pacing are not readily available. Newly designed electrodes have decreased skeletal muscle stimulation and increased both the capture rate and duration of pacing possible.

CATHETER POSITIONING

The ideal catheter position (Fig. 20-15) for ventricular pacing is the right ventricular apex. At the apex the electrode catheter tip becomes wedged in the trabeculae of the right ventricle, and endocardial contact is better maintained. Electrode placement in the right ventricular outflow tract or the free wall is not desirable because of instability. These sites also seem more prone to ventricular perforation, especially if any undue pressure is placed on the

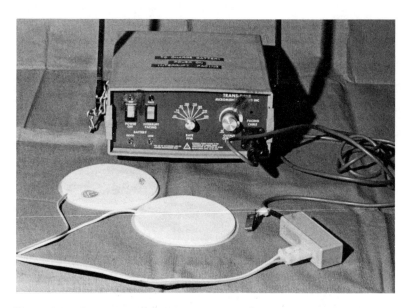

Figure 20-14 External noninvasive pacing. Large electrode patches are attached to the anterior and posterior chest walls, and the output is adjusted upward to obtain ventricular capture. Technically effective pacing can be obtained in nearly 80% of patients; however, patient discomfort used to limit long-term use.

electrode tip. The natural sweep of the electrode catheter from the superior vena cava helps stabilize the lead at the right ventricular apex without undue pressure. As previously stated, it is ideal to position catheters into the right ventricular apex under fluoroscopic control; however, the use of a balloon flotation catheter and electrocardiographic monitoring during catheter insertion can be very successful. In this technique standard limb electrocardiographic leads are attached to the patient. Using an "alligator-to-alligator" connector, the distal electrode of the catheter is connected to one of the precordial chest electrocardiographic leads (usually V_1). Using an electrocardiographic machine that has simultaneous three-channel recording is helpful in that one or two standard limb lead electrocardiograms can be displayed for reference along with the "electrograms" obtained using the unipolar chest lead (Fig. 20-16). When the electrode catheter is in the superior vena cava the atrial deflection is negative, and in the inferior vena cava it is positive. The deflections in the right atrium are more rapid, discrete, and larger than in either vena cava. As the electrode catheter is advanced into the right ventricle, there is a much larger ventricular electrogram and the atrial electrogram becomes exceedingly small. When the electrode catheter touches the right ventricular wall, ST segment elevation ("injury current") is seen. Having a simultaneously recorded limb lead allows an easy reference for recognition of the atrial and ventricular electrograms.

A variety of new electrode catheters are available for atrial pacing. Catheters with several electrodes positioned 10 to 20 cm proximal to the distal tip electrodes have been designed (see Fig. 20-10A). These electrodes are positioned to lie along the lateral right atrial wall, allowing atrial sensing and pacing. An innovative modification of this technique allows for a small atrial J wire to be placed through a luminal opening in the right atrium in a

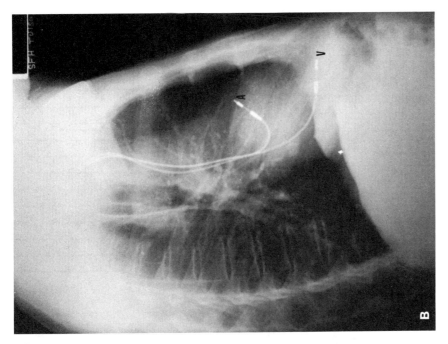

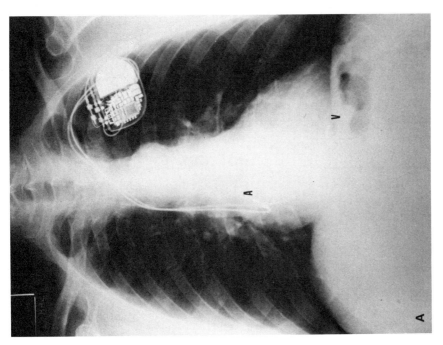

Figure 20-15 Catheter electrode positioning. Although these radiographs are of a patient with a permanent dual chamber pacemaker in place, the correct positioning of both the atrial (A) and ventricular (V) electrodes is shown. **A.** In the AP projection, fluoroscopic evaluation shows the atrial electrode to be moving from a right-to-left direction with atrial contraction and the ventricular lead to have a slight "bend" across the tricuspid valve with right ventricular contraction. **B.** Lateral views should show anterior positioning of both the atrial and ventricular electrodes.

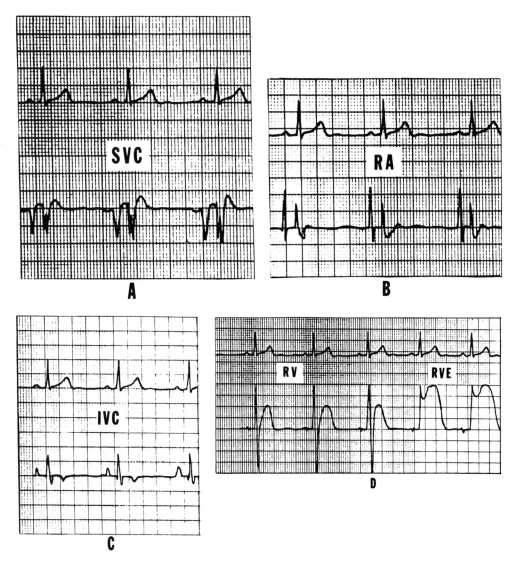

Figure 20-16 Electrocardiographic monitoring during electrode catheter positioning. A unipolar electrogram (*lower tracing in each panel*), obtained by attaching lead V$_1$ of the electrocardiographic machine to the distal pole of the electrode catheter, can be of use in positioning the catheter into the appropriate position. Using an electrocardiographic machine that can give simultaneous limb lead recording (*upper tracing*) is helpful to those unfamiliar with atrial and ventricular electrograms. An electrogram obtained in the superior vena cava (A) shows a negative atrial deflection, whereas in the inferior vena cava (B) the atrial electrogram is positive. The deflections in the right atrium (C) are more rapid, discrete, and larger than in either vena cava. As the catheter is advanced into the right ventricle (D), the ventricular electrogram (RV) is much larger and the atrial electrogram barely detectable. When the electrode catheter is against the right ventricular endocardium (RVE), ST segment elevation is seen (D, last two complexes).

catheter with distal electrodes already positioned in the right ventricular apex (see Fig. 20-10B). Both of these types of catheter adaptations have been developed to allow a "one venous stick" approach to atrioventricular pacing. In my experience, however, those few patients who definitely benefit from temporary AV sequential pacing have significant structural heart disease, and the atrial electrodes provided by these catheters do not *reliably* pace the atrium. Therefore, in patients with significant right ventricular or large anterior myocardial infarctions who require pacing and may benefit from AV synchronous pacing, I prefer to place a second electrode catheter in the atrium. A preformed J-shaped electrode catheter has been developed for transvenous temporary right atrial pacing (see Fig. 20-11). Using the two-access modification of the Seldinger technique previously described, "one stick" can be used to place separate atrial and ventricular leads. In my experience, this approach provides more reliable AV synchronous pacing.

PACING AND SENSING THRESHOLD DETERMINATIONS

After obtaining good anatomic positioning of the pacemaker catheter electrode, a stimulation threshold should be determined. With the pacemaker electrodes connected to the external pulse generator, pacing should begin at a rate at least 10 beats per minute faster than the patient's intrinsic heart rate with the output set at 5 ma. After appropriate pacing is demonstrated by electrocardiographic monitoring, the output of the pacemaker (in milliamps) is gradually decreased until the stimuli fail to produce ventricular (or atrial) capture. The milliampere current setting at which capture fails to occur is called the "pacing threshold." The threshold is usually 0.5 ma and should be less than 1 ma. Because the pacing threshold varies with medications, respiration, sleep, and other physiologic variables, the pacemaker output should be set at three to five times this threshold.

If the pacemaker is to be used in a demand mode, it is also important that adequate sensing of the endocardial electrogram be occurring. The amplitude of the endocardial signal can be recorded using the same precordial chest lead used for positioning as previously described. However, a more common method involves setting the pacemaker at a rate slower than the patient's intrinsic rate. The sensitivity of the pulse generator is then set at its most sensitive level (the lowest amplitude setting), and gradually the sensitivity is decreased (toward higher numbers). When the pacemaker fails to sense and begins pacing competitively with the patient's intrinsic rhythm, the "sensitivity threshold" has been determined. For demand pacing the sensitivity should be set at a more sensitive level (a lower number).

POSTINSERTION CARE

The electrode catheter should be secured externally to the skin preferably at two sites and with 2-0 silk. Antimicrobial ointment should be placed at the electrode insertion site onto the skin and a sterile dressing applied. Some prefer a clear adhesive surgical dressing that allows the insertion site to be inspected easily. If a standard dressing is used, it should be changed daily and the skin inspected for any signs of local infection. Coiling the proximal electrode catheter around the insertion site and firmly securing with tape prevents inadvertent dislodgement of the distal electrode catheter. An extending cable, connecting the proximal electrode pins to the pacemaker generator, should be used. This connecting cable allows the external pulse generator to be securely attached to the patient's bed, free of the patient. The plastic shield provided with the pacemaker generator should be slipped over the controls on the pacemaker unit to prevent inadvertent control movement. Covering of the entire pacemaker unit (including shield) with a plastic see-through glove prevents inadvertent exposure of the generator to liquids.

It is especially important to avoid any electrical hazards, since the patient has an electrically conductive pathway from the outside of the body to the inside of the heart. Any leakage current must be minimized, and thus if the patient is on an electric bed it should be disconnected from the power source except when movement of the bed is required. The safety of all electrical devices in contact with the patient must be assured.

A portable chest radiograph and a 12-lead electrocardiogram should be obtained after pacemaker insertion. The former documents electrode position and, more importantly, excludes the possibility of a pneumothorax, especially if a subclavian approach was used. The electrocardiogram documents QRS morphology produced by pacing at the selected site. This is an important baseline in that a change in the paced QRS morphology can be the first sign of electrode movement. Continuous monitoring of the patient should also be performed.

In addition to daily inspection of the insertion site, a daily physical examination should be performed. The discovery of a pericardial friction rub may indicate catheter perforation. The presence of a clicking noise may imply intercostal muscle stimulation.

The pacing threshold and sensitivity should be checked daily because marked changes in threshold may indicate catheter movement or perforation. Marked changes in threshold generally require repositioning of the electrode catheter. If there is any change in these variables, a chest radiograph and a 12-lead electrocardiogram (during ventricular pacing) should be obtained to ascertain whether the catheter position and the QRS morphology are similar to those obtained immediately after insertion.

At least once each day the rate of the pacemaker generator should be decreased to allow an evaluation of the underlying rhythm. This is important in that it assesses the need for continued pacing. In addition, pacing and sensitivity thresholds should be measured and recorded. Because the electrode catheter presents risks for infection, thromboembolism, and perforation, it should not be kept in place longer than necessary.

COMPLICATIONS

GENERAL

The complications associated with temporary cardiac pacing include cardiac perforation, mechanical stimulation of the heart resulting in arrhythmias, infection, and thromboembolism. Most of these complications have been alluded to earlier in the procedure section; however, they are so important that I believe a separate discussion is warranted.

PERFORATION

Perforation of the ventricular endocardium is suspected when the pacing threshold increases or the pacing sensitivity changes greatly. A more dramatic presentation is that pacing ceases completely, the patient develops severe shoulder or pericardial pain, or diaphragmatic or intercostal muscle stimulation occurs. Supporting physical examination findings include a new pericardial friction rub or extracardiac clicks, or both.

The diagnosis of ventricular perforation can be confirmed by recording intracardiac electrograms (Fig. 20-17). The normal acute unipolar right ventricular endocardial electrogram shows "massive" ST segment elevation. Recording a small unipolar electrogram with-

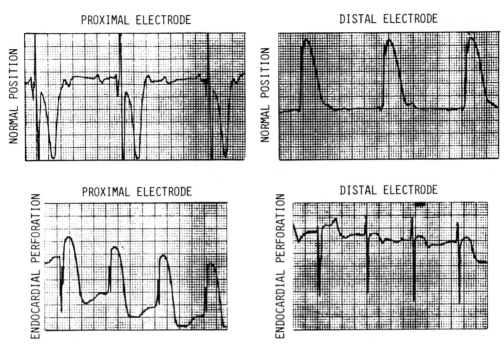

Figure 20-17 Electrocardiographic changes suggestive of endocardial perforation. Normal unipolar electrograms obtained from the proximal *(upper left)* and distal *(upper right)* electrodes at the time of catheter electrode placement are shown. When electrode perforation occurs shortly after electrode placement, the unipolar electrogram from the proximal electrode *(lower left)* resembles the initial electrogram obtained from the distal electrode. The changes shown here are dramatic—more commonly, a small amount of "ST segment elevation" is present on the proximal electrogram, whereas the distal electrogram shows a "flat ST segment" when perforation has occurred.

out or with small ST segment elevation from the distal electrode suggests endocardial perforation. Further, if a unipolar electrogram is obtained from the proximal electrode (usually 10 mm proximal to the distal electrode), an electrogram normally seen with distal electrode may be seen—ST segment elevation. Fortunately, pacemaker withdrawal and repositioning do not usually produce hemopericardium because the site of perforation is sealed by the inflammatory process invoked by the trauma and the contraction of the ventricular myocardium. However, observation for signs of pericardial tamponade is mandatory, and an echocardiogram is recommended.

ARRHYTHMIA INDUCTION

If ventricular premature depolarizations (VPDs) occur more frequently than before pacemaker insertion, and if the morphology of the VPDs resembles that of the paced QRS, mechanical stimulation of the ventricle should be suspected. If excellent pacing and sensing thresholds are still present, the ectopy usually self-dissipates after an hour or two. However, if runs of ventricular tachycardia occur or if threshold changes are marked, catheter repositioning should be attempted to eliminate the possibility that the ventricular ectopy is catheter-related.

THROMBOEMBOLISM

Clinically suspect venous thrombosis and subsequent embolism are uncommon unless the electrode catheter is left in place more than 3 or 4 days or the femoral vein is used for venous access, or both. Because mobility contributes to the risk of thrombosis, the use of the subclavian or internal jugular approaches should minimize the risk of embolism. Prophylactic low-dose heparinization is also useful, as is careful inspection of the venous entry site so that inflammation and infection that predispose to thrombosis can be avoided.

INFECTION

If the electrode catheter is inserted under sterile conditions and appropriate skin care is taken after insertion, infection is a rare complication. Although prophylactic antibiotics are not indicated, once an infection is suspected, systemic antibiotics and catheter removal are imperative.

TROUBLESHOOTING

NONPACING/INCREASING PACING THRESHOLD

Movement or total displacement of the electrode from the endocardium is the most common cause of a marked change in pacing threshold, whereas generator failure or electrode/lead breakage is much less common. The connection of the electrode catheter to the generator and the function of the pacemaker generator and battery can be easily evaluated. A 12-lead electrocardiogram, evaluating axis and QRS morphology, and a chest radiograph are both helpful in accessing electrode movement. Electrode catheter perforation can be verified with endocardial electrograms, as discussed previously.

Abnormalities of the electrode lead are uncommon but can be suspected when there is variation in the pacemaker spikes on the surface electrocardiogram. Recording unipolar electrograms from each electrode (*i.e.,* the distal and the proximal) is useful in diagnosing electrode/lead breakage. For example, inability to record an electrogram or the recording of an intermittent signal indicates electrode or lead disruption. If only one electrode is abnormal, the pacemaker can be converted from a bipolar to a unipolar pacing system (see Fig. 20-9), using the functional electrode and lead.

SENSING ABNORMALITIES

Abnormalities in sensing can be caused by an inadequate endocardial signal, incorrect setting of the generator's sensitivity, and pacemaker generator malfunction. Sensitivity can be evaluated and adjusted as previously discussed. Recording of a bipolar endocardial electrogram from both the proximal and distal electrodes allows evaluation of the amplitude of the sensed endocardial electrogram. If undersensing is occurring even at the most sensitive setting and the bipolar electrogram is small, conversion from bipolar to unipolar sensing (see Fig. 20-9) may have dramatic results. An endocardial electrogram can also be useful in ascertaining whether oversensing of a T wave or ST segment is occurring.

If adjusting the generator's sensitivity or changing to unipolar sensing does not correct the sensing abnormality, then repositioning of the catheter may be needed. If adequate endocardial signals are verified yet abnormalities in sensing occur, generator malfunction should be suspected and another generator connected.

REFERENCES

1. Zipes DP, Duffin EG: Cardiac pacemakers. In Braunwald E (ed): *Heart Disease*, p 744. Philadelphia, WB Saunders, 1984

2. Langendorf R, Pick A: Atrioventricular block type II (Mobitz)—Its nature and clinical significance. *Circulation* 1968; 38:819

3. Atkins J, Leshin S, Blomqvist G, et al: Ventricular conduction blocks and sudden death in acute myocardial infarction. *N Engl J Med* 1973; 288:281

4. Nimitz A, Shubrooks S, Hutter A, et al: The significance of bundle branch block during acute myocardial infarction. *Am Heart J* 1975; 90:439

5. Hindman MD, Wagner GS, JaRo M, et al: The clinical significance of bundle branch block complicating acute myocardial infarction: II. Indications for temporary and permanent pacemaker therapy. *Circulation* 1978; 58:689

6. Batchelder J, Zipes DP: Treatment of tachyarrhythmias by pacing. *Arch Intern Med* 1975; 135:1115

7. Higgins JR: Automatic burst extrastimulus pacemaker to treat recurrent ventricular tachycardia in a patient with mitral valve prolapse: More than 2000 documented successful tachycardia terminations. *J Am Coll Cardiol* 1986; 8:446

8. Smith W, Gallagher J: "Les Torsade de Pointes": An unusual ventricular arrhythmia. *Ann Intern Med* 1980; 93:578

9. Schnitzler RN, Caracta AR, Damato AN: "Floating" catheter for temporary transvenous ventricular pacing. *Am J Cardiol* 1973; 31:351

10. Bilitch M, Berens SC: Insertion techniques and electrode placement. In *Temporary Transvenous Cardiac Pacing: A Clinical Update*, pp 14–19. Pro Clinica, 1981

11. Rosenberg AS, Grossman JI, Escher DJW, Furman S: Bedside transvenous cardiac pacing. *Am Heart J* 1969; 77:697

12. Rao G, Zikria EA: Technique of insertion of pacing electrode through the internal jugular vein. *J Cardiovasc Surg* 1973; 14:294

13. Killip T, Kimball JT: Percutaneous techniques for introducing flexible electrodes for intracardiac pacing. *Ann NY Acad Sci* 1969; 167:597

14. Weinstein J, Gnoj J, Mazzarra JT, et al: Temporary transvenous pacing via the percutaneous femoral vein approach. A prospective study of 100 cases. *Am Heart J* 1973; 85:695

15. Roberts R: Emergency transthoracic pacemaker—Review. *Ann Emerg Med* 1981; 10:600

16. Zoll PM, Zoll RH, Falk RH, et al: External non-invasive temporary cardiac pacing: Clinical trials. *Circulation* 1985; 71:937

17. Littleford PO, Pepine CJ: A new temporary atrial pacing catheter inserted percutaneously into the subclavian vein without fluoroscopy: A preliminary report. *Pace* 1981; 4:458

18. Whalen RE, Starmer CF: Electric shock hazards in clinical cardiology. *Mod Conc Cardiovasc Dis* 1967; 36:7

CHAPTER TWENTY-ONE

LUMBAR PUNCTURE AND EPIDURAL ANALGESIA IN THE ICU

David L. Brown
J. F. Flynn

Peridural analgesia (lumbar puncture and epidural anesthesia) in the intensive care unit (ICU) is made challenging by many factors, including the four "Ps": patient, position, physician, and paraphernalia. Patients are often uncooperative and may have dependent edema obscuring the bony landmarks. Frequently they cannot be positioned properly, and, far too often, the physician performing the procedure is in an early stage of training and unfamiliar with peridural anatomy. Paraphernalia complicate the technique in two ways: First, monitoring and life-support equipment often prevent ideal positioning; and, second, the needles, syringes, and collection tubing used to perform the peridural techniques may be unfamiliar to the operator.

In this chapter we outline the indications and management of peridural techniques in the ICU. The descriptions of lumbar puncture relate to its diagnostic and therapeutic uses, whereas epidural cannulation is used primarily as a route of analgesia administration.

IMMEDIATE CONCERNS

There are three main indications for lumbar puncture: [1] to obtain information about the cellular, chemical, microbiological, and pressure changes of cerebrospinal fluid (CSF) (*e.g.*, bacterial meningitis); [2] as a route of injection in diagnostic procedures (*e.g.*, myelography); and [3] as a route of treatment (*e.g.*, intrathecal antibiotics). Epidural techniques traditionally have been limited to the acute surgical and obstetric settings. Analgesia with local anesthetics and application of narcotics to the neuraxis makes epidural techniques important to the intensivist. Indications include [1] analgesia (either local anesthetic or narcotic) following surgery or trauma and [2] sympathetic blockade (local anesthetic) for pain relief in conditions such as reflex sympathetic dystrophy.

The absolute contraindications to lumbar puncture are similar to those of epidural analgesia. Epidural analgesia mandates considerations of additional relative contraindications. Any listing of indications or contraindications must be tempered with judgment, physician experience, and the clinical situation (Table 21-1).

TABLE 21-1   CONTRAINDICATIONS TO PERIDURAL AND EPIDURAL TECHNIQUES

A. Absolute
   1. Patient refusal
   2. Infection of skin or underlying tissue
   3. Full anticoagulation or severe coagulopathy
   4. Raised intracranial pressure

B. Relative
   1. Hypovolemia (LA)*
   2. Hypotension (LA)*
   3. Fixed cardiac output (mitral, aortic stenosis) (LA)*
   4. Preexisting CNS disease (*e.g.,* multiple sclerosis)
   5. Allergy to drug
   6. Systemic infection (catheter technique)
   7. Spinal deformities (technical difficulty)

*LA = when using local anesthetics.

HOW TO PROCEED

The 12 thoracic and 5 lumbar vertebrae make up the bony reference for peridural techniques. All vertebrae have a similar basic structure, although they vary in shape and size according to position and function. A vertebra is made up of a vertebral body and bony arch, which consists of two pedicles anteriorly and two laminae posteriorly, the junctions of which form the transverse processes (Fig. 21-1). The laminae join to form the spinous process, which varies from almost a horizontal position in the lumbar and lower thoracic region to one of steep caudal angulation in the midthoracic region (Fig. 21-2). Ligamentous structures join the vertebrae and are useful clinically to facilitate needle placement, particularly in epidural applications (Fig. 21-3).

Figure 21-1 Anatomy of the vertebral body and arch.

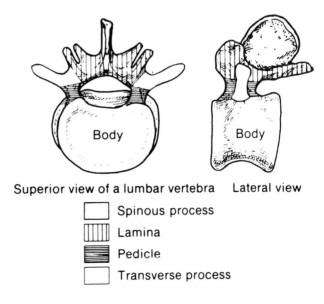

Superior view of a lumbar vertebra   Lateral view

☐ Spinous process

▥ Lamina

▤ Pedicle

☐ Transverse process

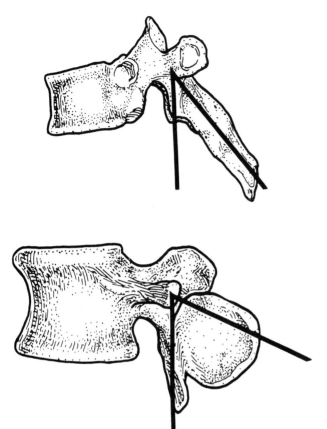

Figure 21-2 Comparison of spinous process angulation; midthoracic (*top*), lumbar (*bottom*) vertebrae.

Figure 21-3 Vertebral ligaments.

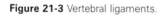

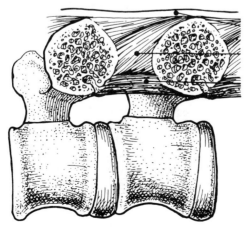

Supraspinous ligament

Interspinous ligament

Ligamentum flavum

The lateral decubitus position is used most frequently during lumbar puncture and epidural catheterization. This position often is the only one a critically ill patient will be able to assume. The fetal position is attained by flexing the knees to the chest and flexing the neck. Every effort should be made to flex the lumbar vertebrae anteriorly while keeping the back perpendicular to the floor (Fig. 21-4a). The sitting position is used less frequently. It is usually chosen in patients who are obese to allow more accurate identification of midline vertebral anatomy (Fig. 21-4b). The patient should sit on the bed, feet supported on a stool and the neck and back maximally flexed. Blood pressure changes may occur during this positioning. A strong, facile assistant is mandatory, as is appropriate monitoring and life-support equipment. Of practical importance is the concept that each of these positions is used in an attempt to increase the vertebral interlaminar gap by forward flexion of the patient.

A hospital-prepared or commercial tray should be used with utmost care to ensure

Figure 21-4 Patient positioning for peridural techniques. **a.** Lateral decubitus position. **b.** Sitting position.

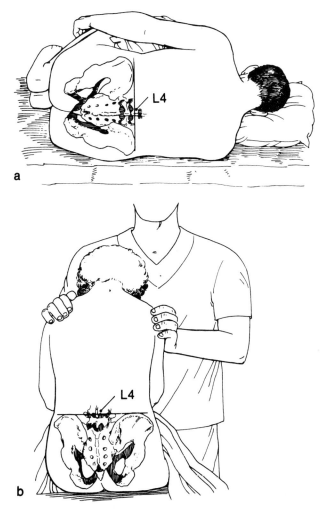

TABLE 21-2 EQUIPMENT NEEDED FOR PERIDURAL TECHNIQUES

Always
1. Skin preparation material
2. Sterile towels for draping
3. Local anesthetic and 25- to 26-gauge needle, and syringe for skin infiltration

Lumbar Puncture
1. CSF collection tubes and manometer tubing
2. Lumbar puncture needle (most commonly 22 gauge, $3\frac{1}{2}''$ (9 cm) in length)

Epidural Catheterization
1. Epidural needle, 18 or 19 gauge (Touhy, Weiss, or Crawford)
2. Epidural catheter
3. Syringe for loss of resistance (preferably ground glass barrel and plunger with Leur-lok connector)

---

asepsis. The choice of tray depends on local preference, use, and the economics of the situation. Whichever tray you may have available, the items listed in Table 21-2 should be included.

LUMBAR PUNCTURE

The lumbar approach is most commonly chosen to obtain CSF. With the patient in the flexed lateral decubitus position, a line drawn between the iliac crests ordinarily bisects the L4 vertebra, or the L4–5 lumbar interspace. Termination of the spinal cord usually is at the level of the space between L1 and L2, although it rarely may extend to the body of L2. Because of this relationship, needle placement below L2 seldom, if ever, causes cord injury.

Midline Approach

A midline approach at the L3–4 or L4–5 interspace is the preferred method. After skin infiltration of local anesthetic, an introducer, which facilitates the use of a small-gauge spinal needle and prevents contact of the needle and skin, is inserted in the interspinous ligament. The spinal needle is passed through the introducer and advanced carefully with a slight cephalad angulation. Be sure that the needle remains midline. Its bevel should be directed to split rather than to cut the longitudinal dural fibers. A characteristic decrease in resistance occurs as the needle traverses the ligamentum flavum and enters the subarachnoid space. When CSF appears in the needle hub, attach a manometer to measure its pressure. The fluid obtained should be "gin clear." Cloudy fluid indicates pleocytosis (meningitis), and bloody CSF may be due to subarachnoid hemorrhage or a traumatic tap. With subarachnoid hemorrhage, no clot forms and a clear supernatant fluid does not develop; after a traumatic lumbar puncture, the CSF should clear with additional flow. After measuring pressure, collect a sample of CSF for cell, protein, and glucose determinations, serology, bacterial culture, and immunoglobins (if clinically indicated).

Paramedian Approach

See epidural technique.

Taylor Approach

The Taylor approach is a special approach used to enter the L5–sacral interspace. The patient is placed in the flexed lateral decubitus position and a 5″ (12 cm) spinal needle inserted 1 cm medial and 1 cm caudal to the most caudad portion of the posterior–superior iliac spine. The needle is directed both medially and cephalad at angles of 45° to 60°.

Cisternal Puncture

Puncture of the Cisterna magna to obtain CSF is a relatively simple technique but should be performed only by experienced personnel. The potential for unintentional needling of the spinal cord or blood vessels makes this a consultant's procedure. Indications include [1] contraindications to lumbar puncture; [2] technical failure to obtain CSF by lumbar puncture; and [3] installation of drugs above an obstruction of the spinal canal.

EPIDURAL PUNCTURE

Whenever epidural nerve blockade is carried out in the ICU, complete monitoring and resuscitative equipment must be available for treatment of complications. Each epidural catheter reinjection should be treated with the care and caution of the original injection. The loss of resistance technique (Fig. 21-5a) is the most common method for identifying the epidural space. Since the epidural space is entered "blindly," the operator's hand must be used to guide the needle. A ground-glass syringe containing saline (preferred) or air is attached

Figure 21-5 Loss of resistance technique for epidural space localization. **a.** Needle seated in interspinous ligament and ligamentum flavum. **b.** Entry of needle into epidural space.

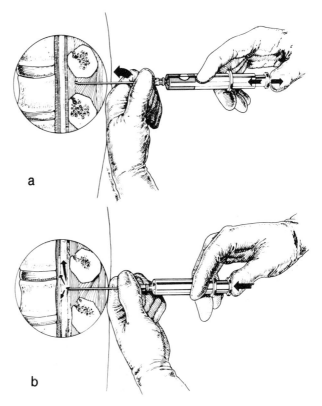

a

b

to an epidural needle once it is placed within the interspinous ligament. Injection of the solution is difficult if the needle tip is within the midline ligament. Place the noninjecting hand firmly against the patient's back, with the thumb and index or middle finger holding the needle hub. Advance the needle slowly with the noninjecting hand while applying constant pressure to the syringe plunger with the other thumb. As the needle enters the ligamentum flavum, an increased resistance to injection is appreciated. As it traverses the ligament and enters the epidural space, injection of solution occurs with ease (Fig. 21-5b).

"Negative" pressure in the epidural space, the magnitude of which is greatest in the thoracic region, is the basis of the hanging drop epidural technique. A drop of fluid is placed in the hub of the epidural needle once the needle is seated within the interspinous ligament. Increased resistance to advancement is noted when the ligamentum flavum is encountered and, as the needle enters the epidural space, the fluid is drawn in by the negative pressure. Many anesthesiologists believe that this method is less reliable than the loss of resistance technique for epidural space identification.

Midline Approach

Position the patient as for a lumbar puncture. Identify the most easily palpable interspace from L2 to L5 and raise an intradermal wheal in its midpoint. After you puncture the skin with a sharp, large-bore needle, advance the epidural needle with care through this skin entry site in the midline of the back. Once the needle is placed in the interspinous ligament, with a 10° to 15° cephalad angulation, remove the stylet and advance the needle to the ligamentum flavum and epidural space using your preferred technique. The usual cause of failure of needle advancement results from striking the lamina when the needle is off the midline. Midline needle placement and modification of cephalocaudad angulation should allow entry through the intralaminar space (Fig. 21-6a).

Paramedian Approach

Patients are encountered in whom a midline approach is difficult. This problem is especially common in older patients with calcification of the supraspinous and interspinous ligaments,

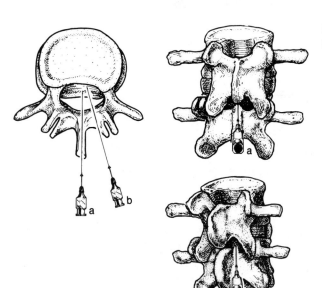

Figure 21-6 Peridural technique. **a.** Midline approach. **b.** Paramedian approach.

in those with rigid spines, and in critically ill patients whose lumbar flexion is limited by life-support equipment. The paramedian approach frees the operator from dependency on patient cooperation, which is needed to produce spinal flexion, and is especially valuable if a midthoracic epidural technique is performed. In the lumbar region, skin infiltration is carried out 1 cm lateral and 1 cm caudad to the cephalad spinous process of the chosen interspace. Advancing the needle parallel to the midline until the bony lamina is reached provides an indication of the depth of the ligamentum flavum. The epidural needle is then withdrawn, reinserted with a medial angulation of 10°, and "walked" off the lamina into the ligamentum flavum (Fig. 21-6b) and finally the epidural space.

Thoracic Approach

A thoracic approach is indicated when a selective local anesthetic block of the thoracic and upper abdominal areas is desired. This technique has the advantage of minimizing the dose of local anesthetic and decreasing the spread of denervation to sacral and lumbar segments, thereby causing less impairment of sympathetic tone. Because of the rare but potential hazard of spinal cord injury, only physicians with considerable experience with other epidural procedures should use this technique. The spinous processes in the midthoracic region have an extreme downward or caudad angulation, making the paramedian approach preferred. The patient is placed in a lateral decubitus position, head on a pillow and thorax bowed toward the operator. The inferior angle of the scapula is at the level of T7. Skin infiltration is made both 1 cm lateral and caudad to the chosen spinous process. Infiltration of local anesthetic to the level of the lamina allows identification of its depth. The epidural needle is inserted with an angulation of 10° to 15° medially and 45° to 60° in the sagittal plane, and again is walked off the lamina into the ligamentum flavum and the epidural space.

Epidural Catheter Technique

Most intensive care unit applications of epidural analgesia require epidural catheter placement. Catheters are biologically inert, radiopaque Teflon or nylon, and pass through a standard thin-walled, 18- or 19-gauge needle. Distance markers are provided to guide depth of insertion, and many have a wire stylet to provide rigidity. If a stylet is used, it should be withdrawn from the catheter tip before insertion in order to decrease the chance of dural puncture. After the needle is placed in the epidural space, the catheter is advanced to the cephalad-directed needle tip, and, as it passes beyond the tip, a slight resistance to further advancement may be felt. Three centimeters to 4 cm of additional catheter length is inserted, the needle withdrawn over the catheter, and the catheter taped securely to the patient's back. As with any through-the-needle technique, the catheter should never be withdrawn through the needle.

PROBLEMS AND RELATED COMPLICATIONS

HEADACHE

Deliberate and inadvertent dural puncture may result in a subsequent headache. The headache is believed to be due to a persistent CSF leak through the dural rent, is characteristically occipital or circumferential, and may have a delayed onset that worsens on rising from the supine position. It usually resolves with conservative therapy, bedrest, fluids, and analgesics; however, in selected cases, an epidural blood patch should be performed. Using strict aseptic technique, 5 to 15 ml of autologous blood, drawn from the patient's arm, is injected into the epidural space at the site of previous dural puncture. This treatment is effective in 90% of patients following one injection; a repeat injection increases the success rate to more than 95%.

NEUROLOGIC DEFICITS

Epidural block or lumbar puncture may rarely be followed by neurologic deficit. The most common cause of neurologic damage is needle trauma and usually involves a single spinal nerve. Danger of direct trauma to the cord is remote if puncture is performed below the level of the conus medullaris. Any patient complaint of pain during insertion of the needle, or with injection of any solution, must be taken as an urgent signal to stop and evaluate the nature of the pain. This warning is masked in patients who are obtunded or sedated.

Epidural Hematoma

Epidural hematomas occur spontaneously in apparently normal patients but are more likely to follow anticoagulant therapy. The principle clinical feature is severe backache associated with progressive paraplegia. This complication constitutes a surgical emergency, and diagnosis followed by surgical decompression is essential. Total systemic anticoagulation and coagulopathy are contraindications to peridural techniques. "Minidose" heparinization heightens concern about the safety of peridural techniques with this therapy. Some authorities consider any form of systemic heparin therapy a contraindication to peridural techniques. Conversely, thousands of cases have been reported with no sequelae under similar circumstances.[1,2] Many anesthesiologists suggest proceeding with the technique if clotting parameters and bleeding time are normal.

Epidural Abscess

Epidural abscess has been reported following uneventful lumbar puncture and epidural block but more frequently is due to hematogenous bacterial spread from distant infectious foci.[3] The usual presentation includes fever and leukocytosis with a progressive backache followed by paraplegia. Again, this complication constitutes a surgical emergency. Unanswered questions include the role of epidural catheterization in the face of systemic infection and whether the catheter can be a focus for epidural infection. Most experts believe that systemic infection is a contraindication to epidural catheterization. Although rare, a subarachnoid infection may occur after a lumbar puncture or epidural technique. Most often, such problems are caused by unusual bacteria that necessitate a meticulous bacteriologic evaluation.

Interruption of Blood Supply

The blood supply of the spinal cord is occasionally tenuous and easily compromised. The anterior spinal artery derives its main lumbar supply from the artery of Adamkiewicz. Interruption of this blood supply, particularly in severe atherosclerotic and low blood flow states, may cause immediate, painless paraplegia. In the critically ill patient, however, interruption of spinal cord blood flow during an abdominal surgical procedure is more common than interruption with use of a peridural technique.

Adhesive Arachnoiditis

Adhesive arachnoiditis is a serious, albeit rare, condition that may progress to disability, accompanied by pain, paralysis, and impairment of bowel function. It usually follows injection of an irritant solution into the CSF. Several compounds, including pyrogen-contaminated dextrose and detergents for cleaning needles, have been implicated. The disorder is characterized by a proliferative reaction of the arachnoid mater, followed by fibrosis and distortion of the arachnoid space. Clinical signs and symptoms may not become apparent for weeks after the precipitating event.

LOCAL ANESTHETICS

Toxicity

The epidural space is highly vascular, and the needle or catheter occasionally can be placed unknowingly within a vessel lumen. Intravascular injection of local anesthetic is the most common cause of serious toxicity, and the central nervous system (CNS) effects, ranging from lightheadedness and circumoral numbness to seizures and coma, are well known. The cardiovascular system may exhibit direct myocardial depression and peripheral vasodilation. Rapid development of severe hypoxemia and acidosis is a result of the seizure activity and is a major factor in myocardial depression. Early and aggressive control of the airway and provision of supplemental oxygen improve outcome.

As a precautionary measure, every needle or catheter injection should include gentle aspiration and an appropriate test dose of 15 µg of epinephrine. A positive test dose is defined as a heart rate increase of 30% in 30 seconds or an increase in blood pressure in β-blocked patients. Incremental injection and constant verbal contact with the patient, in conjunction with a negative test dose of epinephrine, significantly reduce the risk of unrecognized intravascular injection.

Total Spinal Block

Total or high spinal block is most commonly due to the unintentional subarachnoid injection of local anesthetic. Several uneventful injections through an epidural catheter, followed by a subsequent injection that causes a total spinal block, presumably reflect migration of the catheter through the dura. A negative aspiration, followed by a 3- to 5-ml injection of local anesthetic and a 5-minute period of observation, helps to avoid subarachnoid injection. If unintentional subarachnoid injection does occur, a profound degree of sensory and motor blockade develops within 5 minutes. If the block reaches the upper cervical segments, diaphragmatic paralysis may result. Appropriate cardiopulmonary resuscitation, including positive-pressure ventilation, will stabilize the patient until the block recedes.

Hypotension

The most common side-effect of epidural local anesthetic analgesia is a decrease in blood pressure. The decrease is attributed to sympathetic blockade with resultant dilation of both resistance and capacitance vessels. Blockade above the level of T5 not only limits compensatory vasoconstriction, but also affects the cardiac accelerator fibers arising in the T1 to T4 segments. Judicious intravascular volume preload, limiting the extent of the neural blockade, and estimation of preblock volume status minimize the problem.

Inadequate Analgesia

Inadequate analgesia may be due to technical difficulties, the most common problem being catheter malposition. Unilateral analgesia may be seen and is thought to be due to restriction within the epidural space. Local anesthetic tachyphylaxis is indicative of acute tolerance, causing repeated injections to produce successively diminishing effects. To minimize the problem, [1] use the minimum dose possible at initiation (*e.g.*, thoracic epidural); [2] use a long-acting drug (*e.g.*, bupivacaine); [3] add epinephrine to increase the local anesthetic's half-life; and [4] combine epidural opioids with local anesthetics.

UNUSUAL PRESENTATIONS

The subdural space is a potential space because the arachnoid is in close contact with the dural sheath, separated only by a thin film of serous fluid. Cases of massive epidural (total spinal) blocks have followed the injection of small volumes of epidural local anesthetics subdurally. A subdural injection differs from the rapid onset of high spinal block that accompanies unintentional subarachnoid injection. With subdural injection, total block does not occur for 20 to 30 minutes following injection. Management is the same as for high or total spinal block.

Once an epidural catheter is inserted beyond the tip of an epidural needle, do not withdraw it through the needle because catheter shearing may occur. If resistance is encountered during removal of a catheter, increase spinal flexion. Should a catheter break in the epidural space, there is virtually no reason to remove it surgically because of the inert nature of the catheter.

Art is as important as science for successful use of peridural techniques. Nothing substitutes for hands-on experience for lumbar puncture or epidural catheterization.

SPECIAL CONSIDERATIONS

SUBARACHNOID AND EPIDURAL NARCOTICS

Since the discovery of spinal cord opiate receptors, increasing interest has been focused on the selective analgesia available with peridural narcotic administration.[4] Narcotic drugs have a selective spinal action characterized by intense analgesia, absence of motor and sympathetic blockade, and little or no CNS or cardiovascular toxicity sometimes associated with local anesthetic use.

Presynaptic and postsynaptic receptors in the substantia gelatinosa of the dorsal horn are the likely sites of peridural narcotic action. The more lipid soluble agents, fentanyl and sufentanil, diffuse to the opioid receptors more rapidly than does morphine. Morphine, because of the water solubility conferred by its hydroxyl groups, remains in the CSF longer and thus allows rostral CSF spread with the potential for respiratory depression. Its lipid insolubility gives morphine a slower onset but a longer duration of analgesia. Concurrently, the highly lipid-soluble drugs do not spread as far rostrally as morphine, and thus need to be applied closer to the intended level of analgesia.

Respiratory depression was reported shortly after the clinical introduction of peridural narcotic analgesia and remains the most feared complication. This infrequent but potentially devastating problem limits the use of the technique and necessitates careful monitoring. Morphine-induced respiratory depression is a biphasic phenomenon, the initial cause of which is systemic absorption from the epidural space during the first hour. Subsequent depression occurs usually within 6 to 10 hours of administration and represents migration of the narcotic from the epidural space rostrally through the CSF, producing direct depression of the respiratory centers. Reversal with a 5 μg/kg/min intravenous infusion of naloxone prevents peridural narcotic respiratory depression and does not interfere with analgesia in patients undergoing cholecystectomy.[5] Factors associated with an increased likelihood of

TABLE 21-3 FACTORS CONFERRING AN INCREASED RISK OF RESPIRATORY DEPRESSION WITH PERIDURAL NARCOTICS

1. Intrathecal administration
2. Advanced age (> 70 years of age)
3. High doses (> 10 mg morphine)
4. Residual effects of parenteral opioids
5. Residual effects of CNS depressant drugs
6. Lack of tolerance to opioids
7. Preexisting respiratory disease

(Cousins MJ, Mather LE: Intrathecal and epidural administration of opioids. *Anesthesiology* 1984; 61:276)

respiratory depression are listed in Table 21-3. The overall incidence of respiratory depression was < 0.5% in one series of more than 6000 patients.[4]

Nausea and vomiting after peridural narcotic analgesia occur in up to 50% of patients. This figure is similar to that reported with parenteral opioid analgesia. With repeat dosing the incidence decreases; it is extremely low in cancer patients. Nausea usually responds to careful titration of naloxone. Urinary retention, similar to respiratory depression, is more common in the postoperative period or acute care setting, as compared to peridural narcotic analgesia in chronic pain patients. The reported incidence ranges from 25% to 50% and also is reversible with naloxone. Pruritis is one of the most bothersome peridural narcotic side-effects, affecting upward of 50% of patients. Again, it is less of a problem in patients with chronic pain. The itching responds poorly to antihistamine therapy but somewhat better to naloxone.

REFERENCES

1. Odoom JA, Sih IL: Epidural analgesia and anticoagulant therapy. *Anaesthesia* 1983; 38:254
2. Rao TLK, El-Etr AA: Anticoagulation following placement of epidural and subarachnoid catheters. *Anesthesiology* 1981; 55:618
3. Baker AS, Ojemann RG, Swartz MN, et al: Spinal epidural abscess. *N Engl J Med* 1975; 293:463
4. Cousins MJ, Mather LE: Intrathecal and epidural administration of opioids. *Anesthesiology* 1984; 61:276
5. Rawal N, Schott U, Dahlstrom B, et al: Influence of naloxone infusion on analgesia and respiratory depression following epidural morphine. *Anesthesiology* 1986; 64:194

GENERAL BIBLIOGRAPHY

Bromage PR: *Epidural Analgesia.* Philadelphia, WB Saunders, 1978
Covino BG, Scott DB: *Handbook of Epidural Anaesthesia and Analgesia.* New York, Grune & Stratton, 1985
Cousins MJ, Bridenbaugh PO (eds): *Neural Blockade in Clinical Anesthesia and Management of Pain.* Philadelphia, JB Lippincott, 1980
Ellis H, Feldman S: *Anatomy for Anaesthetics,* 4th ed. London, Blackwell Scientific Publications, 1985
Harrison MJG (ed): *Contemporary Neurology.* London, Butterworths Publishing Co, 1984
Katz J: *Atlas of Regional Anesthesia.* Norwalk, Connecticut, Appleton-Century-Crofts, 1985
Moore DC: *Regional Block,* 4th ed. Springfield, Illinois, Charles C Thomas, 1965
Murphy TM: Spinal, epidural and caudal anesthesia. In Miller RD (ed): *Anesthesia,* 2nd ed. New York, Churchill Livingstone, 1986
Pearce JMS: Hazards of lumbar puncture. *Br Med J* 1982; 285:1521
Stevens RA, Stanton–Hicks MDA: Injection of local anesthetic: A complication of epidural anesthesia. *Anesthesiology* 1985; 63:323

CHAPTER TWENTY-TWO

AN APPROACH TO THE FEBRILE ICU PATIENT

Scott H. Norwood

INTRODUCTION

Fever in critically ill patients often creates a sense of urgency to find the etiology. This is understandable because most critically ill surgical patients and many medical intensive care unit (ICU) patients, die of complications of sepsis. The approach to evaluating febrile episodes, however, is often difficult to justify based on existing data from the literature. Infection must always be considered as a cause for fever in critically ill patients, but a rational approach to evaluation should be used rather than rote ordering of expensive and nonspecific laboratory tests and radiographs. An exhaustive treatise on every potential cause for fever is beyond any single textbook chapter. Rather, a rational clinical approach to evaluating fever in critically ill patients is presented.

The evaluation process should be "therapy-directed" so that tests which have no major impact on clinical management are avoided early in the clinical course. An initial febrile episode should be evaluated with a careful review of the patient's history and a thorough physical examination. If this fails to identify a source, then no further procedures are necessary unless the patient is severely immunocompromised or there is a high probability of bacteremia. If a second febrile episode occurs, further testing for various infections must be considered. Figure 22-1 provides guidelines for evaluating infectious sources for fever.

If pneumonia is suspected, then sputum Gram stain should precede any cultures. Urinalysis should always precede urine culture, which should be ordered only if bacteria and more than ten white blood cells per high powered field are present on urinalysis. Venous or arterial catheter-related infection is virtually nonexistent during the first 48 hours of catheter use if the catheter is placed under the usual sterile conditions. Central venous catheters are an infrequent source for fever unless usage exceeds 72 hours. An approach to managing potential catheter-related febrile episodes is outlined in Figure 22-2. Fever in the immediate postoperative period requires careful inspection of all surgical or traumatic wounds. Gas gangrene and necrotizing fasciitis from clostridial or streptococcal organisms can occur within the first 48 hours postoperatively. Other types of infections occur later, but most can usually be diagnosed with careful inspection and palpation of the wound. Crush injury syndrome and tetanus, although infrequent, can be causes for fever in the postoperative trauma patient.

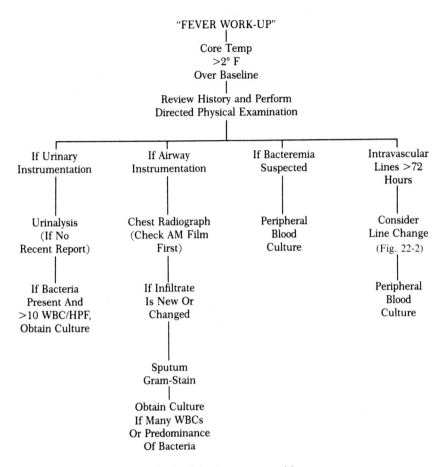

Figure 22-1 Guidelines for evaluating infectious sources of fever.

Meningitis is an infrequent cause of fever in surgical ICU patients, but must be considered in any critically ill patient who develops an altered mental status associated with high fever.

Because of limitations with conventional radiographs, ultrasound, and nuclear scans, computed tomography (CT) has become the preferred method of diagnosing intra-abdominal abscess as a possible cause for fever. However, CT scanning in critically ill patients is not as sensitive, specific, or beneficial as has been reported in general hospital populations. Scanning can be helpful but should not be used as a tool to search blindly for a source of sepsis as part of a fever work-up. Abdominal re-exploration may be necessary in some patients, especially those who develop unexplained single organ system failure.

Other critical etiologies for fever must be considered under certain clinical conditions. Approximately 15% of hospitalized patients experience some type of adverse drug reaction. Fever may be an isolated symptom (drug fever) or the first sign of anaphylaxis or serum sickness. Drugs which are associated with a high probability of allergic reactions should be replaced with other suitable drugs if possible.

About 90% of blood transfusion reactions are allergic or febrile. However, fever may

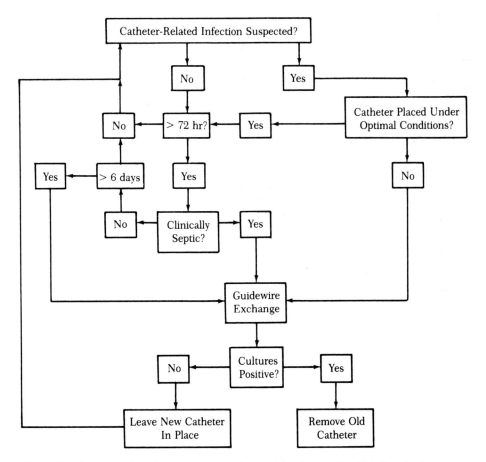

Figure 22-2 An approach to the management of potential catheter-related febrile episodes.

also accompany acute hemolytic reactions, with the first manifestation being sudden diffuse oozing of blood from multiple sites. If fever develops within 20 to 30 minutes after beginning a blood product transfusion, then this potential life-threatening complication must be ruled out.

Malignant hyperthermia, which is classically observed during administration of general anesthesia, may not develop until the patient reaches the ICU. Early symptoms can be confused with thyrotoxicosis, undiagnosed pheochromocytoma, or the neuroleptic malignant syndrome.

Acute adrenocortical insufficiency is a rare cause of fever in critically ill patients. This should be considered in patients who are being weaned from high steroid dosages who suddenly develop fever and hypotension.

Adverse physiologic side-effects of fever cause major alterations in oxygen consumption which may be detrimental to critically ill patients if they are elderly or otherwise have limited ability to increase oxygen delivery. Fever should therefore be treated aggressively in these patients.

DEFINITION, PATHOPHYSIOLOGY, AND PURPOSE

Fever represents a disturbance in normal body thermoregulation. This ancient evolutionary mechanism appears to have evolved in an attempt to combat infection. As with many phylogenic physiologic mechanisms, a useful purpose for fever in many patients has been lost, evolving into a potentially detrimental symptom in the ICU patient. The most important role for fever in critically ill patients is an early warning sign for infection or inflammation.[1]

In humans, thermoregulatory mechanisms are precisely balanced over a narrow range during health so that body temperature is usually maintained at $37 \pm 1°C$, with values lowest in the early morning and highest in the late afternoon.[2] Fever is a disorder of thermoregulation which occurs within the anterior hypothalamus so that the body actively seeks to raise its temperature. Adverse physiologic side-effects of fever include vasoconstriction and shivering, which can dramatically increase oxygen consumption in critically ill patients. For clinical fevers associated with infection, negative feedback mechanisms usually ensure that temperatures rarely exceed $41°C$.[2] However, with disorders such as malignant hyperthermia, negative feedback mechanisms appear to be lost, and body temperatures greater than $41°C$ are common.

Various pathophysiologic mechanisms may induce fever. Substances called "pyrogens" cause fevers in humans and various laboratory models. In addition to infectious pyrogens (viruses, bacteria, fungi), various other substances such as antigen–antibody complexes,[3] steroids,[4] and other inorganic substances[5] can produce experimental fevers. Depending on the agent causing fever, the characteristics vary with respect to time of onset, duration, and character of the fever curve.[2] Despite the vast array of fever-inducing agents, each pyrogen evokes a common mediator, "endogenous pyrogen," a protein produced by leukocytes.[6] Endogenous pyrogen elicits fever by altering the activity of temperature-sensitive neurons located in the anterior hypothalamus. Endogenous pyrogen is an extremely sensitive hormone; as little as 35 ng of the human hormone will produce clinical fevers up to $0.6°C$ above baseline in experimental animals.[7]

It is probable that fever evolved as a mechanism to combat infection. Certain organisms, such as those producing syphilis and gonorrhea, are heat sensitive and can be destroyed *in vivo* by artificially inducing fever. Fever also appears to be protective against infections in lizards and fish.[2] In the ICU patient, however, the detrimental aspects of fever usually outweigh any potential benefits. An elevation in body temperature often creates a sense of urgency and reflex reactions that, when carefully reviewed, are often difficult to justify.

COMMON CAUSES FOR FEVER

Febrile ICU patients can be classified into four groups: patients who are incubating an infection when admitted to the ICU; patients whose fevers are an expression of their underlying disease (*e.g.*, granulomatous infections, tumors of the reticuloendothelial system, connective tissues diseases); patients who develop an endogenous febrile process after admission (*e.g.*, perforated ulcer, appendicitis, gout); and patients who develop fever as a result of medical or surgical therapy or from nosocomial infections.

Common causes for fever in medical and surgical ICU patients are listed in Tables 22-1 and 22-2. Many of these causes are common to both groups of patients and some are

**TABLE 22-1 POTENTIAL CAUSES FOR FEVER IN
MEDICAL ICU PATIENTS**

Infections
    Bacterial
    Fungal
    Viral
Thromboembolism
Drug fevers
Transfusion-related causes
Skin-related problems/decubiti
Neoplasms
    Lymphomas, leukemias
    Pancreatic cancer
    Hypernephroma
    Hepatoma
Central nervous system disorders
    Cerebrovascular accidents
    Tumors
    Hemorrhage
    Hematopoietic disorders
    Connective tissue/immunologic disorders
Metabolic disorders
    Adrenocortical insufficiency
    Thyroid crisis (storm)
    Gout
    Porphyria
Alcohol and drug withdrawal

diagnoses of exclusion. Because there are many potential causes for fever, a rational approach for evaluation must be developed that will direct therapy and eliminate needless expensive laboratory tests and radiographs, thus improving overall efficiency.

There is little doubt that infection is the most common important cause of fever in both medical and surgical ICU patients. Sepsis remains the leading cause of death in critically ill surgical patients[8] and it is certainly high on the list for causes of death in medical ICU patients. Therefore, infection must always be considered; it must be actively, but rationally, eliminated as a source for fever before the more infrequent etiologies are considered.

FEVER AS A PREDICTOR OF INFECTION

Fever can be classified as intermittent, remittent, sustained, and relapsing.[9] Intermittent fever, where the body temperature returns to normal each day, is characteristic of pyogenic infection. Intermittent fevers are the most common type observed in ICU patients, partially because antipyretics are aggressively used. Remittent fevers, where the temperature falls but does not return to normal, is considered the most common febrile response to diseases not specific to ICU patients.[9] Under most clinical situations in the ICU, fever is usually abrupt in onset, but it can vary significantly in degree of elevation per individual.

The primary goal is to separate infection from the many other causes of fever (many of which require no specific therapy). In young, previously healthy patients, fever may not impose any significant harm or great discomfort. However, in older patients, elevated body

TABLE 22-2 POTENTIAL CAUSES FOR FEVER IN SURGICAL ICU PATIENTS

Infections related to surgery or trauma
   Wound infection
   Intra-abdominal abscess
   Crush syndrome
   Tetanus
Nonsurgical related infections
   Pneumonia
   Urinary tract infection
   Catheter-related infection
   Neurologic sources
Adrenocortical insufficiency
Pheochromocytoma (undiagnosed)
Drug fevers
Transfusion related fevers
Malignant hyperthermia

temperatures significantly increase oxygen consumption, which may alter the balance between oxygen delivery and utilization. Fever should therefore be treated aggressively in these patients. Aspirin or acetaminophen can be given rectally to minimize these adverse effects. Occasionally antipyretic agents may cause a sharp decrease in temperature followed by involuntary muscle contractions (a chill).[9] Chills also produce increased oxygen consumption. A sharp reduction in temperature can be avoided by administering antipyretic agents at least every 3 hours around the clock rather than prescribing these agents only for temperature elevations above a certain level. For higher fevers that produce violent muscular contractions, parenteral morphine sulfate or chlorpromazine may be necessary.

The clinical presentation and approach to evaluation of patients with community-acquired causes for fever and sepsis are very different from the approach to the patient who is admitted to the ICU for other reasons and subsequently develops a fever. For purposes of ruling out infection, the approach to evaluation in the medical and surgical patient (with the exception of wound infections and intra-abdominal sepsis) are similar.

One recent study examined 693 patients undergoing surgical procedures to investigate the etiology of postoperative fever (defined as >38°C).[10] The overall rate of fever was 14% for clean, 13.4% for clean–contaminated, and 13.1% for contaminated surgical procedures. Similar rates of postoperative fever have been found in gynecologic[11] and pediatric surgery patients.[12] After clean wound surgery, fever from infectious origins began significantly later (2.7 versus 1.6 days) and lasted significantly longer (5.4 versus 3.5 days) than fever for which no infectious source was determined. Only 50% of the infections in the entire population were associated with fever. Therefore, if fever were used as the only criterion to detect an infection, sensitivity and specificity for this clinical sign were 0.53 and 0.62, respectively. Among the febrile patients in this study for which no source of infection was documented, 94.1% presented with only one episode of temperature elevation. Although not all patients were critically ill, this study suggests that a reasonable approach to evaluating a patient following an initial febrile episode is a thorough physical examination only. Should the physical examination reveal an abnormality, then appropriate tests can be ordered to confirm clinical suspicions.

Postoperative fever is not uncommon during the first 6 days following abdominal operation.[13] In another study, 71 of 464 patients (15%) had rectal temperatures higher than 38.5°C on two consecutive measurements. On analysis, infection was discovered in 27% and in these 19 patients, a correct diagnosis could have been made on clinical findings and confirmed by one single appropriate test in 14 patients (74%).[13] A history and directed physical examination would have revealed the source for fever in most cases, but this did not prevent the usual response of ordering a battery of tests including complete blood cell count (CBC), chest radiograph, and "culturing the patient" (urine, blood, sputum, and wound cultures). The only test with a high positive yield was the undiagnostic and relatively unimportant CBC (44% positive). Frequently used tests had low positive rates in this study. For example, urine cultures were obtained in 86% of patients but were positive in only 10%; chest radiographs were performed in 75% of patients with only one positive result; two blood cultures (only 5% positive) were obtained in 60% of the patients.

A battery of tests seems to be designed to detect the most common causes of postoperative infection. From this perspective, all of the postoperative infections were correctly identified by rote ordering of tests or cultures, except for one patient with a subdiaphragmatic abscess which was ultimately confirmed by CT. However, 3.8 tests were ordered per febrile patient; only 18% (49 of 268) of tests were positive and only 7% (19 of 268) were useful in diagnosing the infection ultimately determined to be the cause of fever.[13] This study clearly demonstrates that a more rational and clinical oriented approach to ordering tests as part of a fever work-up can be done at a significant cost savings without reducing diagnostic accuracy.

RECOMMENDED APPROACH TO FEVER EVALUATION

Rather than using a purely "diagnosis-directed" approach to fever, the evaluation should also be "therapy directed." Tests that have no significant impact on therapeutic interventions should be avoided, or at least postponed, until further clinical changes increase or elevate their true usefulness in the specific patient. Tests that are "low yield" or nonspecific should not be ordered early in the evaluation process. A shotgun approach to evaluation should be discouraged.

The primary goal in evaluating a febrile episode is to determine whether fever is an early warning sign of sepsis, as part of the disease, a developing complication, or from nosocomial infection.

EVALUATING INFECTIOUS SOURCES FOR FEVER

Generally, the first febrile episode (defined as >1.3°C above baseline temperature) should be evaluated with a careful review of the patient's history and a thorough physical examination. If this fails to identify a source, then no further evaluation is necessary. Exceptions to this rule are severely immunocompromised patients or patients with a high probability of bacteremia, where a positive blood culture would significantly affect therapy. A thorough physical examination should always precede any laboratory or radiographic tests. If a second febrile episode occurs, further testing to evaluate for various infections should be considered if clinically appropriate. Figure 22-1 provides guidelines to discourage rote ordering of laboratory tests for determining nosocomial infections.

Respiratory Infections

Pneumonia is one of the most common hospital-acquired infections leading to death, occurring in at least 12% to 15% of all ICU patients.[14] If the clinical setting and physical examination suggest the possibility of pneumonia, a portable chest radiograph should be obtained (upright if possible). The presence of new or significantly different infiltrates should suggest the possibility of bacterial pneumonia. If the patient has been intubated for more than 48 hours, upper airway colonization may have already occurred.[15] A specimen should be obtained for Gram stain. If the Gram stain reveals a large number of white blood cells or a predominant type of organism then appropriate specimens for culture should be taken.

The methods for obtaining a valid culture are notoriously inaccurate in the intubated critically ill patient.[14] The plugged telescopic catheter (PTC) brush, introduced in 1979, has been considered one of the more reliable techniques to improve culture accuracy for directing therapy.[16] Optimal results are achieved only with very careful attention to minor details and quantitative cultures must be performed, with 10^3 colony-forming units per milliliter (CFU/ml) diagnostic for infection.[16] False-positive results with this technique may be as high as 41%,[14] and a more recent study in 12 critically ill intubated patients questioned the superiority and cost-effectiveness of PTC brush cultures over routine cultures obtained by suctioning through the endotracheal tube.[17] Empiric antibiotic therapy must often be started if there is a strong clinical suspicion of pneumonia. Pneumonia may be especially difficult to diagnose in patients with acute respiratory failure and concomitant pulmonary infiltrates (adult respiratory distress syndrome [ARDS]).

Urinary Tract Sources for Fever

Although nosocomial urinary tract infections are a frequent cause for fever in the hospital population collectively, urosepsis is not a frequent source for systemic sepsis in critically ill patients unless significant obstruction or urinary tract instrumentation has occurred. If the urinary tract is suspected (and there has been no recent urinalysis reported) a urinalysis should be obtained. A urine culture is necessary only if bacteriuria and at least ten white blood cells per high powered field are present.[18]

Catheter-Related Febrile Episodes

Strict guidelines concerning the use and maintenance of central venous access catheters, pulmonary artery catheters, and arterial catheters should be developed based on available data specific to ICU patients, individual ICU patient populations, and individual patient risks. If strict aseptic technique and guidelines concerning removal and use of catheters are followed, then catheter-related infection as a source of fever will be infrequent. Civetta and others showed that positive cultures from central catheters accounted for unexplained fever spikes in only 5% of catheters removed from both "clean" and septic patients.[19] These catheter-related infections occurred after the sixth ICU day in 75% of cases in both groups.[19] Catheter-related infection is virtually nonexistent during the first 48 hours of catheter use if the catheter is placed under the usual sterile conditions. Central catheters should not be considered a source for fever unless they have been in place for at least 72 hours.[19] Likewise, arterial catheters are not a common source for sepsis. In a recent study of the incidence of arterial catheter-related infection with prolonged arterial catheterization, no positive semi-quantitative arterial catheter cultures were identified at less than 96 hours.[20] The rate of positive cultures rose to 9.5% at 97 to 120 hours but did not increase thereafter up to 340 hours. There were no associated episodes of bacteremia attributed to the arterial catheter sites.[20] An approach to managing potential catheter-related febrile episodes is outlined in Figure 22-2.

Surgical and Traumatic Wounds

Fever in the immediate postoperative period (within 48 hr) mandates careful inspection of all surgical or traumatic wounds. Surgical dressings should be completely removed and the wounds carefully inspected and palpated for signs of infection. In addition to wound infections, fever can be associated with crush injury syndrome and tetanus.

The crush injury syndrome was first described in 1942 after treating victims of aerial bombings who were trapped for prolonged periods under collapsed buildings.[21] Crushed extremities appear pale and edematous. The skin overlying the crushed muscle is usually pale and tense, often with vesicles. Fluid extravasates from the intravascular space into the osteofascial muscle compartments resulting in a significant rise in hemoglobin and hematocrit levels despite profound hypovolemia. High levels of myoglobin are excreted which can cause acute renal failure. These injuries may be associated with high fevers in the postinjury period despite the relatively benign external appearance of the injured limb.[22]

Tetanus, the clinical syndrome resulting from infection by the anaerobic bacillus *Clostridium tetani*, is relatively uncommon in western countries.[23] Clinical symptoms develop from a potent neurotoxin, tetanospasmin, produced by the bacillus. This high-molecular-weight protein is taken up by the ganglia of the central nervous system (CNS). From the site of the wound the toxin travels directly up the motor network of the peripheral nerves to the spinal cord and the medulla, ultimately producing excessive discharge from motor neurons, resulting in the characteristic tetanic spasms. Trismus and dysphagia are the initial features in most cases.[23] In severe cases, muscular spasms of increasing frequency and duration are superimposed on the muscular hypertonicity resulting in crush fractures of vertebrae and death from respiratory failure. Any wound may be a source of the bacteria, but, in practice, a wound can be identified in only 60% of reported cases of tetanus.[23] Deep penetrating injuries with a focus of necrotic tissue are particularly high-risk injuries. Elevated temperatures may be an early sign, and the interval between the first symptoms and the first severe spasms may vary from less than 24 hours to over 10 days.[23] Patients with a history of parenteral substance abuse, puncture injury, or other traumatic injuries are at risk for developing this rare but lethal disease. Treatment includes large doses of human antitenanus serum and penicillin. Supportive care with mechanical ventilation and complete muscle paralysis may be necessary for as long as 6 to 8 weeks.[23]

Neurologic Sources

Meningitis should be considered in any patient who develops altered mental status associated with high fevers. The prevalence of meningeal infections is higher in patients in medical ICUs. In trauma patients, meningitis is an uncommon finding.

Eighty percent of patients in traumatic coma will have multiple injuries.[24] Brain or spinal cord injury resulting in systemic sepsis in multiple trauma patients has never been specifically addressed, although lumbar puncture with culture of the cerebrospinal fluid is frequently performed if a patient becomes febrile or develops a change in mental status. Anecdotally, meningitis associated with head or spinal cord injury appears to be a very uncommon problem, possibly because many of these patients are treated with broad-spectrum antibiotics for other injuries.

A review of data on 15,000 patients admitted to several large neurosurgical ICUs over an 8-year period identified only 34 (0.2%) cases of bacterial meningitis associated with cranial or spinal cord injury or surgery.[25] More than 70% of these patients developed meningitis after being in the hospital for over 1 week. Sixty-two percent of the infections were associated with contaminated traumatic injuries, the most common organisms being *Pseudomonas aeruginosa* and *Klebsiella* species. Seventy percent of these 34 patients died, 50% as a direct cause of meningitis. Although gram-negative meningitis is a highly lethal disease (mortality rates range from 43%–91%), it is a very uncommon cause of systemic sepsis and death in trauma patients.[24] Lumbar puncture should be considered a part of the fever work-up if there are definite mental status changes that cannot be attributed to other more common causes such as hypoxemia.

Intra-abdominal Sources

Intra-abdominal sepsis must always be considered a potential source for fever in the postoperative period. Diagnosing postoperative intra-abdominal sepsis, however, is a very difficult problem. A clinical diagnosis of sepsis should logically include the abdomen if the patient has sustained blunt or penetrating trauma resulting in intraperitoneal soilage from damage to the colon or the alimentary tract.[26,27] Prolonged elective surgical procedures with enteric anastomoses may also predispose to abdominal abscess. Early diagnosis and drainage is essential for improved survival.[28,29]

Intra-abdominal sepsis begins with the introduction of bacteria into the peritoneal cavity. Fry described three possibilities: a mass of bacteria overwhelms the host's immunologic defense mechanism resulting in death; host defense mechanisms are strong enough, or the size of the inoculum is so small, that complete resolution occurs; and there is a "biologic stand-off" between bacteria and the host, resulting in an abdominal abscess.[30]

A high index of suspicion is crucial for early diagnosis and treatment.[28] If multisystem organ failure (MSOF) develops, it is often too late to change the ultimately fatal outcome. A thorough knowlege of the patient's history and a complete physical examination should precede direct testing to confirm clinical suspicions. A thorough examination may identify an obvious extra-abdominal source such as an old intravenous catheter site, sinusitis caused by the use of a nasotracheal tube,[31] a palpable perirectal abscess, epididymitis induced by prolonged bladder catheterization, or a missed decubitis ulcer. If the physical examination fails to reveal a source, the abdomen, particularly in surgical patients, must be strongly suspected.

Chest radiographs and flat and upright abdominal films are frequently performed but are usually nondiagnostic.[30] A pleural effusion can occur with subphrenic abscess but is often a nonspecific finding in critically ill patients because congestive heart failure, thoracic injury, and ARDS may also be associated with effusions. Barium or Gastrografin studies may be hazardous and are usually not beneficial.

Diagnostic ultrasound has the advantage of being relatively inexpensive compared to other noninvasive imaging techniques. In addition, this study can be performed at the bedside obviating the hazardous and time-consuming transfer of a critically ill patient from the ICU to the radiology suite. Unfortunately, the study is operator dependent in terms of the reliability of interpretation.[32,33] Ultrasonography is frequently not helpful in postoperative patients with ileus and although 85% to 95% accuracy is reported for abdominal abscess,[30] the accuracy specific to critically ill postoperative patients is probably not as good. Ultrasonography is perhaps most useful to confirm acute cholecystitis in critically ill patients, especially when there are physical signs referable to the right upper quadrant.[34] Nuclear imaging studies of the gallbladder and biliary tract are not diagnostic in patients who are not taking food orally or who are receiving total parenteral nutrition.[35] False-positive scintigrams are as high as 60% in alcoholics and 92% in patients receiving total parenteral nutrition secondary to altered bile flow kinetics.[35] Similar problems occur with ^{67}Ga citrate scanning and ^{111}In-tagged leukocyte scans. Gallium scans were originally used to identify neoplasms. The discovery of its uptake by abscesses inspired investigators to use it for identifying occult abdominal abscesses.[30,36,37] Unfortunately, gallium is also concentrated in other areas of inflammation, such as the postoperative surgical wound and the splenic bed. It is excreted by the liver into bile and ultimately into the small bowel.[30,36] The 48-hour delay for optimal localization is a problem since the time required may not be compatible with the more pressing need for therapy in patients with continued clinical deterioration.

Radioactive tagging of endogenous leukocytes with ^{111}In is another approach for diagnosing abdominal abscesses.[38–41] Tagged leukocytes eventually concentrate in an area of inflammation which can be located with scintigraphic scanning. This procedure has similar limitations since all areas of inflammation will concentrate leukocytes and the uptake in the liver and spleen compromises evaluation of these areas.[30] Twenty-four to 48 hours are also required to perform this study.

Because of the limitations associated with conventional radiographs, ultrasound, and nuclear scans, CT has become the preferred method for diagnosing intra-abdominal abscess.[33] Increased availability of CT scans which give more precise definition of anatomic detail allows for successful use of percutaneous drainage methods which have significantly modified the classic approach to the management of intra-abdominal abscesses.[42–47] Unfortunately, clinical criteria for ordering CT scans have not developed as rapidly as technology and, similar to all diagnostic methods without specific indications, misinformation can result. The abdomen postoperatively may contain air, blood, seromas, and areas of tissue necrosis that may present images indistinguishable from collections of pus.[30]

Most CT studies for abscesses report accuracies from a broad selection of patients and do not describe the temporal relationship to intervention or examine the usefulness in arriving at a clinical decision. Further, the accuracy in critically ill patients is not usually addressed. Numerous reports demonstrate that CT is effective in identifying a well-defined abscess. Anecdotal case reports also show that CT scans are useful[48,49] and larger series report overall accuracy rates from 67% to greater than 95%.[50–54] Trunet prospectively examined 31 patients with possible intra-abdominal sepsis during the postoperative period and found an overall accuracy of 94% with a sensitivity of 100% and a specificity of 88%.[55] Only two trauma patients were included in this study. The overall mortality was 29%. Whitley and Shatney reported 92% sensitivity and 79% specificity in 69 trauma patients.[56] Details of the clinical course and timing of the CT scans were not given in either study. Although the accuracy of CT was excellent in the latter study, closer analysis of the data suggests that the information may not have been as helpful clinically. There were 31 true-positive scans and 10 false-positive scans, 7 of which were verified at surgery. Three scans were false negatives, all verified at surgery. The effect of CT in terms of clinical judgment was not addressed in this study. This is very important since 6 of 38 "true negatives" were also explored. Only 7 of 10 false positives had surgery, indicating that at least three patients were not re-explored despite a positive CT scan. Therefore, at least 12 (18%) were either operated or not operated on despite CT findings which suggested the opposite course.

Other studies have reviewed the use of CT in the decision-making process. One study reviewed 135 CT scans in 111 patients and showed that the scan aided or altered the management of patients in only 55% of cases.[57] Another study showed that only 12.5% of CT scans were used as the sole criterion for changing management; in 75% of patients, the decision to operate was based solely on physical examination, regardless of CT results.[58]

A more recent study tried to determine the impact of CT information in 53 critically ill surgical patients who were at risk for developing intra-abdominal abscess.[59] Of the 72 scans obtained, only 17 (23%) provided beneficial information while 55 (77%) provided information that was either not used or detrimental to patient care. Sensitivity and specificity were defined to extend beyond just accuracy of the test and included the impact of the information obtained from CT. Sensitivity in this study was 48% with a specificity of 64%. Calculation of personnel utilization and charges showed a figure of $28,541 for the 55 scans that were of no benefit. These authors observed that CT scanning for sepsis in critically ill patients gave little useful information; even when the scan was positive, the information did not usually influence clinical decision-making. When the information was used to direct the clinical care of the patient, mortality rates did not improve.[59]

This study should not be interpreted to mean that CT scanning is never beneficial in critically ill patients, but CT should not be used as a tool to blindly search for a source of sepsis as part of a fever work-up. Scans were not beneficial during the first week postoperatively; in MSOF patients, the test was generally without benefit unless a negative scan would support a decision to discontinue therapy.[59] Scanning had no effect on outcome in these critically ill patients when used as a final attempt to locate an intra-abdominal abscess. In febrile ICU patients, a CT scan should be done only if there is a reasonable probability that the information obtained will direct or alter clinical decision-making. This probability should be based on a decision-making process in which both negative and positive results actually direct therapy in different directions. As the difficulty to make a clinical diagnosis increases, the likelihood of useful CT information seems to diminish.[59] In febrile ICU patients who are at risk for developing intra-abdominal abscess, CT should by used only to confirm clinical suspicions. This should eventually reduce the number of negative surgical re-explorations.[59]

Abdominal re-exploration may be the only definitive test in some instances, especially in those patients who develop unexplained single organ system failure. However, it is not clear whether reoperation significantly affects outcome in larger populations of critically ill patients with MSOF. Several recent reports have advocated early re-exploration.[60–62]

A retrospective study of 50 patients who underwent reoperation for sepsis evaluated the use of available clinical and laboratory tests to predict findings at reoperation and ultimate outcome.[62] Basic demographic data such as the diagnosis leading to primary operation, interval between primary operation, onset of fever and elevated white blood cell count, highest white blood cell count, serum albumin levels, and other tests did not help to predict findings at re-exploration. In this study, 39 of 50 (78%) patients had positive findings at re-exploration. Thirty-seven patients (74%) survived hospitalization; survivors were significantly younger (41.7 ± 2.8 years) than nonsurvivors (57.0 ± 3.8 years), but there was no significant difference between the groups in terms of time intervals to re-exploration. It is not clear from this study whether all these patients were in fact critically ill and required extensive ICU care. Fifteen patients had no organ system failure while 19 were described as having only one organ system dysfunction. Therefore, 72% of the patients had one or no organ system failure and an 88% survival rate. The 16 patients with MSOF had a 56% mortality rate. The authors concluded that patients should be re-explored before the onset of MSOF, since the risk of negative re-exploration (18.2% mortality) was outweighed by the potential for finding and draining intraperitoneal pus.[62]

Others have reported mortality rates following negative explorations for sepsis ranging from 19% to 71%.[60,61,63] The question is not whether re-exploration is harmful but rather, whether re-exploration significantly affects mortality rates in patients with established MSOF (the majority of critically ill septic surgical patients). There appears to be no question that a properly timed re-exploration may prevent MSOF and significantly improve the chances for survival.[62] The question of whether re-exploration alters the course of established MSOF remains unanswered.

OTHER CRITICAL ETIOLOGIES FOR FEVER

Drug Allergies

It is estimated that 15% of hospitalized patients experience some type of adverse drug reaction.[64] Various drugs produce allergic reactions because of their ability to combine with endogenous molecules, primarily proteins, although polysaccharides and polynucleotides can also serve a similar function. Antibodies in the serum develop to metabolites of various drugs that are capable of existing in covalent linkage with protein.[65,66]

Fever may be the first sign of the two most serious types of allergic drug reactions; anaphylaxis and serum sickness.[64] Anaphylactic drug reactions develop rapidly and reach a maximum within 5 to 30 minutes. In critically ill patients, early symptoms such as nausea, vomiting, pruritus, and dyspnea may be masked or go unrecognized until other systemic signs such as fever, hypotension, and severe respiratory distress develop. Various drugs have been reported to produce fatal anaphylactic reactions (Table 22-3). Anaphylactic sensitivities are primarily mediated by IgE antibodies, although IgG antibodies can also produce the response.[64]

TABLE 22-3   DRUGS ASSOCIATED WITH FATAL ANAPHYLACTIC REACTIONS

Pencillins
Organic mercurials
Opiates
Organic iodides (radiopaque dyes)
Local anesthetics
Streptomycin
Sulfobromophthalein (BSP)
Dehydrocholate sodium (decholin)
Fluorescein
Congo red
Dextran
Aspirin
Heparin
Vitamin B_{12}
Tetracyclines
Cephalosporins

Serum sickness is a systemic allergic reaction to drugs characterized by fever, rash, lymphadenopathy, arthritis, nephritis, edema, and neuritis. Urticarial and maculopapular rashes are particularly common and may occur locally at an earlier drug injection site. This syndrome develops from antigens which remain in the circulation for prolonged periods so that at the time antibody is first formed, intravascular antigen is still present, permitting formation of circulating antigen–antibody complexes.[64] Drugs implicated in the development of serum sickness are listed in Table 22-4.

In addition to these two allergic responses, fever can occur as an isolated manifestation of drug allergy.[67] Other drugs implicated in causing fever are listed in Table 22-5.

If drug allergy is the suspected source for fever in a critically ill patient, then all drugs should be carefully reviewed, and those which are known to be associated with a high incidence of allergic reactions should be discontinued or replaced with another suitable drug if possible. Determining the exact cause of a drug allergy in patients who are on multiple medications can be very difficult. The likelihood of an allergic reaction to any drug increases with the duration and number of courses of therapy.[68] There is no single universally applicable test for drug allergy since a number of different pathogenic mechanisms lead to allergic symptoms.[69] Most allergic reactions can be easily managed simply by withdrawing the drug. However, if the patient develops severe systemic side-effects, such as vasculitis, interstitial nephritis, severe dermatitis, or hepatitis, then high-dose corticosteroid therapy may be necessary.[70]

Blood Transfusion Reactions

Approximately 90% of reactions to blood products are allergic or febrile.[71] Allergic reactions may also produce a febrile response, with reactions varying from hives to acute anaphylaxis.[72] Most allergic reactions are mild and self-limited. Treatment consists of stopping the blood product infusion and administering antihistamines, usually diphenhydramine hydrochloride.[72]

Febrile reactions are usually caused by antibodies to white blood cells. These reactions are usually harmless and self-limited, but further evaluation is mandatory since fever may also accompany hemolysis or may be caused by blood products that have been contaminated with bacteria.[72] Febrile reactions generally begin within 30 minutes to 2 hours after a blood product transfusion is begun. The fever generally lasts between 2 and 24 hours and may be preceded by chills.[72]

TABLE 22-4   DRUGS ASSOCIATED WITH SERUM SICKNESS AND OTHER CYTOTOXIC REACTIONS

Serum Sickness	Thrombocytopenia	Hemolytic Anemia
Penicillins	Quinine	Quinine
Sulfonamides	Quinidine	Quinidine
Thiouracils	Meprobamate	Dipyrone
Cholecystographic dyes	Chlorthiazide	Aminosalicylic acid
Diphenylhydantoin	Thiouracils	Mephenytoin
Aminosalicylic acid	Chloramphenicol	Stibophen
Streptomycin	Sulfonamides	Cephalothin
		Phenacetin
		Methyldopa
		Mefenamic acid

TABLE 22-5 OTHER DRUGS IMPLICATED IN
CAUSING DRUG FEVERS

Allopurinol	Methyldopa
Antihistamines	Nitrofurantoin
Azathioprine	Pentazocine
Barbiturates	Phenytoin
Cimetidine	Procainamide
Diazoxide	Procarbazine
Folic acid	Propylthiouracil
Hydralazine	Sulindac
Ibuprofen	Trimaterine
Isoniazid	

It is estimated that hemolytic transfusion reactions occur in 1 of every 6000 units of blood transfused.[73] Approximately 80% of these reactions are a result of clerical identification errors resulting in the patient receiving ABO-incompatible blood. In critically ill patients, severe agitation due to chest, back, or infusion site pain accompanied by chills and fever may be the first sign. Severe reactions are accompanied by hypotension and hemoglobinuria. The patient may develop sudden diffuse oozing of blood from multiple sites. If a hemolytic transfusion reaction is suspected as a source for fever, the blood transfusion must be immediately stopped since the severity of the reaction is directly related to the number of incompatible red blood cells transfused.[72] The suspected blood unit and all attached tubing and solutions should be returned to the laboratory for verification of all clerical work. Blood should be drawn from a site remote to the transfusion site and checked for free hemoglobin. A direct antiglobulin (direct Coombs') test should be performed. The urine is checked for hemoglobin, and, if positive, a brisk diuresis is maintained.

Hemolytic transfusion reactions may be delayed, often up to 2 weeks.[74] In these situations, patients with no detectable antibody to red blood cell antigens at the time of transfusion develop a titer of antibodies sufficient to destroy transfused red blood cells several days after transfusion. If enough donor red blood cells are still in circulation, and if the antibody titer rises rapidly, clinically significant hemolysis can occur. The symptoms of delayed hemolysis include fever, jaundice, and an unexplained fall in hematocrit. Antibodies against antigens in the Rh, Kidd, and Kell blood groups are involved with this type of reaction.[72] The direct antiglobulin test is usually positive with these reactions.

Malignant Hyperthermia

Malignant hyperthermia is a clinical syndrome in which skeletal muscle activity suddenly and unexpectedly increases its oxygen consumption and lactate production resulting in increased heat production, with severe respiratory and metabolic acidosis. This syndrome is classically observed during administration of general anesthesia. The body temperature rapidly increases, usually as high as 1°C/5 min.[75] The syndrome is triggered by a decrease in the control of intracellular calcium within the skeletal muscle resulting in the release of free, unbound, ionized calcium from the sites in the skeletal muscle that normally maintain relaxation.[76] The onset of malignant hyperthermia is usually in the operating room, often with induction of general anesthesia. However, it is not unusual for the onset to be delayed for several hours, and therefore, the symptoms may not develop until the patient has reached the recovery room or the ICU. Anesthetics and muscle relaxants that trigger malignant hyperthermia include halothane, enflurane, isoflurane, sevoflurane, methoxyflurane, cyclopropane, ether, succinylcholine, and decamethonium.[75] Other anesthetic agents and muscle relaxants have also been implicated in various case reports.

Early diagnosis is more difficult than the treatment. Signs of increasing metabolism may be masked or subtle. Other clinical signs develop before the rise in temperature, which may be as high as 43°C (109.4°F). Onset of symptoms may be delayed until the patient begins to emerge from general anesthesia.[77] Early symptoms can mimic thyrotoxicosis,[78] pheochromocytoma, or the neuroleptic malignant syndrome.[79]

Malignant hyperthermia should be suspected if there is sudden onset of sinus tachycardia, tachypnea, dysrhythmias, cyanosis, muscle rigidity, and an unstable blood pressure. These symptoms can develop before the onset of fever. Arterial blood gases will show a severe mixed metabolic and respiratory acidosis. Mixed venous oxygen tension ($P\bar{v}_{O_2}$) and carbon dioxide tension ($P\bar{v}_{CO_2}$) generally change more dramatically than arterial blood gases.[75] Normally, $P\bar{v}_{CO_2}$ should be only about 5 mm Hg higher than Pa_{CO_2}. If Pa_{CO_2} is greater than 60 mm Hg and the patient has an acute base deficit of -5 to -7 meq/liter, the diagnosis is made (assuming that hypoventilation as a cause for hypercapnea has been eliminated). The Pa_{CO_2} may rise as high as 100 mm Hg with pH decreasing to 7.00. Treatment must be immediate or onset of fever or death will rapidly ensue. Early mortality rates were reportedly as high as 70%.[75] However, with development of dantrolene, mortality rates have decreased to less than 10%.[75]

Treatment includes discontinuance of all anesthetic agents and hyperventilation with 100% oxygen. Dantrolene is administered in 2 mg/kg boluses every 5 minutes for a total dose of 10 meq/kg. The dose may be repeated every 4 to 8 hours for a total of three doses.[75] Sodium bicarbonate is initially given at a rate of 2 to 4 meq/kg and titrated to maintain normal acid base balance. Fever should be controlled with surface cooling blankets and iced intravenous saline if necessary. Cooling is stopped at 38°C to 39°C to prevent hypothermia.

Patients can develop myoglobinuria and a brisk diuresis should be maintained to avoid acute renal failure. Continued use of all the above drugs will depend on the clinical course. If ventricular dysrhythmias develop, procainamide is the drug of choice.[75]

Adrenocortical Insufficiency

Acute adrenocortical insufficiency is a rare cause of fever in the critically ill patient. The availability and effective use of complete steroid replacement therapy have virtually eliminated hypotensive crises due to lack of corticosteroids following most elective surgical procedures.[80] However, adrenocortical crisis can still occasionally develop in the ICU patient, usually manifested by a sharp rise in body temperature with hypotension.

Adrenocortical crisis should be considered in patients who are being weaned from high steroid dosages and suddenly develop fever. This is especially true in patients who may have abdominal abscesses or other remote infections where more than just a maintenance dose of hydrocortisone is required.

In elective surgical patients, acute adrenal insufficiency will usually develop within the first 72 hours postoperatively. The syndrome presents with sinus tachycardia, fever, and hypotension.[80] Acute adrenocortical crisis results from an abrupt disparity between the metabolic need for glucocorticoids and the amount of these hormones available. Thus, severe metabolic stress, which can result from systemic sepsis or MSOF, may produce acute adrenocortical insufficiency even when the hormone supply that is available is adequate during the patient's normal basal state.[80]

If the diagnosis is suspected clinically, the patient should receive therapy immediately. Hydrocortisone (100 mg) is administered intravenously to most patients unless there is a question of underlying sepsis or the patient has MSOF. Higher doses may be necessary in these situations. The patient will show dramatic clinical improvement within minutes of receiving steroids if adrenocortical insufficiency is the cause for fever and hypotension.

Pulmonary Embolization Syndromes

Pulmonary embolus can cause fever in critically ill patients. This etiology should be considered in patients who are at risk for developing pulmonary thromboembolism.[81] The diagnosis is often extremely difficult in critically ill patients, however.

REFERENCES

1. Majeski JA, Alexander JW: Complications of wound infections. In Greenfield LJ (ed): *Complications in Surgery and Trauma*, p 27. Philadelphia, JB Lippincott, 1984
2. Bernheim HA, Block LH, Atkins E: Fever: Pathogenesis, pathophysiology, and purpose. *Ann Intern Med* 1979; 91:261
3. Root RK, Wolff SM: Pathogenetic mechanisms in experimental immune fever. *J Exp Med* 1968; 128:309
4. Bodel P, Dillard M: Steroids and steroid fever. I. Production of leukocyte pyrogen in vitro etiocholanolene. *J Clin Invest* 1968; 47:107
5. Petersdorf RG, Bennett IL: Studies on the pathogenesis of fever. VIII. Fever-producing substance in the serum of dogs. *J Exp Med* 1957; 106:293
6. Atkins E, Bodel PT: Fever. In Zweifach BW, Grant L, McClusky RT (eds): *The Inflammatory Process*, 2nd ed, p 467. New York, Academic Press, 1974
7. Dinarello CA, Golden NP, Wolff SM: Demonstration and characterization of two distinct human leukocytic pyrogens. *J Exp Med* 1974; 139:1369
8. Shires GT, Dineen P: Sepsis following burns, trauma, and intra-abdominal infections. *Arch Intern Med* 1981; 142:2012
9. Petersdorf RG: Chills and fever. In Petersdorf RG, Adams RD, Braunwauld E, et al (eds): *Harrison's Principles of Internal Medicine*, 10th ed, p 57. New York, McGraw-Hill, 1983
10. Galicier L, Richet H: A prospective study of postoperative fever in a general surgery department. *Infect Control* 1985; 6:487
11. Ledger WJ, Child MA: The hospital care of patients undergoing hysterectomy: An analysis of 12,026 patients from the professional activity study. *Am J Obstet Gynecol* 1973; 117:423
12. Young RSW, Buck JR, Filler RM: The significance of fever following operations in children. *J Pediatric Surg* 1982; 17:347
13. Freischlag J, Busuttil RW: The value of postoperative fever evaluation. Surgery 1983; 94:358
14. Tobin MJ, Grenvik A: Nosocomial lung infection and its diagnosis. *Crit Care Med* 1984; 12:191
15. Wanner A, Amikam B, Robinson MJ, et al: Comparison between the bacteriologic flora of different segments of the airways. *Respiration* 1973; 30:561
16. Wimberly N, Faling JC, Bartlett JG: A fiberoptic bronchoscopy technique to obtain uncontaminated lower airway secretions for bacterial culture. *Am Rev Respir Dis* 1979; 119:337
17. Baigelman W, Bellin S, Cupples A, Berenberg MJ: Bacteriologic assessment of the lower respiratory tract in intubated patients. *Crit Care Med* 1986; 14:864
18. Martinez OV, Civetta JM, Anderson K, et al: Bacteriuria in the catheterized surgical intensive care patient—a prospective study of 100 patients. *Crit Care Med* 1986; 75:1298
19. Civetta JM, Hudson–Civetta JA, Dion L, et al: Duration of illness effects, catheter-related infection and bacteremia (abstr). Interscience Conference on Antimicrobial Agents and Chemotherapy, 1987; 27 (in press)
20. Norwood SH, Cormier BA, Moss AM, Anderson VA: An evaluation of catheter-related infection during prolonged arterial catheterization. Unpublished data.
21. Bywaters EGL: War medicine series: Crushing injury. *Brit Med J* 1942; 2:643

22. Weiner SL, Barrett J: Explosions and explosive device-related injuries. In Weiner SL, Barrett J (eds): *Trauma Management for Civilian and Military Physicians*, p 23. Philadelphia, WB Saunders, 1986
23. Westaby S: Tetanus and antibiotic prophylaxis. In Westaby S (ed): *Wound Care*, p 91. St. Louis, CV Mosby, 1986
24. Rosner MJ, Berker DP: Complications of craniotomy and trauma. In Greenfield LJ (ed): *Complications in Surgery and Trauma*, p 663. Philadelphia, JB Lippincott, 1983
25. Mombelli G, Klastersky J, Coppens L, et al: Gram-negative bacillary meningitis in neurosurgical patients. *J Neurosurg* 1983; 59:634
26. Dellinger EP, Oreskovich MR, Wertz MJ, et al: Risk of infection following laparotomy for penetrating abdominal injury. *Arch Surg* 1984; 119:20
27. Goris RJA, Draaisma J: Causes of death after blunt trauma. *J Trauma* 1982; 22:141
28. Pitcher WD, Musler DM: Critical importance of early diagnosis and treatment of intra-abdominal infection. *Arch Surg* 1982; 117:328
29. Doberneck RC, Mittelman J: Reappraisal of the problems of intra-abdominal abscess. *Surg Gynecol Obstet* 1982; 154:875
30. Fry DE: The diagnosis of intra-abdominal infection in the postoperative patient. *Prob Gen Surg* 1984; 1:558
31. Deutschman CS, Wilton P, Sinow J, et al: Paranasal sinusitis associated with nasotracheal intubation: A frequently unrecognized and treatable source of sepsis. *Crit Care Med* 1986; 14:111
32. Clark RA, Tobin R: Abscess drainage with CT and ultrasound guidance. *Radiol Clin North Am* 1983; 21:445
33. Mueller PR, Simeone JF: Intra-abdominal abscesses: Diagnosis by sonography and computed tomography. *Radiol Clin North Am* 1983; 21:425
34. Laing, FC: Diagnostic evaluation of patients with suspected acute cholecystitis. *Radiol Clin North Am* 1983; 21:447
35. Shuman WP, Gibbs P, Rudd TG, Mack LA: PIPIDA scintigraphy for cholecystitis: False positives in alcoholism and total parenteral nutrition. *Am J Radiol* 1982; 138:1
36. Caffee HH, Watts G, Mena I: Gallium-67 citrate scanning in the diagnosis of intra-abdominal abscess. *Am J Surg* 1977; 133:665
37. Moir C, Robins RE: Role of ultrasonography, gallium scanning, and computed tomography in the diagnosis of intra-abdominal abscess. *Am J Surg* 1982; 143:582
38. Segal AW, Arnot RN, Thakur ML, et al: Indium-111 labeled leukocytes for localization of abscesses. *Lancet* 1976; 1:1056
39. Coleman RE, Black RE, Welch DM, Maxwell JG: Indium-111 labeled leukocytes in the evaluation of suspected abdominal abscesses. *Am J Surg* 1980; 139:99
40. Dutcher JP, Schiffer CA, Johnson GS: Rapid migration of 111-indium-labeled granulocytes to sites of infection. *N Engl J Med* 1981; 304:586
41. Ascher NL, Ahrenholz DH, Simmons RL, et al: Indium-111 autologous tagged leukocytes in the diagnosis of intraperitoneal sepsis. *Arch Surg* 1979; 114:386
42. Gerzof SG, Robbins AH, Johnson WC, et al: Percutaneous catheter drainage of abdominal abscesses. *N Engl J Med* 1981; 305:653
43. Gobien RP, Young JWR, Curry NS, et al: Computed tomography guidance of percutaneous needle aspiration and drainage of abdominal abscesses. *J Comp Tomog* 1982; 6:127
44. Martin EC, Karlson KB, Fankuchen EI, et al: Percutaneous drainage of postoperative intra-abdominal abscesses. *Am J Radiol* 1982; 138:13
45. Mandel SR, Boyd D, Jaques PF, et al: Drainage of hepatic, intra-abdominal, and mediastinal abscesses guided by computerized axial tomography. *Am J Surg* 1983; 145:120
46. Sunshine J, McConnell DB, Weinstein CJ, et al: Percutaneous computerized axial tomography. *Am J Surg* 1983; 145:120
47. Aeder MI, Wellman JL, Haaga JR, Hau T: Role of surgical and percutaneous drainage in the treatment of abdominal abscesses. *Arch Surg* 1983; 118:273
48. Daffner RH, Halber MD, Morgan CL, et al: Computed tomography in the diagnosis of intra-abdominal abscesses. *Am J Surg* 1983; 145:136
49. Shin MS, Ho KJ, Heald C, et al: Computed tomographic evaluation of intra-abdominal abscess in immunocompromised hosts. *South Med J* 1981; 74:1277
50. Norton L, Eule J, Burdick D: Accuracy of techniques to detect intraperitoneal abscess. *Surgery* 1978; 84:370
51. Koehler PR, Moss AA; Diagnosis of intra-abdominal and pelvic abscesses by computed tomography. *JAMA* 1980; 244:49
52. Robinson JG, Pollock TW: Computed tomography in the diagnosis and localization of intra-abdominal abscesses. *Am J Surg* 1980; 140:783
53. Saini S, Kellum JM, O'Leary MO, et al: Improved localization and survival in patients with intra-abdominal abscesses. *Am J Surg* 1983; 145:136
54. Knochel JQ, Koehler PR, Lee TG, Welch DM: Diagnosis of abdominal abscesses with computed tomography, ultrasound, and In-111 luekocyte scans. *Radidology* 1980; 137:425

55. Trunet P, LeGall JR, Fagniez PL, et al: Computed tomography and post-laparotomy intra-abdominal abscesses. *Intensive Care Med* 1982; 8:193

56. Whitley NO, Shatney CH: Diagnosis of abdominal abscesses in patients with major trauma: The use of computed tomography. *Radiology* 1982; 147:179

57. Roche J: Effectiveness of computed tomography in the diagnosis of intra-abdominal abscess. *Med J Aust* 1981; 25:85

58. Wright HK, Dunn E, MacArthur JD, Pelliccia O. Specific but limited role of new imaging techniques in decision-making about intra-abdominal abscesses. *Am J Surg* 1982; 143:456

59. Norwood SH, Civetta JM: Abdominal CT scanning in critically ill surgical patients. *Ann Surg* 1985; 202:166

60. Ferraris VA: Exploratory laparotomy for potential abdominal sepsis in patients with multiple-organ failure. *Arch Surg* 1983; 118:1130

61. Hinsdale JG, Jaffe BM: Reoperation for intra-abdominal sepsis. *Ann Surg* 1984; 199:31

62. Machiedo GW, Tikellia J, Suval W, et al: Reoperation for sepsis. *Am Surg* 1985; 51:149

63. Driver T, Kelly GL, Eiseman B: Reoperation after abdominal trauma. *Am J Surg* 1978; 135:747

64. Parker CW: Drug allergy: Part I. *N Engl J Med* 1975; 292:511

65. Schneider CH, deWeck AL: The reaction of benzylpenicillin with carbohydrates at neutral *p*H with a note on the immunogenicity of hapten polysaccharide conjugates. *Immunochemistry* 1967; 4:331

66. Parker CW: Pencillin allergy. *Am J Med* 1963; 34:747

67. Tabor PA: Drug induced fever. *Drug Intell and Clin Pharm* 1986; 20:413

68. Parker CW: Drug allergy: Part II. *N Engl J Med* 1975; 292:732

69. Parker CW: Drug allergy: Part III. *N Engl J Med* 1975; 292:957

70. Sheffer AL, Pennoyer DS: Management of adverse drug reactions. *J Allergy Clin Immunol* 1984; 74:580

71. Rush B, Lee N: Clinical presentation of nonhemolytic transfusion reactions. *Anaesth Intensive Care* 1980; 8:125

72. Rutledge R, Sheldon GF, Collins ML: Massive transfusion. *Crit Care Clin* 1986; 2:791

73. Pineda A, Brzica S, Taswell H: Hemolytic transfusion reaction. Recent experience in a large blood bank. *Mayo Clin Proc* 1978; 53:378

74. Patten E, Reddi C, Riglin H, et al: Delayed hemolytic transfusion reaction caused by a primary immune response. *Transfusion* 1982; 22:248

75. Gronert GA: Malignant hyperthermia. In Miller RD (ed): *Anesthesia*, p 1971. New York, Churchill Livingstone, 1986

76. Gronert GA: Malignant hyperthermia. *Semin Anesth* 1983; 2:197

77. Schulte–Sasse U, Hess W, Eberlein HJ: Postoperative malignant hyperthermia and dantrolene therapy. *Can Anaesth Soc J* 1983; 30:635

78. Stevens JJ: A case of thyrotoxic crisis that mimicked malignant hyperthermia. *Anesthesiology* 1983; 59:263

79. Weinberg S, Twersky RS: Neuroleptic malignant syndrome. *Anesth Analg* 1983; 62:848

80. Hardy JD: Endocrine emergencies. In Hardy JD (ed): *Critical Surgical Illness*, p 154. Philadelphia, WB Saunders, 1980

81. Hyers TM, Hull RD, Weg JG: Antithrombotic therapy for venous thromboembolic disease. *Chest (Suppl)*: 89:26S

INDEX

Page numbers followed by *f* indicate illustrations; those followed by *t* indicate tabular material.